Lecture Notes in Mathematics 1497

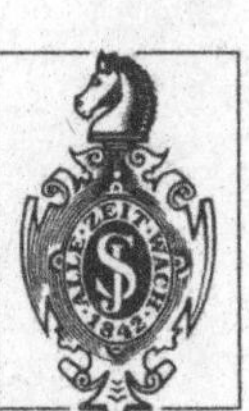

G. T. Herman A. K. Louis F. Natterer (Eds.)

Mathematical Methods in Tomography

Proceedings of a Conference held in Oberwolfach, Germany, 5-11 June, 1990

Springer-Verlag
Berlin Heidelberg New York
London Paris Tokyo
Hong Kong Barcelona
Budapest

Editors

Gabor T. Herman
University of Pennsylvania
Department of Radiology
Philadelphia, PA 19104, USA

Alfred K. Louis
Fachbereich Mathematik
Universität des Saarlandes
6600 Saarbrücken, Germany

Frank Natterer
Institut für Numerische und Instrumentelle Mathematik
Universität Münster
Einsteinstraße 62, 4400 Münster, Germany

Mathematics Subject Classification (1991): 44-02, 44A15, 65R10, 44-06, 92-08

ISBN 3-540-54970-6 Springer-Verlag Berlin Heidelberg New York
ISBN 0-387-54970-6 Springer-Verlag New York Berlin Heidelberg

Typesetting: Camera ready by author
Printing and binding: Druckhaus Beltz, Hemsbach/Bergstr.
46/3140-543210 - Printed on acid-free paper

PREFACE

The word *tomography* means "a technique for making a picture of a plane section of a three-dimensional body." For example, in x-ray computerized tomography (CT), the picture in question is a representation of the distribution in the section of the body of a physical property called x-ray attenuation (which is closely related to density). In CT, data are gathered by using multiple pairs of locations (in the plane of the section) of an x-ray source and an x-ray detector (with the body between them) and measuring for each pair of locations the total attenuation of x-rays between the source and the detector. Mathematically speaking, each measurement provides an approximate value of one sample of the Radon transform of the distribution. (Roughly, the Radon transform of a two-dimensional distribution is a function which associates with any line in the plane the integral of the distribution along that line.) Therefore, the mathematical essence of CT is the *reconstruction* of a distribution from samples of its Radon transform.

Over the years, "tomography" became to be used in a wider sense, namely for any technique of reconstructing internal structures in a body from data collected by detectors (sensitive to some sort of energy) outside the body. Tomography is of interest to many disciplines: physicists, engineers, bioscientists, physicians, and others concern themselves with various aspects of the underlying principles, of equipment design, and of medical or other applications. Mathematics clearly enters in the field where inversion methods are needed to be developed for the various modes of data collection, but we also find mathematicians busily working in many other diverse aspects of tomography, from the theoretical to the applied.

This book contains articles based on selected lectures delivered at the August 1990 conference on Mathematical Methods in Tomography held at the Mathematisches Forschungsinstitut (Mathematical Research Center) at Oberwolfach, Germany. The aim of the conference was to bring together researchers whose interests range from the abstract theory of Radon transforms to the diverse applications of tomography. This was the third such conference at Oberwolfach, with the first one held just over ten years earlier [5]. Much has happened in the field of tomography since that first meeting, including the appearance of a number of books (such as [3, 2, 7, 6]) and many special issues (including [4, 1]).

Oberwolfach is a remote place in the Black Forest with excellent conference and housing facilities. Mathematical conferences of one week duration take place there nearly every week.

Participation is by invitation only and there are usually 20–60 participants. The meeting on which this book is based had 41 participants; seventeen came from the USA, seven from Germany, five from France, two from each of Brazil, Sweden, and USSR, and one from each of Belgium, Hungary, Israel, Italy, Japan, and the Netherlands. The lively international scientific atmosphere of the conference resulted in many stimulating discussions; some of which are reflected in the papers that follow.

Thus our book is a collection of research papers reporting on the current work of the participants of the 1990 Oberwolfach conference. Those desiring to obtain an overview of tomography, or even only of its mathematical aspects, would be better served by looking at the already cited literature [3, 2, 4, 7, 6]. However, the collection that follows complements this literature by presenting to the reader the current research of some of the leading workers in the field.

We have organized the articles in the book into a number of sections according to their main topics. The section entitled *Theoretical Aspects* contains papers of essentially mathematical nature. There are articles on Helgason's support theorem and on singular value decomposition for Radon transforms, on tomography in the context of Hilbert space, on a problem of integral geometry, and on inverting three-dimensional ray transforms. The section entitled *Medical Imaging Techniques* is devoted to the mathematical treatment of problems which arise out of trying to do tomography with data collected using various energies and/or geometrical arrangements of sources and detectors. Thus, there are articles on using backscattered photons, on cone-beam 3D reconstruction, and on tomography for diffraction, for diffusion, for scattering, and on biomagnetic imaging. The section on *Inverse Problems and Optimization* discusses mainly the algorithmic aspects of inversion approaches for tomographic data collections. This section contains articles on various formulations of the inverse problems in terms of optimization theory, as well as on iterative approaches for solving the problems. Finally, the section on *Applications* contains articles that have been closely motivated by some practical aspect of tomography; for example, on the determination of density of an aerosol, on nondestructive testing of rockets, and on evaluating the efficacy of reconstruction methods for specific tasks.

Finally, we would like to thank Prof. Martin Barner, the director of the Mathematisches Forschungsinstitut, and his splendid staff for providing us with all the help and just the right ambiance for a successful mathematical conference. We are also grateful to Springer-Verlag for their kind cooperation in publishing this volume.

REFERENCES

[1] Y. Censor, T. Elfving, and G. Herman, *Special issue on linear algebra in image reconstruction from projections*, Linear Algebra Appl., 130 (1990), pp. 1–305. Guest Eds.

[2] S. Deans, *The Radon Transform and Some of Its Applications*, John Wiley & Sons, New York, 1983.

[3] G. Herman, *Image Reconstruction from Projections: The Fundamentals of Computerized Tomography*, Academic Press, New York, 1980.

[4] ——, *Special issue on computerized tomography*, Proc. IEEE, 71 (1983), pp. 291–435. Guest Ed.

[5] G. Herman and F. Natterer, eds., *Mathematical Aspects of Computerized Tomography*, Springer-Verlag, Berlin, 1981.

[6] G. Herman, H. Tuy, K. Langenberg, and P. Sabatier, *Basic Methods of Tomography and Inverse Problems*, Adam Hilger, Bristol, England, 1987.

[7] F. Natterer, *The Mathematics of Computerized Tomography*, John Wiley & Sons, Chichester, England, 1986.

Gabor T. Herman
Department of Radiology, University of Pennsylvania
Philadelphia, PA 19104, USA

Alfred K. Louis
Fachbereich Mathematik, Universität des Saarlandes
D-6600 Saarbrücken, Germany

Frank Natterer
Institut für Numerische und Instrumentelle Mathematik, Universität Münster
D-4400 Münster, Germany

Table of Contents

Theoretical Aspects

Helgason's support theorem for Radon transforms – a new proof and a generalization
J. Boman 1

Singular value decompositions for Radon transforms
P. Maaß 6

Image reconstruction in Hilbert space
W.R. Madych 15

A problem of integral geometry for a family of rays with multiple reflections
R.G. Mukhometov 46

Inversion formulas for the three – dimensional ray transform
V.P. Palamadov 53

Medical Imaging Techniques

Backscattered Photons — are they useful for a surface – near tomography
V. Friedrich 63

Mathematical framework of cone beam 3D reconstruction via the first derivative of the Radon transform
P. Grangeat 66

Diffraction tomography : some applications and extension to 3D ultrasound imaging
P. Grassin, B. Duchene, W. Tabbara 98

Diffuse tomography : a refined model
F.A. Grünbaum 106

Three dimensional reconstructions in inverse obstacle scattering
R. Kress , A. Zinn 112

Mathematical questions of a biomagnetic imaging problem
A.K. Louis 126

Inverse Problems and Optimization

On variable block algebraic reconstruction techniques
Y. Censor 133

On Volterra – Lotka differential equations and multiplicative algorithms for monotone complementary problems
P.P.B. Eggermont 141

Constrained regularized least squares problems
T. Elfving 153

Multiplicative iterative methods in computed tomography
A. de Pierro 167

Remark on the informative content of a few measurements
P.C. Sabatier 187

Applications

Theorems for the number of zeros of the projection radial modulators of the 2D – exponential Radon transform
W.G. Hawkins, N.C. Yang, P.K. Leichner 194

Evaluation of reconstruction algorithms
G.T. Herman, D. Odhner 215

Radon transform and analog coding
H. Ogawa, I. Kumazawa 229

Determination of the specific density of an aerosol through tomography
L.R.Oudin 242

Computed tomography and rockets
E.T. Quinto 261

Helgason's support theorem for Radon transforms – a new proof and a generalization

Jan Boman

Department of Mathematics, University of Stockholm
Box 6701, S-11385, Stockholm, Sweden

1. Denote by Rf the Radon transform of the function f, i. e. $Rf(H) = \int_H f ds_H$ for, say, continuous functions f on $\mathbb{R}^n$ that decay at least as $|x|^{-n}$ as $|x| \to \infty$, and $H \in G_n$, the set of hyperplanes in $\mathbb{R}^n$; the surface measure on H is denoted ds_H. The well-known support theorem of Helgason [**He1**], [**He2**] states that if $Rf(H) = 0$ for all H not intersecting the compact convex set K and $f(x) = O(|x|^{-m})$ as $|x| \to \infty$ for all m, then f must vanish outside K. In [**He3**] Helgason extended this theorem to the case of Riemannian manifolds with constant negative curvature. Helgason's proofs depend in an essential way on the strong symmetry properties of the Radon transform. Here we will extend the theorem just cited to the case when a real analytic weight function depending on H as well as x is allowed in the definition of the Radon transform (see below), a situation without symmetry. For C^∞ weight functions analogous theorems are not true in general [**B2**]. Our method depends on the microlocal regularity properties of the Radon transform, a method we have already used in [**BQ1**] and [**BQ2**]. The case when f is assumed to have compact support was considered in [**BQ1**]. For rotation invariant (not necessarily real analytic) Radon transforms support theorems were given by E. T. Quinto [**Q3**].

2. Let $\rho = \rho(x, H)$ be a smooth function on the set Z of all pairs (x, H) of $H \in G_n$ and $x \in H$. We define the generalized Radon transform R_ρ by

$$R_\rho f(H) = \int_H f(\cdot)\rho(\cdot, H) ds_H, \quad H \in G_n.$$

If ρ is constant, R_ρ is of course the classical Radon transform. To describe our assumptions on ρ we shall consider $\mathbb{R}^n$ as sitting inside the projective space $\mathbb{P}^n(\mathbb{R})$ in the usual way:

$$\mathbb{R}^n \ni (x_1, \ldots, x_n) \mapsto (1, x_1, \ldots, x_n) \in \mathbb{P}^n(\mathbb{R}). \tag{1}$$

The manifold Z then becomes imbedded in the manifold

$$\tilde{Z} = \{(x, H); x \in H, \ H \text{ hyperplane in } \mathbb{P}^n(\mathbb{R})\}.$$

Note that $\mathbb{P}^n(\mathbb{R})$ and $\tilde{Z}$ are compact real analytic manifolds. Our assumption will be that ρ can be extended to a positive real analytic function on $\tilde{Z}$. This assumption is of course fulfilled for the constant function, which is the case considered by Helgason in [**He1**].

THEOREM. *Assume ρ is a positive, real analytic function on Z that can be extended to a positive, real analytic function on $\tilde{Z}$. Let K be a compact, convex subset of $\mathbf{R}^n$. Let f be continuous on $\mathbf{R}^n$ and*

$$f(x) = O(|x|^{-m}) \quad \text{as} \quad |x| \to \infty \tag{2}$$

for all m, and assume $R_\rho f(H) = 0$ for all H disjoint from K. Then $f = 0$ outside K.

As pointed out by Helgason, the assumption that f tends to zero rapidly as $|x| \to \infty$ cannot be omitted, even in the case of constant ρ.

The assumption that ρ is analytic at infinity cannot be omitted, even if the decay assumption is considerably strengthened. In fact, using ideas from [B2] one can construct examples where ρ is real analytic on Z, $1 \leq \rho \leq C$, f not identically zero, $R_\rho f = 0$, and, for instance, $f(x) = \mathcal{O}(\exp(-e^{|x|}))$ as $|x| \to \infty$.

The approach adopted here is suggested by the following facts. First, if ρ is analytic and different from zero, it is known that any solution f to $R_\rho f = 0$ must be real analytic, hence vanish if it vanishes in some open set [B1], [BQ1]. Second, if one could prove that f, considered as a function on the projective space $\mathbf{P}^n(\mathbf{R})$, must be analytic at infinity, then the assumption that f decays rapidly at infinity would imply that f vanishes identically. Third, the examples showing that the decay assumption cannot be omitted, in two dimensions the functions $\mathrm{Re}(x_1 + ix_2)^{-m}$, are in fact analytic at infinity. An advantage with this approach is, in addition to the fact that the weight function ρ is allowed to be non-constant, that the role of the decay assumption on f is "explained".

We prove the theorem by considering R_ρ as an operator on functions on $\mathbf{P}^n(\mathbf{R})$. The crucial fact is that f, considered as a function on $\mathbf{P}^n(\mathbf{R})$, must have a certain regularity property along the hyperplane at infinity, H_∞; in precise terms, the conormal manifold to H_∞, $N^*(H_\infty)$, must be disjoint from the analytic wavefront set of f (Proposition 1).

3. We are now going to express R_ρ in terms of a Radon transform on $\mathbf{P}^n(\mathbf{R})$. For this purpose we need to introduce some more notation. Set $X = \mathbf{R}^n$, $Y = G_n$, denote $\mathbf{P}^n(\mathbf{R})$ by $\tilde{X}$ and the set of hyperplanes in $\mathbf{P}^n(\mathbf{R})$ by $\tilde{Y}$. Denote the map (1) from X to $\tilde{X}$ by α. This map induces maps $Y \to \tilde{Y}$ and $X \times Y \to \tilde{X} \times \tilde{Y}$, which we will also denote by α. As models for $\tilde{X}$ and $\tilde{Y}$ we shall use the unit sphere S^n with opposite points identified. Thus a model for $\tilde{Z} \subset \tilde{X} \times \tilde{Y}$ will consist of all pairs $(u, \omega) \in S^n \times S^n$ such that $u \cdot \omega = 0$, all four pairs $(\pm u, \pm\omega)$ identified. On the plane $L(\omega) = \{u;\ u \cdot \omega = 0\}$ we choose the measure ds_L equal to the (push-forward of) $n-1$-dimensional surface measure on S^n. We use the notation $\omega = (\omega_0, \omega')$, and we note that the plane at infinity, L_∞, is represented by $\omega = (\pm 1, 0, \ldots, 0)$.

Examples of functions ρ satisfying the hypothesis of the theorem can easily be constructed as follows. Let $a(z, \omega)$ be real analytic and positive on $\{(z, \omega); z \cdot \omega = 0\} \subset \mathbf{R}^{2n+2}$, even and homogeneous of degree zero in both variables (separately), let $H_{\theta,p}$ be the plane $x \cdot \theta = p$, $\theta \in S^{n-1}$, and set

$$\rho(x, H_{\theta,p}) = a(1, x, -p, \theta), \tag{3}$$

for $x \in H_{\theta,p}$. Then a (restricted to $S^n \times S^n$) represents the extension, $\tilde{\rho}$, of ρ. Conversely, every ρ satisfying our assumptions can obviously be represented in the form (3).

Let τ be a positive real analytic function on $\tilde{Z}$. For continuous functions g on $\tilde{X}$ we define the generalized Radon transform $\tilde{R}_\tau$ by

$$\tilde{R}_\tau(g)(L) = \int_L g(\cdot)\tau(\cdot, L)\, ds_L, \quad L \in \tilde{Y}.$$

If f is a function on X, sufficiently small at infinity, $\tilde{f} = f \circ \alpha^{-1}$, $\tilde{\rho} = \rho \circ \alpha^{-1}$, and $L = \alpha(H)$, then

$$R_\rho f(H) = \int_H f(\cdot)\rho(\cdot, H)\, ds_H = \int_L \tilde{f}(\cdot)\tilde{\rho}(\cdot, L)\, \alpha_*(ds_H)$$

$$= \int_L \tilde{f}(\cdot)\tilde{\rho}(\cdot, L) b(\cdot, L)\, ds_L; \tag{4}$$

here $\alpha_*(ds_H) = b(u, L) ds_L$ is the push-forward of the measure ds_H under α. It is very important for us that the density $b(u, L)$ can be factored, $b(u, L) = b_0(u) b_1(L)$, into a function depending only on u and one depending only on the plane L. This fact is well known; see e. g. [GGG], pp. 64-66.

LEMMA 1. *The measure $\alpha_*(ds_H)$ is equal to $b(u, L)\, ds_L$, where*

$$b(u,\omega) = b(u, L(\omega)) = c|u_0|^{-n}\sqrt{1-\omega_0^2} = c|u_0|^{-n}|\omega'|, \quad u_0 \neq 0, \quad |\omega'| \neq 0. \tag{5}$$

for some positive constant c.

Formula (5) shows that the measure $\alpha_*(ds_H)$ has a strong singularity along the plane at infinity. However, the fact that the density function $b(u, L)$ factors as expressed by (5), $b(u, L) = b_0(u) b_1(L)$, implies that this singularity is harmless in our context. In fact, using (4) and (5) we can write

$$R_\rho f(H) = b_1(L) \int_L \tilde{f}(u) b_0(u) \tilde{\rho}(u, L)\, ds_L = b_1(L)(\tilde{R}_\tau g)(L),$$

where $g(u) = \tilde{f}(u) b_0(u) = \tilde{f}(u)|u_0|^{-n}$, and $\tau(u, L) = \tilde{\rho}(u, L)$. Note that $g(u)$ tends to zero as $u_0 \to 0$, since f is rapidly decreasing; hence g is extendible to a continuous function on all of $\tilde{X}$, which vanishes on L_∞. Thus, in particular, if $R_\rho f(H) = 0$ for all H not intersecting K, then $\tilde{R}_\tau g$ must vanish in some neighbourhood of L_∞.

4. We will now turn our attention to the microlocal regularity properties of solutions to the equation $\tilde{R}_\tau g = 0$. The result that we shall need, Proposition 1 below, is well known, but it is not easy to find it in the literature. The analogous statement for the C^∞ category is clearly contained in the very general theory in [H1] as well as in [GS]. The additional arguments needed for the real analytic case can be found for instance in [Bj], ch. 4. Generalized Radon transforms as Fourier integral operators are discussed in [GS]; see also [GU] and [Q2]. In particular, Radon transforms on projective spaces are considered in [Q1]. For definition and basic properties of the analytic wavefront set, see [H2], ch. 8. If E is a smooth submanifold of the manifold M, one denotes by $N^*(E)$ the conormal manifold to E, that is, the set of all $(x, \xi) \in T^*(M) \setminus 0$ such that $x \in E$ and ξ is conormal to the tangent space to E at x.

PROPOSITION 1. *Assume $\tau(u, L)$ is real analytic and positive on $\tilde{Z}$ and that*

$$\tilde{R}_\tau g(L) = 0$$

for all L in some neighbourhood of $L_0 \in \tilde{Y}$. Then

$$N^*(L_0) \cap \mathrm{WF_A}(g) = \emptyset.$$

We finally need the following lemma, related to an important theorem of Hörmander, Kawai, and Kashiwara ([**H2**], Theorem 8.5.6.).

LEMMA 2. *Let S be the spherical surface $\{x;\ |x| = 1\}$ in $\mathbf{R}^m$, and let f be continuous in some neighbourhood of S. Assume*

$$f(x) = O((|x| - 1)^N) \quad \text{as} \quad |x| \to 1 + 0 \quad \textit{for all} \quad N, \tag{6}$$

(or as $|x| \to 1 - 0$), and

$$N^*(S) \cap \mathrm{WF_A}(f) = \emptyset. \tag{7}$$

Then $f = 0$ in some neighbourhood of S.

PROOF: Let S_t be the sphere with radius t and define the function h by

$$h(t) = \int_{S_t} f\, ds,$$

where ds is surface measure on S_t. By basic facts about the wavefront set it follows from (7) that none of the elements above $t = 1$ can be contained in $\mathrm{WF_A}(h)$, i. e. h is analytic at $t = 1$. But (6) implies that h is rapidly decreasing as $t \to 1 + 0$. Hence h must vanish in some neighbourhood of $t = 1$.

Let $\varphi(x)$ be any real analytic function defined on a neighbourhood of S. Multiplying f by φ clearly preserves the properties (6) and (7). Applying our reasoning to φf we conclude that

$$\int_{S_t} \varphi f\, ds = 0$$

for t near 1 and for all bounded and analytic functions φ. This implies that $f = 0$ in some neighbourhood of S. The lemma is proved.

PROOF OF THE THEOREM: Let f be a function satisfying the hypotheses of the theorem, and consider again the function g on $\tilde{X}$ defined by

$$g(u) = |u_0|^{-n} \tilde{f}(u) = |u_0|^{-n} f(\alpha^{-1}(u)).$$

We have seen that $\tilde{R}_\tau g(L)$ must vanish for L near L_∞. But then Proposition 1 implies that

$$N^*(L_\infty) \cap \mathrm{WF_A}(g) = \emptyset. \tag{8}$$

Now we want to use Lemma 2 to infer that g vanishes near L_∞. The fact that L_∞, considered as a hypersurface in $\tilde{X}$, is non-orientable is a slight inconvenience for us; we therefore move up to S^n, the double cover of $\tilde{X}$. We will use the same notation on S^n as on $\tilde{X}$, so that points will be denoted by u and the function g pulled back to S^n will again be denoted g; this will cause no confusion. Thus g is an even function defined in a neighbourhood of the equator $\Sigma = \{u;\ u_0 = 0\} \subset S^n$. It is clear that (8) holds with Σ in place of L_∞. Now, the stereographic map takes S^n with the north pole removed into $\mathbf{R}^n$ and Σ into an $n-1$-sphere in $\mathbf{R}^n$. An application of Lemma 2 now proves that $g = 0$ in a neighbourhood of Σ, hence $f = 0$ outside some compact set in $\mathbf{R}^n$. An application of the theorem in [**BQ1**] therefore finishes the proof. We prefer, however, to complete the proof with another application of the arguments already used here. Since a compact, convex set is equal to the intersection of all closed balls that contain it, we may assume that K is a ball. We may also assume that its center is the origin; let R be its radius. Let S_r be the sphere with radius r, centered at the origin, and let r_0 be the smallest r for which $f = 0$ outside S_r. Assume $r_0 > R$. Applying Proposition 1 (or the analogous statement for the Radon transform R_ρ on $\mathbf{R}^n$) to all tangentplanes to S_{r_0} we find that $N^*(S_{r_0}) \cap \mathrm{WF_A}(f)$ must be empty. Lemma 2 now shows that f must vanish in some neighbourhood of S_{r_0}. This contradicts the definition of r_0, hence the proof is complete.

References

[**B1**]. *Uniqueness theorems for generalized Radon transforms*, in "Constructive Theory of Functions '84," Sofia, 1984, pp. 173-176.

[**B2**]. J. Boman, *An example of non-uniqueness for a generalized Radon transform*, Dept. of Math., University of Stockholm 1984:13.

[**Bj**]. J.-E. Björk, "Rings of Differential Operators," North-Holland Publishing Comp., Amsterdam, 1979.

[**BQ1**]. J. Boman and E. T. Quinto, *Support theorems for real-analytic Radon transforms*, Duke Math. J. **55** (1987), 943-948.

[**BQ2**]. J. Boman and E. T. Quinto, *Support theorems for real-analytic Radon transforms on line complexes in three-space*, to appear in Trans. Amer. Math. Soc.

[**GS**]. V. Guillemin and S. Sternberg, "Geometric Asymptotics," Amer. Math. Soc., Providence, RI, 1977.

[**GU**]. A. Greenleaf and G. Uhlmann, *Nonlocal inversion formulas for the X-ray transform*, Duke Math. J. **58** (1989), 205-240.

[**H1**]. L. Hörmander, *Fourier integral operators I*, Acta Math. **127** (1971), 79-183.

[**H2**]. L. Hörmander, "The analysis of linear partial differential operators, vol. 1," Springer-Verlag, Berlin, Heidelberg, and New York, 1983.

[**He1**]. S. Helgason, *The Radon transform on Euclidean spaces, compact two-point homogeneous spaces and Grassmann manifolds*, Acta Math. **113** (1965), 153-180.

[**He2**]. S. Helgason, "The Radon transform," Birkhäuser, Boston, 1980.

[**He3**]. S. Helgason, *Support of Radon transforms*, Adv. Math. **38** (1980), 91-100.

[**Q1**]. E. T. Quinto, *On the locality and invertibility of Radon transforms*, Thesis, M.I.T., Cambridge, Mass. (1978).

[**Q2**]. E. T. Quinto, *The dependence of the generalized Radon transforms on the defining measures*, Trans. Amer. Math. Soc. **257** (1980), 331-346.

[**Q3**]. E. T. Quinto, *The invertibility of rotation invariant Radon transforms*, J. Math. Anal. Appl. **91** (1983), 510-522.

Singular Value Decompositions for Radon Transforms

Peter Maass

Department of Mathematics,
Tufts University
Medford, MA 02155,
U. S. A.

1 Introduction

In this paper simple techniques are developed for the construction of singular value decompositions (SVD) for rotationally invariant Radon transforms in euclidean spaces. First we introduce the definition of a SVD.

Definition 1. Let A be a linear operator between (separable) Hilbert spaces X, Y

$$A : X \rightarrow Y \quad .$$

The triple $\{u_n, v_n, \sigma_n\}_{n\geq 0}$ is called a **Singular Value Decomposition (SVD)** of the operator A if

$\{u_n\}_{n\geq 1}$ is a complete orthonormal system in X,
$\{v_n\}_{n\geq 1}$ is an orthonormal system in Y,
$\{\sigma_n\}$ is a set of non-negative real numbers,

$$Au_n = \sigma_n v_n \quad and \quad A^* v_n = \sigma_n u_n \quad .$$

The singular values σ_n are usually ordered such that $\sigma_1 \geq \sigma_2 \geq .. \geq 0$.

Sometimes one refers to the singular functions $\{u_n\}$ as generalized Eigenfunctions, since

$$(A^* A) u_n = \sigma_n^2 u_n \quad .$$

The importance of a SVD comes form its ability to express the action of A by orthogonal series expansions, $f = \sum f_n u_n$ with $f_n = < f, u_n >_X$:

$$Af = A(\sum f_n u_n) = \sum f_n \sigma_n v_n \quad .$$

From this one immediately obtains an inversion formula, range characterizations and results on the ill posedness of the inverse problem.

SVD's for Radon transforms have a long history in computerized tomography. The early results of Marr [6] and Cormack [2] show that the 2-dimensional Radon transform maps a set of certain orthogonal functions to products $U_m(s)e^{il\omega}$ of Tchebycheff polynomials with trigonometric functions. Subsequently these results have been extended to arbitrary dimensions, weighted L_2-spaces, functions of unbounded support and Radon transforms modelling limited data problems in tomography, see Perry [8], Quinto [9], Louis [3,4], Maass [5]. Quite different techniques have been used in these papers. Our aim is to demonstrate two elementary and general ways of obtaining SVD's for Radon transform with rotational symmetry, e.g. for full, exterior and interior Radon transforms.

It will be more convenient to work with the adjoint of the Radon transform, the backprojection operator, and to translate the results to the original Radon transform at the end. The next section recalls the invariance of the spherical harmonics under the action of the backprojection operator for rotationally invariant Radon transforms. This reduces the original problem posed for the n-dimensional Radon transform to finding SVD's for 1-dimensional integral operators.

Even in a simple construction of a SVD we must be able to define the sets of orthogonal functions $\{u_n\}$ and $\{v_n\}$. Since they are built from special functions, e.g. orthogonal polynomials, they are usually defined by either 3-term recurrence relations or differential equations.

Chapter 3 starts with the definition of the functions $\{u_n\}$ as solutions of differential equations $D_1 u_n = 0$. From there a second differential operator D_2, intertwining with the action of the adjoint Radon transform, is constructed. This determines the images of $\{u_n\}$ as solutions of differential equations and immediately gives the desired orthogonality properties. The procedure is examplified by carrying out the computations for the full Radon transform.

At the beginning of Chapter 4 the functions $\{u_n\}$ are introduced by 3-term recurrence relations. The corresponding recurrence relations for the functions $\{v_n\}$ can be obtained in a surprisingly simple way. Examples include a SVD for the interior Radon transform.

2 The adjoint operator $\mathcal{R}^*$

We use the standard notation for the Radon transform as a map between weighted L_2-spaces, i.e. a real valued function f is mapped to its integrals over hyperplanes, which are parametrized by a normal unit vector ω and the signed distance s from the origin. The function f may either be defined on $\mathbb{R}^n$ or on a subset, e.g. the unit ball. For the full Radon transform, the integrals over all hyperplanes are measured. For limited data problems, the integrals over some hyperplanes are missing.

$$\begin{aligned} \mathcal{R} \ &: L_2(\Omega, W^{-1}) \to L_2(Z, w^{-1}) \\ f \ &\mapsto \int_{\omega^\perp} f(s\omega + y)\, dy \quad . \end{aligned}$$

There are many meaningful choices for Ω and Z. We are interested in Radon transforms where the set of accessible hyperplanes is rotationally invariant, i.e.

$$\Omega = \mathbb{R}^n \quad or \quad \Omega = B_a := \{\, x \in \mathbb{R}^n \mid \| x \| \le a \,\}$$

$$and \ \mathbf{Z} = S^{n-1} \times I \quad , I \subset \mathbb{R} \quad .$$

The following cases are of particular importance.

$\Omega = I\!R^n$, $I = I\!R$: the full Radon transform for functions with unbounded support,

$\Omega = B_1$, $I = [-1,1]$: the full Radon transform for functions with compact support,

$\Omega = I\!R^n$, $I = \{s \in I\!R \mid \mid s \mid \geq 1\}$: the exterior Radon transform,

$\Omega = I\!R^n$, $I = [-1,1]$: the interior Radon transform .

Since Ω, Z are both invariant under rotations it is natural to assume that the weight functions W, resp. w, only depend on $|x|$, resp. s. It will be more convenient to work with the adjoint operator. Obviously a SVD for the adjoint operator also gives a SVD for the operator itself.
The adjoint Radon transform is a continuous linear operator hence we can compute the transform of g for each term in the sum separately. The following Lemma states the well known property that spherical harmonics are invariant under the action of $\mathcal{R}^*$.

Lemma 2. *Let $g_l \in L_2(I, w)$ then*

$$\mathcal{R}^*(wg_lY_l)(x) = |S^{n-2}|\ W(|x|)f_l(|\ x\ |)\ Y_l(\frac{x}{|\ x\ |})$$

where

$$f_l(r) = \int_{-1}^{1} g_l(rs)(w_\nu C_l^\nu)(s)ds \quad ,$$

the integral extending over those values of s where $g_l(|\ x\ |\ s)$ is defined. Here $(w_\nu C_l^\nu)$ is the weighted Gegenbauer polynomial with $\nu = (n-2)/2$.

This Lemma is a direct consequence of the Funk-Hecke Theorem, e.g. see [7]. We will call T_l the radial operators of the Radon transform. The orthogonality relations for spherical harmonics of different degree reduce the problem of finding a SVD for $\mathcal{R}^*$ to the construction of SVDs for the integral opertors transforming the radial parts in the expansion $g = \sum wg_lY_l$. The weight function W will be choosen appropriately later and we ignore the constant factor $|\ S^{n-2}\ |$. The radial tranforms are then given by

$$(T_lg)(r) := \int_{-1}^{1} g(rt)(w_\nu C_l^\nu)(t)dt \quad .$$

Again the integration extends only over those values of s where the integrand is defined. For the interior Radon transform this yields

$$(T_lg)(r) := \int_{max(-1/r,-1)}^{min(1/r,1)} g(rt)(w_\nu C_l^\nu)(t)dt \quad ,$$

and for the exterior Radon transform

$$(T_lg)(r) := \int_{1/r\leq|t|\leq 1} g(rt)(w_\nu C_l^\nu)(t)dt \quad .$$

In any of these cases the Radon transform decomposes into a series of 1-dimensional integral operators.

Corollary 3. *Let* $g \in L_2(\mathbf{Z}, w^{-1})$, *i.e.* $g(\omega, s) = \sum w(s) g_l(s) Y(\omega)$, *then*

$$(\mathcal{R}^* g)(x) = W(x) \mid S^{n-2} \mid \sum (T_l g_l)(\mid x \mid) Y_l(\frac{x}{\mid x \mid}) \quad ,$$

this implies that given SVD's $\{u_{ml}, v_{ml}, \sigma_{ml}\}$ *for the radial transforms* T_l *we have a SVD for the adjoint Radon transform by,* $\{Y_{lk}\}$ *enumerates an orthonormal basis for the spherical harmonics,*

$$\{u_{ml}(s) Y_{lk}(\omega), v_{ml}(\mid x \mid) Y_{lk}(\frac{x}{\mid x \mid}), \mid S^{n-2} \mid \sigma_{ml}\} \quad .$$

3 Intertwining differential operators

In the previous chapter the original problem, i.e. how to find a SVD for Radon transforms, was reduced to the construction of SVD's for the integral transforms T_l, see Corollary 4. The idea is to construct intertwining pairs of differential operators (D_1, D_2) such that

$$T_l D_1 = D_2 T_l \quad .$$

Then given a function g, which satisfies $D_1 g = 0$, its transform $T_l g$ is the solution of $D_2 f = 0$ with appropriate boundary conditions. Thus if we can find a complete set of intertwining differential operators, i.e. a pair (D_1, D_2) for any element of an orthogonal basis $\{u_m\}$; the images $\{T_l u_m\}$ are characterized as solutions of ordinary differential equations. The structure of these differential equations will not only allow to compute $T_l u_m$ explicitly it will also determine the weight function $W(\mid x \mid)$ for which the transformed functions are orthogonal. This procedure was used to obtain a SVD for the interior Radon transform; see [5]. We will demonstrate this technique with the full Radon transform. The operator T_l is defined by

$$(T_l g)(r) = \int_{-1}^{1} g(rt)\, C_l^{(n-2)/2}(t)(1-t^2)^{(n-3)/2} dt \quad .$$

Functions g which have a parity opposite to the parity of l are mapped to zero. Let us start with a general class of differential operators D_1 :

$$(D_1 g)(t) = (1-t^2) g''(t) + \alpha t g'(t) + \beta g(t) \quad . \tag{1}$$

For example all classical polynomials obey differential equations built with operators of this kind. We aim to combine derivatives of $T_l g$ in such a way that $D_1 g$ occurs under the integral. From the definition of $T_l g$ it follows

$$\frac{d}{dr}[(T_l g)](r) = (1/r)[T_l(t g')](r) \quad , \tag{2}$$

and

$$\frac{d^2}{dr^2}[(T_l g)](r) = (1/r^2)[T_l(t^2 g'')](r) \quad . \tag{3}$$

The difficult part is the construction of a term involving only g'' under the integral. To this end we use the differential equation for the Gegenbauer polynomials $C_l^{(n-2)/2}(s)$, see 22.6.6 [1], all formulae for special functions used in this paper are taken from [1] :

$$l(l+n-2)\,(T_l g)(r) = \int_{-1}^{1} g(rt)\,[(n-1)t(C_l^\nu)'(t)-(1-t^2)(C_l^\nu)''(t)]\,(1-t^2)^{(n-3)/2}\,dt\ .$$

Integration by parts, in order to lift the second derivative of the Gegenbauer polynomial, yields :

$$l(l+n-2)(T_l g)(r) = (n-1)r\frac{d}{dr}[T_l g](r) + r^2\frac{d^2}{dr^2}[T_l g](r) - r^2(T_l g'')(r)\ . \quad (4)$$

Theorem 4. *Let T_l denote the radial operator for the full Radon transform and let D_1 denote the differential operator (1). Then the intertwining differential operator D_2, i.e. the operator fulfilling $D_2T_l = T_lD_1$, is given by*

$$(D_2 f)(r) = (1-r^2)f''(r) + (\alpha r + \frac{n-1}{r})f'(r) + (\beta - \frac{l(l+n-2)}{r^2})f(r)\ . \quad (5)$$

Proof. The proof follows from combining formulae (2)-(4) such that $(T_lD_1g)(r)$ is obtained.

Remark: Symmetrizing the differential operator D_2 shows that two solutions $f, \bar{f}$ of $D_2 f = 0$ for different parameters β are orthogonal in

$$L_2([0,1], r^{n-1}(1-r^2)^{-(n+\alpha+1)/2}).$$

This gives rise to the weight function $W^{-1}(|\ x\ |) = (1-\ |\ x\ |)^{-(n+\alpha+1)/2}$ in Corollary 2.

Lemma 5. *Let $\{U_m\}$ denote the Tchebycheff polynomials of the second kind, i.e. they fulfill a differential equation with $\alpha = -3$, $\beta = m(m+2)$.*
Then their transforms $f_{ml} := T_lU_m$, $m+l$ even, are the bounded solutions of the differential equation $D_2 f = 0$ with boundary conditions

$$f_{ml}(0) = \begin{cases} 0 \neq c_{ml} < \infty & \text{for } l = 0 \\ 0 & \text{for } l > 0 \end{cases} \quad or \quad |\ f_{ml}(1)\ | = \begin{cases} d_{ml} < \infty & \text{for } m \geq l \\ 0 & \text{for } m < l\ . \end{cases}$$

$m < l$ leads to the trivial solution $f = 0$, for $m \geq l$ these differential equations are solved by

$$f_{ml}(r) = r^l P_{(m-l)/2}^{(1-n/2,\,l+n/2-1)}(2r^2-1)\ . \quad (6)$$

$P_l^{\alpha,\beta}(x)$ denotes the Jacobi polynomial of order l.

Proof. The boundary conditions follow from the orthogonality properties of the Gegenbauer polynomials
For $m \geq l, m+l$ even, we compute $D_2 f_{ml}$ with f_{ml} defined in (6). To abbreviate notation we use $p_{ml}(r) := P_{(m-l)/2}^{(1-n/2,l+n/2-1)}(r)$:

$$(D_2 f_{ml})(r) = 4r^l \ \{(4r^2 - 4r^4)\, p''_{ml}(2r^2-1) + (2l+n-(2l+4)r^2)\, p'_{ml}(2r^2-1) + \frac{m^2-2m-l^2-2l}{4} p_{ml}(2r^2-1)\ \} \ .$$

This is the differential equation for the Jacobi polynomials with shifted argument, see formula 22.6.1 [1], hence $D_2 f_{ml} = 0$.
The second linear independent solution of (5) is unbounded.

Except for the computation of the singular values σ_{ml} we have found a SVD for the operators T_l, and therefore also for the full Radon transform. For the computation of the singular values we observe that $T_l U_m$ has a zero of order l at $r = 0$. This again follows from the orthogonality of the Gegenbauer polynomials. The exact value of $A := [\frac{1}{r^l}(T_l U_m)(r)](0)$ can be obtained from the explicit representation for the l-th coefficient of U_m, see 22.3.7 [1], and the normalizing constant of the Gegenbauer polynomials. Then σ_{ml} is calculated by comparing A with $P_{(m-l)/2}^{(1-n/2,l+n/2-1)}(-1)$. This leads to the standard SVD for the full Radon transform, see [3], as a mapping

$$\mathcal{R} \ : \ L_2(B_1) \longrightarrow L_2(Z, (1-s^2)^{-1/2}) \ .$$

The computation of intertwining differential operators for the exterior and the interior Radon transform can be obtained in the same way, but the calculations of the derivatives are technically more involved since the boundaries in the integral $(T_l g)(r)$ also depend on r.

4 Recurrence relations

In this chapter we will obtain SVD's for the radial operators T_l by exploiting 3-term recurrence relations. Whenever possible we will not state explicitly whether the transform T_l refers to the interior, the exterior or the full Radon transform, anyhow they differ only in the interval over which the integral $(T_l g)$ extends. In all cases the integral extends over a symmetric interval. The parity of the Gegenbauer polynomials, i.e. $C_l^{(n-2)/2}(s)(1-s^2)^{(n-3)/2}$ inherits its parity from the index l, yields that functions $g(s)$ with different parity are elements of the Nullspace of T_l.

Therefore we assume that the basis functions $\{u_m\}$ fulfill a 3-term recurrence relation of the following kind :

$$u_{m+1}(s) = s a_m \ u_m(s) + b_m u_{m-1}(s) \ . \qquad (7)$$

Inserting this relation under the integral in the definition on T_l immediately gives

$$T_{l+1}u_{m+1} = b_m T_{l+1}u_{m-1} + a_m T_{l+1}(su_m) \ . \tag{8}$$

Only the last term needs further simplification. Here we use the 3-term recurrence relation obeyed by the Gegenbauer polynomials $C_l^{(n-2)/2}(s), \nu = (n-3)/2$:

$$T_{l+1}(su_m)(r) = \int ru_m(rs) \underbrace{sC_{l+1}^{(n-2)/2}(s)}_{=1/(2l+n)\{(l+2)C_{l+2}^{(n-2)/2}(s)-(l+n-2)C_l^{(n-2)/2}(s)\}} (1-s^2)^\nu \, ds$$

$$= \frac{r}{2l+n}\{(l+2)(T_{l+2}u_m)(r) + (l+n-2)(T_l u_m)(r)\} \ .$$

By combining the formulae above we obtain

Lemma 6. *Let $\{u_m\}$ fulfill the recurrence relation (7) then their transforms $\{T_l u_m\}$ obey the following recurrence relation :*

$$T_{l+1}u_{m+1} = b_m T_{l+1}u_{m-1} + rc_{ml}T_{l+2}u_m + rd_{ml}T_l u_m \ , \tag{9}$$

where

$$c_{ml} = a_m \frac{l+2}{2l+n} \quad and \quad d_{ml} = a_m \frac{l+n-2}{2l+n} \ .$$

Remark : the complete set of functions $\{T_l u_m\}$ can be constructed via this recurrence relation from $\{T_l u_0 \mid l \geq 0, \ l \ even\}$.

Example 1: Let us consider the full 2-dimensional Radon transform for functions with compact support and assume that we started with the Legendre polynomials, i.e. $u_m(s) = P_m(s)$. The coefficients in the recurrence relations are

$$a_m = \frac{2m+1}{m+1} \, , \ b_m = -\frac{m}{m+1} \, , \ c_{ml} = \frac{(2m+1)(l+2)}{(m+1)(2l+2)} \, , \ d_{ml} = \frac{l(2m+1)}{(m+1)(2l+2)} \, .$$

Due to the orthogonality of the Gegenbauer polynomials the starting values for the recurrence relation are

$$(T_0 P_0)(r) = const. \ \ and \ \ (T_l P_0)(r) = 0 \ \ for \ l > 0 \ .$$

Corollary 7. *The recurrence relation (10) for the functions $\{T_l P_m\}$ is solved by*

$$(T_l u_m)(r) = r^l P_{(m-l)/2}^{(-1/2,l)}(2r^2 - 1) \quad m \geq l \ .$$

Proof. We insert the Jacobi polynomials in the recurrence relation (10). This involves polynomials $P_k^{(\alpha,\beta)}$ with $\beta = l, l+1, l+2$. By applying formula 22.7.16 [1] we obtain a recurrence relation for Jacobi polynomials with $\beta = l$ only. This results in the standard recurrence relation 22.7.1 for the Jacobi polynomials.

These shifted Jacobi polynomials are orthogonal in $L_2([0,1],(1-r^2)^{-1/2})$. Hence choosing $W(x) = (1-|x|^2)^{-1/2}$ and applying Corollary 4 results in a SVD for the full Radon transform, compare [3].

Example 2: If we consider the 2-dimensional interior Radon transform, then the functions $(T_l P_m)(r)$ coincide for $|r| \leq 1$ with Example 1. For $|r| > 1$ we have to solve the recurrence relation (4) with starting functions

$$(T_l P_0)(r) = \int_{-1/r}^{1/r} \frac{C_l^0(t)}{\sqrt{1-t^2}} dt \ .$$

But $(C_l^0)(r) = const * \cos(l \ \arccos(r))$, since it is a Tchebycheff polynomial of the first kind, and we can integrate directly :

$$(T_0 P_0)(r) = 2 \ \arcsin(1/r) \ ,$$

$$(T_l P_0)(r) = 2 \ \sin(l \ \arcsin(1/r)) = const. \frac{1}{\sqrt{r}} P_{l-1/2}^{-1/2}\left(\sqrt{1-\frac{1}{r^2}}\right) \ .$$

P_μ^ν denotes a Legendre function see chapter 8 [1].

Corollary 8. *The recurrence relation (10) for the interior Radon transform is solved by* $(n = 2, u_m = P_m)$:

$$(T_l P_m)(r) = \begin{cases} r^l P_{(m-l)/2}^{-1/2,l}(2r^2-1) & for \ |r| \leq 1 \\ const. \ \frac{1}{\sqrt{r}} P_{l-1/2}^{-1/2-m}\left(\sqrt{1-\frac{1}{r^2}}\right) & for \ |r| > 1 \end{cases}$$

These functions are orthogonal in $L_2(\mathbb{R}, W^{-1})$ *with*

$$W(r) = \begin{cases} 1/\sqrt{1-r^2} & for \ |r| \leq 1 \\ 1/\sqrt{r^2-1} & for \ |r| > 1 \ . \end{cases}$$

The proof needs only basic but lengthy operations involving the recurrence relations for Legendre functions. For the final result compare with [5].

References

1. M. Abramovitz and I.A. Stegun, *Handbook of Mathematical Functions*, Dover, New York, 1965.
2. A. Cormack, *Representation of a function by its line integrals with some radiological applications II*, J. Appl. Phys., 43(1964) pp.2908-13.
3. A.K. Louis, *Orthogonal function series expansions and the nullspace of the Radon transform*, SIAM J. Math. Anal., 15(1984), pp.621-633.
4. A.K. Louis, *Incomplete data problems in X-ray computerized tomography. I: Singular value decomposition of the limited angle transform*, Numer. Math., 48(1986), pp.251-262.

5. P. MAASS, *The interior Radon transform*, accepted for publication in SIAM J. on Applied Mathematics.
6. R.B. MARR, *On the reconstruction of a function on a circular domain from a sampling of its line integrals* , J. Math. Anal. Appl. 45(1974), pp. 357-374.
7. F. NATTERER, *The Mathematics of Computerized Tomography*, Teubner, Stuttgart, 1986.
8. R.M. PERRY, *On reconstructing a function on the exterior of a disc from its Radon transform*, J. Math. Anal. Appl., 59(1977), pp.324-341.
9. E.T. QUINTO, *Singular value decompositions and inversion methods for the exterior Radon transform and a spherical transform* J. Math. Anal. Appl., 95(1985), pp. 437-448.

Image Reconstruction in Hilbert Space

W. R. Madych*

Abstract

We outline a general procedure for reconstructing images and certain features from measurements based on a linear model. Roughly speaking, the method involves the construction of a Hilbert space on which the measurement functionals are continuous; the desired quantities can then be determined by variants of established techniques. In certain cases this construction results in a reproducing kernel Hilbert space. The basic ideas are illustrated by familiar examples, including certain models in tomography.

In short, the primary goal of this paper is to indicate a natural framework for the application of classical Hilbert space methods to the problem of reconstruction of images from indirect measurements.

1 Introduction.

In various circumstances one obtains measurements concerning a given quantity with the objective of determining certain features of that quantity. If the desired features cannot be determined or measured directly then these features must be determined or approximated from indirect measurements. The case of indirect measurement raises a host of interesting questions and problems, some of which can be roughly summarized as follows:

- Do the measurements determine the desired features uniquely?

*Department of Mathematics, U-9; University of Connecticut; Storrs, CT 06269. Partially supported by a grant from the Air Force Office of Scientific Research, AFOSR-90-0311

- If not, then how well can one approximate the desired features from the measurements?
- Is there a constructive method for determining or approximating the desired features from the measurements?

It is the purpose of this note to address the third question on this list when the relationship between the desired quantities and the measurements is linear. The first two questions are treated only incidentally.

Observe that the above questions are essentially mathematical in nature and cannot be effectively addressed without a precise mathematical model relating the measurements to the desired features. The general setup is as follows:

The measurements are a collection of scalars, $f_1, \ldots, f_n$, which are functionals of an image or phantom f. In particular if we call these functionals $\ell_1, \ldots, \ell_n$, then $f_1 = \ell_1(f), \ldots, f_n = \ell_n(f)$. The desired quantity may be the image or phantom f itself or certain features of f which may be modeled by other functionals $\{\ell_\alpha(f)\}$ of f. Of course in most instances one can only hope to reconstruct an approximation of f or such functionals. In what follows we will denote such approximations of f or certain functionals by $\tilde{f}$ and $\{\widetilde{\ell_\alpha(f)}\}$ respectively.

In the case when the functionals $\ell_1, \ldots, \ell_n$ are linear and are continuous on some Hilbert space $\mathcal{H}$, which presumably contains the image or phantom, a popular and natural choice for $\tilde{f}$ is the orthogonal projection of f onto the subspace generated by these functionals. See the example in Subsection 1.1 below. This projection can be computed from the given data by well known methods and has several interesting properties. Perhaps the most significant of these is the fact that the mapping $(f_1, \ldots, f_n) \rightarrow \tilde{f}$ is linear. Furthermore this projection is that unique element of minimal $\mathcal{H}$ norm which satisfies the data and the resulting approximation is optimal in a certain sense, see [4] and [17].

Unfortunately, in many circumstances, the linear functionals are not continuous on some obvious Hilbert space nor is the phantom necessarily a member of such a space. See the examples in Subsections 1.2 and 1.3 below. In this paper we address a fairly common situation of this type which may be described abstractly as follows:

The phantom f is an element of some ambient linear space $\mathcal{W}$ and the set $\{\ell_1, \ldots, \ell_n\}$ is a collection of linearly independent linear functionals defined on a linear subspace of $\mathcal{W}$ which contains f. The collection $\{\phi_j\}$, $j = 1, \ldots$, is a complete orthonormal set in some Hilbert space $\mathcal{H}$ such that $\ell_k(\phi_j)$ is a well defined scalar for all j and k. Of course $\mathcal{H}$ is assumed to be a subspace of $\mathcal{W}$ but the linear functionals are not assumed to be continuous on $\mathcal{H}$. The values $\ell_1(f), \ldots, \ell_n(f)$ are known and the problem is to find an approximation $\tilde{f}$ of f or approximations $\{\widetilde{\ell_\alpha(f)}\}$ of the linear functionals $\{\ell_\alpha(f)\}$. In this paper we introduce and elaborate on the following algorithm for computing the desired approximant:

- Construct a Hilbert space $\mathcal{H}^\natural$ on which the linear functionals are continuous. The details of this construction are given in Subsection 2.3.
- In $\mathcal{H}^\natural$ we can apply various Hilbert space methods for computing an approximation for f or $\ell(f)$. Here we consider the following recipes which are outlined in Subsections 2.4 and 2.5 respectively: (i) Orthogonal projection of f and (ii) Orthogonal projection of ℓ.

The above algorithm is very versatile and can be manipulated to yield many diverse results. For example, it should be clear that in certain instances it reduces to a routine procedure leading to familiar approximants. Nevertheless, even in such instances, ingenious application of the algorithm can lead to results which are less familiar. We will use three well-known concrete scenarios to illustrate this versatility, see Subsections 1.1, 1.2, and 1.3. These examples are further developed in Subsections 3.1, 3.2, and 3.3 after the basic algorithm is outlined.

Section 2 is devoted to the development of the general ideas; certain perturbations are indicated in Subsection 2.6 which allow measurement inaccuracies and prior knowledge to be taken into account. Various comments which are relevant but not specifically germane to the development are recorded in Section 4.

1.1 The basic example

This first example is one of the most basic problems treated by classical approximation theory. It is also one of the simplest examples of the general scenario under consideration in this paper. Here is the problem:

Given the constants

$$f_k = \int_0^1 f(x) \cos k\pi x \, dx \,, \qquad k = 0, 1, \ldots, n, \tag{1}$$

find a good approximant for f.

A natural choice of $\mathcal{W}$ and $\mathcal{H}$ seems to be the following: $\mathcal{W} = L^1([0,1])$, the space of Lebesgue integrable functions on the interval $[0,1]$ and $\mathcal{H} = L^2([0,1])$, the space of Lebesgue square integrable functions on $[0,1]$ with scalar product given by

$$\langle \phi, \psi \rangle = \int_0^1 \phi(x)\overline{\psi(x)}dx$$

where the overline denotes the complex conjugate. Of course f is the phantom in this case and the linear functionals are defined by

$$\ell_k(f) = \int_0^1 f(x) \cos k\pi x \, dx \ , \qquad k = 0, \ldots, n.$$

These functionals are continuous on $\mathcal{H}$.

There are many well-known classical methods to produce approximants $\tilde{f}$. Recall that the method of orthogonal projection goes as follows:

- Identify $\ell_k(f)$ with the scalar product $\langle f, g_k \rangle$ where $g_k(x) = \cos k\pi x$.
- Take the approximant $\tilde{f}$ to be

  $$\tilde{f} = \sum_{k=0}^{n} a_k g_k$$

  where the coefficients a_k are given by the solution of the system of equations

  $$\sum_{k=0}^{n} a_k \langle g_k, g_m \rangle = \langle f, g_m \rangle \ , \qquad m = 0, \ldots, n \ .$$

- The resulting approximant is the unique element in $\mathcal{H}$ which minimizes the quadratic form $\langle \phi, \phi \rangle$ and satisfies

  $$\langle \tilde{f}, g_k \rangle = f_k \ , \qquad k = 0, \ldots, n \ .$$

  Specifically in this case $\tilde{f}$ is given by

$$\tilde{f} = \sum_{k=0}^{n} 2 f_k \cos k\pi x \ . \tag{2}$$

Of course there are many other well established methods for finding approximants to problems like the one presented above. In this paper however we will concentrate on extensions of the method of orthogonal projection.

1.2 Extrapolation

The following is a classical extrapolation problem: Given numbers $x_1, \ldots, x_n$ and the corresponding values of a 2π periodic function $f(x_1), \ldots, f(x_n)$, extrapolate f to all of $R = \{-\infty < x < \infty\}$. In other words, the problem is to find a 2π periodic function $\tilde{f}$ which approximates f on all of R from knowledge of only the values $f(x_1), \ldots, f(x_n)$.

In this case a reasonable choice of $\mathcal{W}$ and $\mathcal{H}$ appears to be $\mathcal{W} = \mathcal{H} = L^2(R/2\pi Z)$, the class of 2π periodic functions which are locally Lebesgue square integrable. The scalar product in $\mathcal{H}$ is given by

$$\langle \phi, \psi \rangle = \frac{1}{2\pi} \int_0^{2\pi} \phi(x) \overline{\psi(x)}\, dx \,.$$

The linear functionals are defined by $\ell_j(f) = f(x_j)$, $j = 1, \ldots, n$.

Since functions in $L^2(R/2\pi Z)$ are defined only up to sets of measure zero, pointwise evaluation of such functions does not make sense. In short, the mappings $f \to f(x_j)$, $j = 1, \ldots, n$, are not well defined on all of $\mathcal{H}$. Nevertheless, these mappings are well defined on the class of continuous functions $C(R/2\pi Z)$; indeed, if $\Phi = \{\ldots \phi_{-1}, \phi_0, \phi_1, \ldots\}$ is the complete orthonormal sequence $\phi_k(x) = \exp(ikx)$, $k = 0, \pm 1, \pm 2, \ldots$, then

$$\ell_j(\phi_k) = \exp(ikx_j) \,.$$

Thus it is quite reasonable to assume that the phantom f is in $C(R/2\pi Z)$ and that its approximant can be computed from the values $f(x_j)$ and $\ell_j(\phi_k)$, $j = 1, \ldots, n$, $k = 0, \pm 1, \ldots$.

1.3 Tomography

A typical model which arises in tomography is the following:

The measurements $f_1, \ldots, f_n$ are the integrals of a function $f(\vec{x})$ along certain lines in the plane. Here $\vec{x}$ is variable in some planar region Ω. The main objective, of course, is to reconstruct f from these measurements.

If we parametrize the j-th line by

$$\vec{x}_j(t) = \vec{u}_j t + \vec{p}_j \,, \qquad -\infty < t < \infty, \tag{3}$$

where $\vec{p}_j$ is a point on the line and $\vec{u}_j$ is a unit tangent, then these measurements can be expressed as

$$(4) \qquad f_j = \ell_j(f) = \int_{-\infty}^{\infty} f(\vec{x}_j(t))dt\,, \qquad j = 1,\ldots,n.$$

For completeness we mention that $\ell_j(f)$ can be viewed as a sampling of the Radon transform of f. This point of view is very useful in certain instances. However we will have no occasion to use it here.

Typically $\mathcal{W}$ is the class of measurable functions with support in Ω and

$$\mathcal{H} = L^2(\Omega,\omega) = \{f \in \mathcal{W} : \int_\Omega |f(\vec{x})|^2\omega(\vec{x})d\vec{x} < \infty\}$$

where ω is a positive integrable weight function and $d\vec{x}$ is the "element of area" for planar Lebesgue measure.

Note that with this choice of model the functionals $\ell_1,\ldots,\ell_n$ are not continuous on $\mathcal{H}$. Indeed, $\ell_j(f)$ need not be well-defined! On the other hand, if $\phi_1,\phi_2,\ldots$ is a collection of orthogonal polynomials in $L^2(\Omega,\omega)$ then, taking ϕ_k to be 0 outside of Ω, $\ell_j(\phi_k)$ is a well defined scalar for each j and k.

2 Details.

First we recall the basic definitions.

Suppose $\Phi = \{\phi_1,\phi_2,\ldots\}$ is a complete orthonormal system in a Hilbert space $\mathcal{H}$. As is customary, the symbols $\langle f,g\rangle$ denote the inner product of two elements, f and g, in $\mathcal{H}$ and $\hat{f}_j = \langle f,\phi_j\rangle$, $j = 1,2,\ldots$. Thus $\{\hat{f}_1,\hat{f}_2,\ldots\}$ is the sequence of Fourier coefficients of f with respect to the complete orthonormal system Φ. $\mathcal{H}$ may be regarded as a collection of such sequences via the standard identification. The norm $\|f\|$ of an element f of $\mathcal{H}$ is defined by $\|f\|^2 = \langle f,f\rangle$ of course. In the discussion below, we assume the field of scalars to be the complex numbers.

Suppose $\mathcal{W}$ is a linear space which contains the Hilbert space $\mathcal{H}$. If ℓ is a linear functional whose domain $\mathcal{V}$ is a subspace of $\mathcal{W}$ we say that ℓ is *compatible* with the complete orthonormal system $\Phi = \{\phi_1,\phi_2,\ldots\}$ if

- Φ is in the domain of ℓ. In other words, $\ell(\phi_j)$ is a well defined scalar for each j, $j = 1,2,\ldots$.

- If $f = \sum_{j=1}^{\infty} a_j \phi_j$ is in $\mathcal{H}$ and $\sum_{j=1}^{\infty} |a_j||\ell(\phi_j)| < \infty$ then f is in the domain of ℓ and $\ell(f) = \sum_{j=1}^{\infty} a_j \ell(\phi_j)$.

2.1 The basic setup and problem

The basic setup can be summarized as follows:

- $\mathcal{W}$ is a linear space which contains the phantom f.
- $\Phi = \{\phi_1, \phi_2, \ldots\}$ is a complete orthonormal set in a separable Hilbert space $\mathcal{H}$. $\mathcal{H}$ is a subspace of $\mathcal{W}$.
- $\ell_1, \ldots, \ell_n$ is a collection of linearly independent linear functionals each of which is compatible with Φ. In particular, we assume that the n sequences $\{\ell_k(\phi_1), \ell_k(\phi_2), \ldots\}$, $k = 1, \ldots, n$, are linearly independent.
- The phantom f is in the domain of each ℓ_j, $j = 1, \ldots, n$.

We emphasize that the functionals ℓ_j are not necessarily defined on all of $\mathcal{W}$ or $\mathcal{H}$ and of course they are not necessarily continuous on $\mathcal{H}$. Also, f is not assumed to be in $\mathcal{H}$.

Suppose the values $\ell_1(f), \ldots, \ell_n(f)$ are given. The problems we address below are the following:

- Find an approximant $\tilde{f}$ of f.
- Suppose ℓ is another linear functional whose domain contains f and which is compatible with Φ. Find an approximant $\widetilde{\ell(f)}$ of $\ell(f)$.

In what follows, for simplicity, we assume that the collection $\ell_1, \ldots, \ell_n$ of linear functionals (or measurements) is finite. This is the case in most practical applications. However it is not difficult to see that this is not an essential restriction and with minor modifications the development given below holds in the case when the collection is infinite. This may be of some academic interest.

2.2 Simple interpolation.

Consider the matrix

$$M = (\ell_i(\phi_j)) \; , \quad i,j = 1,\ldots,n. \tag{5}$$

This matrix is not necessarily invertible in the general case. However, in view of the fact that the sequences $\{\ell_j(\phi_1), \ell_j(\phi_2), \ldots\}$, $j = 1, \ldots, n$, are linearly independent, it should be clear that, by reordering the ϕ_j's if necessary, we can and do assume that M is invertible.

Since M is not singular, we can always find an element $\tilde{f}$ which satisfies

$$\ell_k(\tilde{f}) = \ell_k(f) \; , \quad k = 1,\ldots,n, \tag{6}$$

by simply setting

$$\tilde{f} = \sum_{j=1}^{n} a_j \phi_j \tag{7}$$

where the a_j's are scalars which satisfy the system of equations

$$\sum_{j=1}^{n} a_j \ell_k(\phi_j) = \ell_k(f) \; , \quad k = 1,\ldots,n. \tag{8}$$

Since M is invertible, a unique set of such a_j's exists.

Note that this method can be applied even if the basis elements $\phi_1, \ldots, \phi_n$ are not necessarily orthogonal as long as the corresponding matrix M given by (5) is not singular. The resulting approximant, $\tilde{f}$ is a simply a linear combination of $\phi_1, \ldots, \phi_n$ which interpolates the data $\ell_1(f), \ldots, \ell_n(f)$, namely, $\ell_1(\tilde{f}) = \ell_1(f), \ldots, \ell_n(\tilde{f}) = \ell_n(f)$. The properties of such a solution depend on the relationship between f, the ℓ's, and ϕ's. In certain instances it results in excellent approximants; the general case, however, is not well documented.

In the development below we present a natural Hilbert space method for computing an approximant $\tilde{f}$ in the general case.

2.3 Constructing a Hilbert space for the problem

Let h_j, $j = 1, 2, \ldots$, be a sequence of non-negative real numbers such that

$$\sum_{j=1}^{\infty} h_j |\ell_k(\phi_j)|^2 < \infty \tag{9}$$

for all k. Set $w_j = h_j^{-1}$ and consider the subspace $H^\natural$ of $\mathcal{H}$ consisting of those elements f for which

$$\|f\|_\natural = \left(\sum_{j=1}^{\infty} |\hat{f}_j|^2 w_j \right)^{1/2} \tag{10}$$

is finite. (In the case $h_j = 0$ the term $|\hat{f}_j|^2 w_j$ is taken to be zero if $\hat{f}_j$ is zero; otherwise it fails to be finite.) The Hilbert space $\mathcal{H}^\natural$ is the completion of $H^\natural$ in the norm $\|f\|_\natural$ defined by (10). We assume that $\mathcal{W}$ is sufficiently large that it contains $\mathcal{H}^\natural$. The inner product in $\mathcal{H}^\natural$ is given by

$$\langle f, g \rangle_\natural = \sum_{j=1}^{\infty} \hat{f}_j \overline{\hat{g}_j} w_j . \tag{11}$$

Proposition 1 *The linear functionals $\ell_1, \ldots, \ell_n$ are well defined and continuous on $\mathcal{H}^\natural$.*

Proof That $\ell_k(f)$ is well defined for f in $\mathcal{H}^\natural$ follows from the fact that we may write

$$\begin{aligned} |\ell_k(f)| &= |\sum_{j=1}^{\infty} \hat{f}_j \ell_k(\phi_j)| \\ &\le \left(\sum_{j=1}^{\infty} |\hat{f}_j|^2 w_j \right)^{1/2} \left(\sum_{j=1}^{\infty} |\ell_k(\phi_j)|^2 h_j \right)^{1/2} . \end{aligned}$$

and $c_k^2 = \sum_{j=1}^{\infty} |\ell_k(\phi_j)|^2 h_j$ is finite. The last inequality may be re-expressed as

$$|\ell_k(f)| \le c_k \|f\|_\natural$$

which implies continuity of ℓ_k. ∎

Proposition 2 *If the sequence h_j, $j = 1, 2, \ldots$, is bounded then $\mathcal{H}^\natural$ is a subspace of $\mathcal{H}$. If, in addition, all the h_j's are non-zero, then $\mathcal{H}^\natural$ is dense in $\mathcal{H}$ and the set $\ell_1^\natural, \ldots, \ell_n^\natural$ is linearly independent in $\mathcal{H}^\natural$.*

Proof To see the first statement simply write

$$\|f\|^2 = \sum_{j=1}^{\infty} |\hat{f}_j|^2 \le \sup_j \{h_j\} \sum_{j=1}^{\infty} |\hat{f}_j|^2 w_j = \sup_j \{h_j\} \|f\|_\natural^2 .$$

The second statement follows from the fact that the subspace consisting of those f's which have only a finite number of non-zero Fourier coefficients is dense in both $\mathcal{H}^\natural$ and $\mathcal{H}$. ∎

Recall that if ℓ is a continuous linear functional on $\mathcal{H}^\natural$ then there is an element $\ell^\natural$ of $\mathcal{H}^\natural$ so that $\ell(f) = \langle f, \ell^\natural \rangle_\natural$. In fact we may identify ℓ with $\ell^\natural$. However, they may differ as elements of $\mathcal{W}$ and in order to keep this difference clear we will always use the notation $\ell^\natural$ to denote the representative of the continuous linear functional ℓ on $\mathcal{H}^\natural$. Thus for f in $\mathcal{H}^\natural$ we have

$$\ell(f) = \langle f, \ell^\natural \rangle_\natural = \sum_{j=1}^{\infty} \hat{f}_j \overline{\hat{\ell}^\natural_j} w_j \tag{12}$$

and it is clear that

$$\ell^\natural_k = \sum_{j=1}^{\infty} h_j \overline{\ell_k(\phi_j)} \phi_j \tag{13}$$

for $k = 1, \ldots, n$. These series converge in $\mathcal{H}^\natural$ by virtue of (9). Furthermore, if the h_j's are bounded then these series also converge in $\mathcal{H}$. The scalar product of $\ell^\natural_k$ and $\ell^\natural_m$ in $\mathcal{H}^\natural$ is given by

$$\langle \ell^\natural_k, \ell^\natural_m \rangle_\natural = \sum_{j=1}^{\infty} \overline{\ell_k(\phi_j)} \ell_m(\phi_j) h_j. \tag{14}$$

Note that the collection $\ell^\natural_1, \ldots, \ell^\natural_n$ is not necessarily linearly independent as a subset of $\mathcal{H}^\natural$; this depends on the choice of the h_j's. However the h_j's can always be chosen so that $\ell^\natural_1, \ldots, \ell^\natural_n$ is linearly independent and, in what follows, we always assume that this is the case. In particular the matrix

$$L = (\langle \ell^\natural_k, \ell^\natural_m \rangle_\natural) \tag{15}$$

whose elements are defined by (14) is not singular and is positive definite.

2.4 Orthogonal projection of f

Let $s(f)$ be defined by the formula

$$s(f) = \sum_{k=1}^{n} a_k \ell^\natural_k \tag{16}$$

where the coefficients a_k are computed from the data $\ell_1(f),\ldots,\ell_n(f)$ by solving the system of linear equations

$$\sum_{k=1}^{n} a_k \langle \ell_k^\natural, \ell_m^\natural \rangle_\natural = \ell_m(f)\ , \ m = 1,\ldots,n. \tag{17}$$

Since the matrix L defined by (15) is not singular there is a unique set of a_k's which satisfies (17) and thus $s(f)$ is well defined. Observe that

$$\ell_m(s(f)) = \langle s(f), \ell_m^\natural \rangle_\natural = \ell_m(f) \tag{18}$$

for $m = 1,\ldots,n$.

Suppose $\mathcal{L}$ is the subspace of $\mathcal{H}^\natural$ spanned by $\ell_1^\natural,\ldots,\ell_n^\natural$. If we choose to regard the phantom f as an element of $\mathcal{H}^\natural$ formulas (16), (17), and (18) imply the following:

Proposition 3 *The element $s(f)$ defined by (16) is the orthogonal projection of f onto $\mathcal{L}$ in $\mathcal{H}^\natural$. As a consequence we have*

$$\|f\|_\natural^2 = \|f - s(f)\|_\natural^2 + \|s(f)\|_\natural^2\ . \tag{19}$$

In view of the last proposition we now have a method for constructing an approximant $\tilde{f}$ of f, namely $\tilde{f} = s(f)$.

2.4.1 A biorthogonal representation

A particularly elegant way of representing the orthogonal projection $s(f)$ is in terms of elements $\lambda_1,\ldots,\lambda_n$ which are biorthogonal to $\ell_1^\natural,\ldots,\ell_n^\natural$ in $\mathcal{L}$.

Recall that a collection $\lambda_1,\ldots,\lambda_n$ is said to be biorthogonal or dual to $\ell_1^\natural,\ldots,\ell_n^\natural$ in $\mathcal{L}$ if it is a subset of $\mathcal{L}$ and

$$\langle \lambda_j, \ell_k^\natural \rangle_\natural = \delta_{jk}\ , \quad j,k = 1,\ldots,n \tag{20}$$

where δ_{jk} is the Kronecker delta. Here $\mathcal{L}$, the subspace spanned by $\ell_1^\natural,\ldots,\ell_n^\natural$, is regarded as a closed subspace of $\mathcal{H}^\natural$ whose inner product coincides with that of $\mathcal{H}^\natural$.

If $\lambda_1,\ldots,\lambda_n$ is biorthogonal to $\ell_1^\natural,\ldots,\ell_n^\natural$ in $\mathcal{L}$ then it is easy to check that

$$\lambda_k = \sum_{j=1}^{n} b_{kj} \ell_j^\natural\ , \quad k = 1,\ldots,n. \tag{21}$$

The coefficients b_{kj} can be found by solving

$$\sum_{j=1}^{n} b_{kj}\langle \ell_j^\natural, \ell_m^\natural\rangle_\natural = \delta_{km}\,, \quad k,m = 1,\ldots,n, \tag{22}$$

in other words, the matrix (b_{kj}) is simply L^{-1} where L is given by (15). In terms of such λ_k's the orthogonal projection $s(f)$ has the representation

$$s(f) = \sum_{k=1}^{n} \ell_k(f)\lambda_k. \tag{23}$$

It should be mentioned that in spite of the fact that representation (23) is elegant, in specific examples it may be awkward to use and other representations may be more convenient. On the other hand, in certain cases the ℓ_k's and λ_k's may be conveniently related making it unnecessary to solve (22) and easy to evaluate (23). See Subsection 3.2.1.

2.4.2 A general error estimate.

The following proposition gives an estimate of the error in the $\mathcal{H}$ norm whenever $\mathcal{H}^\natural$ is a subspace of $\mathcal{H}$

Proposition 4 *Suppose the sequence $\{h_j\}$ is bounded and f is in $\mathcal{H}^\natural$. Then*

$$\|f - s(f)\| \le \epsilon\|f\|_\natural \tag{24}$$

where

$$\epsilon \le \left\{\max_{j\ge n+1}\{h_j\} + \rho^2\left(\sum_{k=1}^{n}\sum_{j=n+1}^{\infty} |\ell_k(\phi_j)|^2 h_j\right)\right\}^{1/2}$$

and ρ^{-2} is the smallest eigenvalue of the matrix L defined by (15).

Proof First observe that it suffices to prove the proposition in the case

$$\ell_k(f) = 0\,, \quad k = 1,\ldots,n. \tag{25}$$

For if the result holds in this case then it holds in the general case, since $\ell_k(f - s(f)) = 0$ for all k and $s(f - s(f)) = 0$, we may write

$$\|f - s(f)\| \le \epsilon\|f - s(f)\|_\natural. \tag{26}$$

Now, by virtue of (19) we have $\|f - s(f)\|_{\natural} \leq \|f\|_{\natural}$ which together with inequality (26) imply the desired result.

Now suppose that f satisfies (25). In other words

$$\sum_{j=1}^{\infty} \hat{f}_j \ell_k(\phi_j) = 0 \, , \, k = 1, \ldots, n$$

or

$$\sum_{j=1}^{n} \ell_k(\phi_j)\hat{f}_j = - \sum_{j=n+1}^{\infty} \ell_k(\phi_j)\hat{f}_j \, , \, k = 1, \ldots, n. \tag{27}$$

If we denote the right hand side of (27) by y_k, set $\vec{y} = (y_1, \ldots, y_n)^T$, and set $\vec{x} = (\hat{f}_1, \ldots, \hat{f}_n)^T$ then (27) may be rewritten as

$$M\vec{x} = \vec{y} \tag{28}$$

where M is the matrix defined by (5). From (28) it follows that

$$|\vec{x}|^2 = |M^{-1}\vec{y}|^2 \leq \rho^2 |\vec{y}|^2 \tag{29}$$

where $|\vec{x}|^2$ denotes the sum of the squares of the components of $\vec{x}$ and, since $M^*M = L$, ρ^{-2} is the smallest eigenvalue of L. An application of the Schwartz inequality gives

$$|\vec{y}|^2 \leq \sum_{k=1}^{n} \left\{ \left(\sum_{j=n+1}^{\infty} |\hat{f}_j|^2 h_j^{-1} \right) \left(\sum_{j=n+1}^{\infty} |\ell_k(\phi_j)|^2 h_j \right) \right\}$$

and since term in the first set of parentheses is dominated by $\|f\|_{\natural}^2$ we may write

$$|\vec{y}|^2 \leq \left(\sum_{k=1}^{n} \sum_{j=n+1}^{\infty} |\ell_k(\phi_j)|^2 h_j \right) \|f\|_{\natural}^2. \tag{30}$$

Finally

$$\sum_{j=n+1}^{\infty} |\hat{f}_j|^2 \leq \max_{j \geq n+1} \{h_j\} \sum_{j=n+1}^{\infty} |\hat{f}_j|^2 h_j^{-1} = \max_{j \geq n+1} \{h_j\} \|f\|_{\natural}^2. \tag{31}$$

Since

$$\|f\|^2 = \sum_{j=1}^{n} |\hat{f}_j|^2 + \sum_{j=n+1}^{\infty} |\hat{f}_j|^2 \tag{32}$$

the desired result follows from (32) together with (29), (30), and (31). ■

We remark that in many cases this estimate is far from optimal. Better estimates can usually be derived based on the specific model under consideration. See [4] for examples of tight bounds.

2.5 Orthogonal projection of ℓ

Suppose ℓ is a linear functional which is compatible with Φ and whose domain contains f. Assume that $\mathcal{H}^\natural$ is chosen so that ℓ is well defined and continuous on $\mathcal{H}^\natural$. We wish to find an approximant $\widetilde{\ell(f)}$ of $\ell(f)$ in terms of $\ell_1(f), \ldots, \ell_n(f)$.

One immediate solution to this problem is given by

$$\widetilde{\ell(f)} = \ell(\tilde{f}) \tag{33}$$

where $\tilde{f}$ is an approximant of f. Under certain conditions the optimal approximant of $\ell(f)$ is given when $\tilde{f} = s(f)$, namely,

$$\widetilde{\ell(f)} = \ell(s(f)) \tag{34}$$

where $s(f)$ is the orthogonal projection of f onto $\mathcal{L}$ as described in Subsection 2.4; see [4].

Alternate approximations can be derived in terms of weighted averages of $\ell_1(f), \ldots, \ell_n(f)$. Such expressions are of the form

$$\widetilde{\ell(f)} = \sum_{j=1}^{n} a_j \ell_j(f) \,. \tag{35}$$

There are many ways one can determine acceptable coefficients a_j in (35). Some of these depend on the specifics of the particular model at hand. A straightforward method which is also quite general goes as follows:

Using the notation established in Subsection 2.3 let $\ell^\natural$ be the representative of ℓ in $\mathcal{H}^\natural$, recall that $\ell_j(f) = \langle f, \ell_j^\natural \rangle_\natural$, $j = 1, \ldots, n$, and write

$$|\ell(f) - \sum_{j=1}^{n} a_j \ell_j(f)| = |\langle f, \ell^\natural - \sum_{j=1}^{n} a_j \ell_j^\natural \rangle_\natural| \leq \|f\|_\natural \|\ell^\natural - \sum_{j=1}^{n} a_j \ell_j^\natural\|_\natural \,. \tag{36}$$

Inequality (36) suggests choosing the coefficients a_j in such a way so that $\|\ell^\natural - \sum_{j=1}^n a_j \ell_j^\natural\|_\natural$ is minimized. Doing so results in the choice

(37) $$s(\ell^\natural) = \sum_{j=1}^{n} a_j \ell_j^\natural$$

where $s(\ell^\natural)$ is the orthogonal projection of $\ell^\natural$ onto $\mathcal{L}$; in other words the a_j's satisfy

(38) $$\sum_{j=1}^{n} a_j \langle \ell_j^\natural, \ell_k^\natural \rangle_\natural = \langle \ell^\natural, \ell_k^\natural \rangle_\natural \qquad k = 1, \ldots, n\,.$$

The resulting approximation is given by

(39) $$\widetilde{\ell(f)} = \langle f, s(\ell^\natural) \rangle_\natural\,.$$

Proposition 5 *The approximations given by (34) and (39) are identical. In other words,*

$$\ell(s(f)) = \langle f, s(\ell^\natural) \rangle_\natural\,.$$

Proof The proposition follows from the facts that $\ell(f) = \langle f, \ell^\natural \rangle_\natural$ and that the mapping $f \to s(f)$ is an orthogonal projection in $\mathcal{H}^\natural$. ■

In essence (34) and (39) represent the same quantity computed in two different ways. Formula (34) requires the solution of the system (17) and then the evaluation of (35). Whereas formula (39) requires the solution of the system (38) followed by the evaluation of (35). In other words, if one is interested in the approximation of one linear functional for many sets of data arising from a family of phantoms then (39) seems more efficient; on the other hand, if one is interested in approximating many linear functionals $\ell_x(f)$, where x is in some index set Ω, then (34) seems more efficient. Of course much depends on the specific model. For instance, the linear functionals ℓ_x may be related to one another in some convenient way which gives rise to efficient formulas for the a_j's in

$$s(\ell_x^\natural) = \sum_{j=1}^{n} a_j(x) \ell_j^\natural$$

so that multiple solutions of (38) may not be necessary.

2.6 Noise and prior knowledge

Here we indicate several modifications one may wish to adopt in cases where there are errors in the measurements or one wishes to take advantage of certain prior knowledge. Of course we allow for the possibility of both senarios being present simultaneously.

First we stress that the method outlined in Subsections 2.3 and 2.4 is not a regularization method. The resulting approximant $\tilde{f}$ satisfies $\ell_j(\tilde{f}) = \ell_j(f)$, $j = 1, \ldots, n$. No attempt is made to compensate for possible errors in the data. The whole point of the procedure outlined above is to indicate how to construct a natural framework to solve for potential approximants $\tilde{f}$.

If the data is corrupted by noise, that is to say, the actual data $f_1, \ldots, f_n$ is given by $f_j = \ell_j(f) + \eta_j$ where η_j denotes the possible error in the measurement of $\ell_j(f)$ then, given the framework outlined in Subsections 2.3 and 2.4, there are well known and accepted procedures for approximating the phantom f. For example, one could compute approximants $\tilde{f}_\alpha$ which minimize the expression

$$\left\{ \sum_{j=1}^{n} |f_j - \langle f, \ell_j^\natural \rangle_\natural|^2 \right\} + \alpha \|f\|_\natural^2 \tag{40}$$

over all f in $\mathcal{H}^\natural$. Here the parameter α is a positive real number. Note that for small values of α the solution $\tilde{f}_\alpha$ should be close to $s(f)$, whereas for large values of α it may not be so closely related. For more details concerning regularization see [7, 8, 16] and the pertinent references listed there.

There are many ways of taking prior knowledge which is independent of the data into account when computing an approximant. Of course the specific method will generally depend on the nature of this knowledge. For example, the choice of orthogonal set used to construct $\mathcal{H}^\natural$ could reflect such knowledge; see 3.1.3. Another way that such knowledge can be implemented in the construction of $\tilde{f}$ is in terms of *a priori* bounds on certain functionals of f. If $\{\ell_x\}$ where x is in some index set Ω is a family of such functionals then the reconstruction problem would take the form of finding an approximant $\tilde{f}$ which satisfies the data

$$\ell_j(\tilde{f}) = f_j \qquad j = 1, \ldots, n,$$

together with the constraints

$$a(x) \le \ell_x(\tilde{f}) \le b(x) \qquad x \in \Omega\,.$$

We do not deal with such constraints in the examples below and will treat this matter within the framework established here in more detail elsewhere.

3 Examples

Before getting down to specific cases we first record several observations of a general nature.

In order to guarantee that the space $\mathcal{H}^\natural$ is contained in the ambient space it is clear that $\mathcal{W}$ should be chosen sufficiently large. Essentially $\mathcal{W}$ should consist of all feasible phantoms f for which $\langle f, \phi_j \rangle$ is well defined for all j. For example, the case where Φ is the class of complex exponentials namely,

$$\Phi = \{\exp(ikx) : k = 0, \pm 1, \ldots \text{ and } -\infty < x < \infty\},$$

then it is quite natural to take $\mathcal{W}$ to be a class of periodic distributions.

On the other hand, in the cases where the sequence h_j is taken to be bounded then $\mathcal{H}^\natural \subset \mathcal{H}$ and it suffices to choose $\mathcal{W} = \mathcal{H}$.

An obvious choice for h_j which will guarantee convergence of (9) is the sequence

$$h_j = \begin{cases} 1 & \text{if } j = 1, \ldots, N \\ 0 & \text{otherwise} \end{cases}$$

where N is some finite positive integer. Clearly a necessary condition for matrix L defined by (15) to be non-singular is that N be $\geq n$. In the case $N \geq n$ it is clear that the invertibility of the matrix M which is defined by (5) is sufficient to guarantee the invertibility of L. Indeed, in the case $N = n$ the approximants given by (7) and (16) are identical.

3.1 Return to the basic example

We continue making observations of a somewhat general nature by first looking at the abstract version of this problem.

3.1.1 The abstract version

Suppose the linear functionals $\ell_1, \ldots, \ell_n$ are bounded on $\mathcal{H}$ so we may write

$$\ell_j(f) = \langle f, g_j \rangle \tag{41}$$

Let $\Phi = \{\phi_1, \phi_2, \ldots\}$ be the complete orthonormal system under consideration and choose the sequence h_j so that $\sum_{j=1}^{\infty} h_j |\hat{g}_{ij},|^2$ is finite for $i = 1, \ldots, n$. Recall that

$$\ell_i^\natural = \sum_{j=1}^{\infty} h_j \hat{g}_{ij} \phi_j, \qquad i = 1, \ldots, n,$$

and that $\mathcal{L}$ is the subspace spanned by $\ell_1^\natural, \ldots, \ell_n^\natural$. To compute the orthogonal projection $s(f)$ of f into $\mathcal{L}$ in $\mathcal{H}^\natural$, we consider two scenarios.

Case 1: The span of $\{g_1, \ldots, g_n\}$ = the span of $\{\phi_1, \ldots, \phi_n\}$.

In this case the sequence h_j plays essentially no role in the determination of $s(f)$. To see this, let $G = (\hat{g}_{ij})$ be the $n \times n$ matrix of Fourier coefficients of g_i, $i = 1, \ldots, n$, with respect to ϕ_j, $j = 1, \ldots, n$. Since G is invertible, setting $G^{-1} = (b_{ij})$ we have

$$g_i = \sum_{j=1}^{n} \hat{g}_{ij} \phi_j \,, \qquad i = 1, \ldots, n$$

and

$$\phi_i = \sum_{j=1}^{n} b_{ij} g_j \,, \qquad i = 1, \ldots, n.$$

Hence, for $i = 1, \ldots, n$,

$$\hat{f}_i = \langle f, \phi_i \rangle = \sum_{j=1}^{n} \bar{b}_{ij} \langle f, g_j \rangle = \sum_{j=1}^{n} \bar{b}_{ij} \ell_j(f). \tag{42}$$

By virtue of (42) and the fact that $\{\sqrt{h_j}\phi_j\}_{j=1}^{n}$ is an orthonormal basis for $\mathcal{L}$ in $\mathcal{H}^\natural$ we may write

$$s(f) = \sum_{j=1}^{n} \langle f, \sqrt{h_j}\phi_j \rangle_\natural \sqrt{h_j}\phi_j$$

which reduces to

$$s(f) = \sum_{j=1}^{n} \hat{f}_j \phi_j \tag{43}$$

As a consequence of (43) we may conclude the following: *If $h_j > 0$ for all $j = 1, \ldots, n$ and the span of $\{g_1, \ldots, g_n\}$ = the span of $\{\phi_1, \ldots, \phi_n\}$ then $s(f)$ is simply the orthonormal projection of f onto the span of $\{\phi_1, \ldots, \phi_n\}$ in $\mathcal{H}$. Thus $s(f)$ is essentially independent of the sequence $\{h_j\}$ in this case.*

Case 2: The span of $\{g_1, \ldots, g_n\} \neq$ the span of $\{\phi_1, \ldots, \phi_n\}$.

Here the role played by the sequence $\{h_j\}$ is more significant. For example, if $h_j = 1$ for all j then it is clear that $s(f)$ is the orthogonal projection of f onto the subspace spanned by $\{g_1, \ldots, g_n\}$ in $\mathcal{H}$. On the other hand, if $h_j = 0$ for $j \geq n+1$ then $\mathcal{H}^h$ is an n dimensional subspace of $\mathcal{H}$ and $s(f)$ is the simple interpolant described in Subsection 2.2.

3.1.2 The concrete version

Here we return to the specific example introduced in Subsection 1.1. The observations made in 3.1.1 show that when the span of $\{g_0, \ldots, g_n\} =$ the span of the first $n+1$ terms in Φ then $s(f)$ is independent of the choice of $\{h_j\}$ and the situation reduces to the very familiar classical senario outlined in Subsection 1.1. We compare this with the case when the span of $\{g_0, \ldots, g_n\} \neq$ the span of the first $n+1$ terms in Φ. In particular we take Φ to be the classical Haar system on the interval $[0,1]$. We remind the reader that this system is doubly indexed and is defined by

$$\phi_{00}(x) = 1$$

and if $k = 0, 1, 2, \ldots,\ j = 1, \ldots, 2^k$ then

$$\phi_{kj}(x) = \begin{cases} 2^{k/2} & \text{if } 2(j-1)/2^{k+1} \leq x < (2j-1)/2^{k+1} \\ -2^{k/2} & \text{if } (2j-1)/2^{k+1} \leq x < 2j/2^{k+1} \\ 0 & \text{otherwise.} \end{cases}$$

In the numerical experiments whose results are illustrated by Figures 1 and 2 the classical approximant given by (2) is compared with the approximant $s(f)$ which results when Φ is the Haar system. In each case the data is described by (1), $n = 15$, and $h_{kj} = 1$ if $k \leq 3$ and $h_{kj} = 0$ otherwise. In Figure 1 the phantom is the indicator function of the interval $[1/4, 3/4]$; note the familiar behavior of the classical approximant whereas the approximant based on the Haar system is indistinquishable from the phantom. In Figures 2 the phantom is described by

$$f(x) = \pi^2 \left\{ \frac{(x-1)^2}{2} - \frac{1}{6} \right\}.$$

In this case the classical approximant is almost indistinquishable from the phantom.

3.2 Point evaluation functionals

Suppose that the ambient space $\mathcal{W}$ is a collection of functions defined on some set Ω. If x is an element of Ω then the point evaluation functional ℓ_x is defined by $\ell_x(f) = f(x)$ and generally makes sense for some, but not necessarily all, f in $\mathcal{W}$. In many such instances there are readily available collections of functions, $\phi_1, \phi_2, \ldots$, which are orthonormal with respect to appropriate scalar products $\langle \phi, \psi \rangle$ and for which $\ell_x(\phi_j)$ is well defined, for all j. Whenever this is the case one can take $\mathcal{H}$ to be the closed linear span of such a sequence. One can then follow the procedure outlined in Subsection 2.3 to obtain a Hilbert space $\mathcal{H}^\natural$ on which ℓ_x is a continuous linear functional.

If $\mathcal{H}^\natural$ is such that ℓ_x is continuous for all x in Ω then it is a reproducing kernel Hilbert space. The theory of such spaces is well documented and has found wide application; a detailed account of the basic theory may be found in [2], examples and various applications may be found in [1, 3, 4, 12] and the references cited there. In our setup the reproducing kernel K is given by

$$K(x,y) = \sum_{j=1}^{\infty} h_j \overline{\ell_x(\phi_j)} \ell_y(\phi_j) \,. \tag{44}$$

3.2.1 Periodic extrapolation

Recall the periodic extrapolation problem and the corresponding setup introduced in Subsection 1.2. The measurement or data functionals are point evaluation functionals and the desired information is the pointwise behavior of the approximant $\tilde{f}$. In view of this the sequence $\{h_j\}$ should be chosen so that all such functionals are continuous on $\mathcal{H}^\natural$. In short, it is appropriate that $\mathcal{H}^\natural$ be a reproducing kernel Hilbert space.

It should be clear that $\mathcal{H}^\natural$ *is a reproducing kernel Hilbert space if and only if the sequence* $\{h_j\}_{j\in Z}$ *satisfies*

$$\sum_{j\in Z} h_j < \infty \,. \tag{45}$$

Here Z denotes the set of all integers. If $\{h_j\}_{j\in Z}$ is a sequence which satisfies (45) then the representative of ℓ_k in $\mathcal{H}^\natural$ is the function

$$\ell_k^\natural(x) = \sum_{j\in Z} h_j e^{-ijx_k} e^{ijx} = \sum_{j\in Z} h_j e^{ij(x-x_k)} \,.$$

Note that $\ell_k^\natural$ may be re-expressed as

$$\ell_k^\natural(x) = h(x - x_k) \tag{46}$$

where

$$h(x) = \sum_{j \in Z} h_j e^{ijx} \tag{47}$$

is in $C(R/2\pi Z)$. Furthermore, in view of (44), the reproducing kernel for $\mathcal{H}^\natural$ is given by

$$K(x, y) = h(x - y)\,. \tag{48}$$

It should be clear that (46), (47), and (48) allow for a rather wide choice of such kernels K. By choosing the sequence $\{h_j\}_{j \in Z}$ appropriately one can recover many of the classical kernels use in the theory of Fourier series and classical approximation theory. For example if

$$h_j = \begin{cases} 1 & \text{if } |j| = 1, \ldots, N \\ 0 & \text{otherwise} \end{cases}$$

then

$$h(x) = \frac{\sin(N + \frac{1}{2})x}{\sin \frac{1}{2}x}$$

and $K(x, y)$ is the familiar Dirichlet kernel $D_N(x, y)$. If

$$h_j = \begin{cases} 1 - \frac{|j|}{N+1} & \text{if } |j| \le N \\ 0 & \text{otherwise} \end{cases}$$

then

$$h(x) = \frac{1}{N+1} \left\{ \frac{\sin \frac{N+1}{2} x}{\sin \frac{1}{2} x} \right\}^2$$

and $K(x, y)$ is the familiar Fejer kernel $F_N(x, y)$. In the case when the knots $x_1, \ldots, x_n$ satisfy

$$x_k = x_1 + 2\pi(k-1)/n, \qquad k = 2, \ldots, n\,, \tag{49}$$

the classical theory of extrapolation, i.e. trigonometric interpolation, is well developed in terms of such kernels. See [13] or [18].

Returning to the general case and computing $s(f)$ we see that

$$s(f,y) = \sum_{j=1}^{n} a_j h(y - x_j)$$

where the coefficients a_j satisfy

$$\sum_{j=1}^{n} a_j h(x_k - x_j) = f(x_k) , \qquad k = 1, \ldots, n .$$

This leads to

$$\tilde{f}(x) = \sum_{j=1}^{n} a_j h(x - x_j) \tag{50}$$

as the extrapolated value of f at x.

On the other hand, computing $s(\ell_x^\natural)$ we see that

$$s(\ell_x^\natural, y) = \sum_{j=1}^{n} b_j(x) h(y - x_j)$$

where the coefficients $b_j(x)$ satisfy

$$\sum_{j=1}^{n} b_j(x) h(x_k - x_j) = h(x_k - x) , \qquad k = 1, \ldots, n .$$

This leads to

$$\tilde{f}(x) = \sum_{j=1}^{n} b_j(x) f(x_j) \tag{51}$$

as the extrapolated value of f at x. In view of the results in Subsection 2.5 the values produced by formulas (50) and (51) are identical.

A dual basis To find a basis $\lambda_1, \ldots, \lambda_n$ which is biorthogonal or dual to $\ell_1^\natural, \ldots \ell_n^\natural$ in $\mathcal{L}$ in the general case one must solve (22). However if the knots $x_1, \ldots, x_n$ satisfy (49) convenient formulas for the λ_k's can be derived avoiding (22).

To see this suppose $x_1, \ldots, x_n$ satisfy (49), let

$$B_m = \sum_{j \in Z} h_{m+nj} \text{ for all } m \in Z , \tag{52}$$

and observe that

(53) $$B_{m+n} = B_m \text{ for all } m \in Z\ .$$

Note that h_m/B_m is well defined; namely if $h_m > 0$ then $B_m > 0$ and if $h_m = 0$ then the ratio h_m/B_m is taken to be 0. Finally let

(54) $$\lambda(x) = \frac{1}{n}\sum_{m\in Z}\frac{h_m}{B_m}e^{imx}\ .$$

Proposition 6 *If $x_1, \ldots, x_n$ satisfy (49) and λ is the function defined by (54) then*

$$\lambda(x - x_1), \ldots, \lambda(x - x_n)$$

is a basis dual to $\ell_1^\natural, \ldots \ell_n^\natural$ in $\mathcal{L}$. In other words

(55) $$\lambda(x_k - x_l) = \delta_{kl}$$

where δ_{kl} is the Kronecker delta.

Proof To see (55) observe that $e^{i(m+n)(x_k-x_l)} = e^{im(x_k-x_l)}$, recall (53) and write

$$\lambda(x_k - x_l) = \frac{1}{n}\sum_{m=0}^{n-1}\left(\sum_{j\in Z}\frac{h_{m+nj}}{B_m}\right)e^{im(x_k-x_l)}$$

The desired result follows from the fact that the term in parenthesis in the above expression equals one and

$$\sum_{m=0}^{n-1} e^{im(x_k-x_l)} = n\delta_{kl}\ .$$

■

Some particular examples Consider the sequence $\{h_j\}_{j\in Z}$ defined by

$$h_j = \begin{cases} 1 & \text{if } j = 0 \\ j^{-2} & \text{otherwise.} \end{cases}$$

In this case it should be clear that $\mathcal{H}^\natural$ consists of those 2π periodic functions which are absolutely continuous and whose derivative is locally square integrable. Moreover the corresponding norm of an element f can be expressed in terms of the derivative f' of f, namely,

(56) $$\|f\|_\natural^2 = \frac{1}{2\pi}\int_{-\pi}^{\pi}|f'(x)|^2dx + \left(\frac{1}{2\pi}\int_{-\pi}^{\pi}f(x)\,dx\right)^2\ .$$

The corresponding function h is given by

$$h(x) = \frac{(x - \pi(2j-1))^2}{2} + (1 - \frac{\pi^2}{6}) \qquad \text{whenever } 2(j-1)\pi \le x \le 2j\pi$$

for all j in Z; its plot is given in Figure 3. The plot of the function λ defined in the previous paragraph is indicated in Figure 4 in the case $n = 17$.

Finally, consider the sequence $\{h_j\}_{j\in Z}$ defined by

$$h_j = (1 + j^2)^{-1}$$

In this case $\mathcal{H}^\natural$ also consists of those 2π periodic functions which are absolutely continuous and whose derivative is locally square integrable. Furthermore the corresponding norm of an element f is can also be expressed in terms of the derivative f' of f. The exact expression however is slightly different, namely,

$$\|f\|_\natural^2 = \frac{1}{2\pi}\int_{-\pi}^{\pi} \left\{|f'(x)|^2 + |f(x)|^2\right\} dx \,. \tag{57}$$

Nevertheless it should be clear the norms defined by (56) and (57) are equivalent. In this case the corresponding function h is given by

$$h(x) = \pi\frac{\cosh(x - \pi(2j-1))}{\sinh\pi} \qquad \text{whenever } 2(j-1)\pi \le x \le 2j\pi$$

for all j in Z; its plot is given in Figure 5. The plot of the corresponding function λ is indicated in Figure 6 in the case $n = 17$.

3.3 Tomography revisited

Recall the model introduced in Subsection 1.3. Assume that Ω is a bounded convex subset of the plane. In this case the only ℓ_j's of interest are those that correspond to lines which intersect Ω. In view of this, we may parametrize these functionals by pairs of boundary points of Ω. Since such a parametrization is very convenient for the material which follows, we shall adopt it. Thus if $\vec{x}_0$, $\vec{x}_1$ is a pair of distinct points on the boundary of Ω we write

$$\ell_{\vec{x}_0,\vec{x}_1}(f) = \int_{-\infty}^{\infty} f(\vec{x}(t))dt \tag{58}$$

where

(59)
$$\vec{x}(t) = \frac{\vec{x}_1 - \vec{x}_0}{|\vec{x}_1 - \vec{x}_0|}t + \vec{x}_0 .$$

Next we restrict our attention to the case where Ω is the square $[0,1]\times[0,1]$ and $\omega(x) \equiv 1$. However we stress that the development outlined below can be adapted to include many other Ω's and ω's.

There are many natural choices for the orthonormal set Φ in this instance. We consider the orthonormal set $\Phi = \{\phi_{kl}\}$, where $k,l = 1,2,\ldots$, which doubly indexed for convenience and defined by

$$\phi_{kl}(x,y) = \psi_k(x)\psi_l(y)$$

where

$$\psi_k(x) = \sqrt{2}\sin k\pi x .$$

This is a familiar orthonormal set. Note that ϕ_{kl} may be expressed as

(60)
$$\phi_{kl}(x,y) = \cos\pi(kx - ly) - \cos\pi(kx + ly)$$

which is useful for evaluating (58) with $f = \phi_{kl}$ in closed form. Indeed, if $f(\vec{x}) = \cos\langle\vec{u},\vec{x}\rangle$, where $\langle\vec{u},\vec{x}\rangle = u_1x_1 + u_2x_2$ is the scalar product of $\vec{u} = (u_1,u_2)$ and $\vec{x} = (x_1,x_2)$, then

(61)
$$\ell_{\vec{x}_0,\vec{x}_1}(f) = \int_0^{|\vec{x}_1-\vec{x}_0|}\cos\langle\vec{u},\vec{x}(t)\rangle\,dt = \sigma(\vec{u},\vec{x}_0,\vec{x}_1)$$

where

$$\sigma(\vec{u},\vec{x}_0,\vec{x}_1) = |\vec{x}_1 - \vec{x}_0|\left\{\frac{\sin\langle\vec{u},\vec{x}_1\rangle - \sin\langle\vec{u},\vec{x}_0\rangle}{\langle\vec{u},\vec{x}_1 - \vec{x}_0\rangle}\right\}$$

if $\langle\vec{u},\vec{x}_1 - \vec{x}_0\rangle \neq 0$ and

$$\sigma(\vec{u},\vec{x}_0,\vec{x}_1) = |\vec{x}_1 - \vec{x}_0|\cos\langle\vec{u},\vec{x}_0\rangle$$

if $\langle\vec{u},\vec{x}_1 - \vec{x}_0\rangle = 0$. In view of (60) and (61) it follows that

(62)
$$\ell_{\vec{x}_0,\vec{x}_1}(\phi_{kl}) = \sigma(\vec{u}_{kl},\vec{x}_0,\vec{x}_1) - \sigma(\vec{v}_{kl},\vec{x}_0,\vec{x}_1)$$

where $\vec{u}_{kl} = \pi(k,-l)$ and $\vec{v}_{kl} = \pi(k,l)$.

Observe that

$$\sum_{(k,l)\in Z_+^2}|\ell_{\vec{x}_0,\vec{x}_1}(\phi_{kl})|^2$$

fails to converge; here the sum is take over all (k,l) in positive cone Z_+^2 of the integer lattice Z^2. On the other hand, if the sequence $\{h_{kl}^\alpha\}_{(k,l)\in Z_+^2}$ is defined by

(63) $$h_{kl}^\alpha = (k^2+l^2)^{-\alpha}$$

then

(64) $$\sum_{(k,l)\in Z_+^2} h_{kl}^\alpha |\ell_{\vec{x}_0,\vec{x}_1}(\phi_{kl})|^2 \text{ converges whenever } \alpha > 1/2.$$

Let $\mathcal{H}_\alpha$ be the Hilbert space defined via the recipe outlined in Subsection 2.3 with the h's given by (63). In other words,

$$\mathcal{H}_\alpha = \{f \in L^2(\Omega) : \sum_{(k,l)\in Z_+^2} |\hat{f}_{kl}|^2 w_{kl}^\alpha\}$$

where

$$\hat{f}_{kl} = \int_\Omega f(\vec{x})\phi_{kl}(\vec{x})d\vec{x} \text{ and } w_{kl}^\alpha = \frac{1}{h_{kl}^\alpha}.$$

Then in view of (64) the linear functionals $\ell_{\vec{x}_0,\vec{x}_1}$ are continuous on $\mathcal{H}_\alpha$ whenever $\alpha > 1/2$.

Note that if $\alpha > 1$ then $\mathcal{H}_\alpha$ is a reproducing kernel Hilbert space. On the other hand $\mathcal{H}_\alpha$ fails to be such a space if $\alpha \le 1$. Also observe that in the case $\alpha = 1$ the space $\mathcal{H}_\alpha$ may be described as the closure of the class of infinitely differentiable functions with compact support in Ω with respect to the norm

$$\|f\|_1^2 = \int_\Omega |\text{grad} f(\vec{x})|^2 d\vec{x}$$

Thus $\mathcal{H}_1$ is a familiar Hilbert space. Similar descriptions of $\mathcal{H}_\alpha$ in terms of f and its derivatives are also possible for other integer values of α.

If $\alpha > 1/2$ the linear functional defined by (58) enjoys the representation

(65) $$\ell_{\vec{x}_0,\vec{x}_1}^\alpha = \sum_{(k,l)\in Z_+^2} h_{kl}^\alpha \ell_{\vec{x}_0,\vec{x}_1}(\phi_{kl})\phi_{kl}$$

on $\mathcal{H}_\alpha$. In addition to converging in the $\mathcal{H}_\alpha$ sense, this series converges absolutely and uniformly on Ω which implies that $\ell_{\vec{x}_0,\vec{x}_1}^\alpha$ is a continuous function on Ω. Thus if the data consists of the measurements of (65) corresponding to selected pairs of points $\vec{x}_0$, $\vec{x}_1$ then the approximant $s(f)$ is a linear combination of the corresponding $\ell_{\vec{x}_0,\vec{x}_1}^\alpha$'s. Figure 7 shows the surface plot of $\ell_{\vec{x}_0,\vec{x}_1}^\alpha$ in the case $\vec{x}_0 = (0,1/4)$, $\vec{x}_1 = (1,1/4)$, and $\alpha = 7/8$.

A well known example of the model described by (65) with $\Omega = [0,1] \times [0,1]$ or a scaled variant is the so-called linearized well to well model used in seismic borehole tomography. See [6, 15]. We will present detailed numerical examples based on this model using the reconstruction method outlined above in another report.

4 Miscellaneous remarks

We again emphasize that the ideas and examples outlined above are not variants of some regularization method. The resulting approximants interpolate the data. The main point is to construct a natural framework in which to find potential approximants. For remarks concerning regularization see Subsection 2.6.

We also bring to the reader's attention the fact that the application of these ideas to tomography, as done in Subsection 3.3, does not result in a variant of the so-called convolution method. Again, the resulting approximants interpolate the data whereas reconstructions produced via any convolution method in general do not.

The simple interpolants mentioned in Subsection 2.2 are sometimes referred to as reconstructions via the series expansion method in X-ray tomography; see [5]. For more information concerning tomography, the Radon transform, and convolution methods see [5, 9, 10, 14] and the pertinent references cited there. References [9, 14] also contain discussions concerning regularization methods in this context.

Several acknowledgements are in order. First, I would like to thank Peter Maass for making the preprint [8] available to me. This motivated me to rewrite and expand the technical report [11] resulting in this paper. Next, I thank Hans Weinberger who brought the important work [4] to my attention and made it possible for me to participate in a workshop on inverse problems held at the IMA in Minnesota in January of 1987. The workshop certainly broadened my outlook on the subject and indirectly led to the present work. Finally, I would like to express my sincere appreciation to Gabor Herman, Alfred Louis, and Frank Natterer for initiating my slow acceptance into the mathematical tomography community by inviting me to participate in the 1986 Oberwolfach conference.

References

[1] J. H. Ahlberg, E. N. Nilson, and J. L. Walsh, *The Theory of Splines and Their Applications*, Academic, New York, 1967.

[2] N. Aronszajn, Theory of Reproducing Kernels, *Trans. Amer. Math. Soc.*, 68 (1950), 337-404.

[3] P. J. Davis, *Interpolation and Approximation*, Dover, New York, 1975.

[4] M. Golomb and H. F. Weinberger, Optimal Approximation and Error Bounds, in *On Numerical Approximation*, R. E. Langer, ed. Madison, 1959, 117-190.

[5] G. T. Herman, *Image Reconstruction from Projections. The Fundamentals of Computerized Tomography*, Academic Press, 1980.

[6] S. Ivanson, Seismic Borehole Tomography - Theory and Computational Methods, *Proc. IEEE*, 74 (1986), 328-338.

[7] A. K. Louis, *Inverse und schlecht gestellte Probleme*, Teubner Studienbücher, Stuttgart, 1989.

[8] A. K. Louis and P. Maass, Smoothed projection methods for the moment problem, preprint, 1990.

[9] A. K. Louis and F. Natterer, Mathematical Problems of Computed Tomography, *Proc. IEEE.*, 71 (1983), 379-389.

[10] W. R. Madych, Summability and approximate reconstruction from Radon transform data, in *Integral Geometry and Tomography*, E. Grinberg and E. T. Quinto, eds., Vol. 113 in Contemporary Mathematics, American Math. Soc., Providence, 1990.

[11] W. R. Madych, Hilbert spaces for estimators, BRC/MATH-TR-88-5.

[12] J. Meinguet, Surface spline interpolation: basic theory and computational aspects, in *Approximation Theory and Spline Functions*, S. P. Singh, J. Burry, and B. Watson, eds., Reidel, Dordrecht, 1984, 124-142.

[13] I. P. Natanson, *Constructive Function Theory*, Vol. III, Frederick Ungar Publishing Co., New York, 1965.

[14] F. Natterer, *The Mathematics of Computerized Tomography*, John Wiley & Sons, Stuttgart, 1986.

[15] J. E. Peterson, B. N. P. Paulson, and T. V. McEvilly, Application of algebraic reconstruction techniques to crosshole seismic data, *Geophysics*, 50 (1985), 1566-1580.

[16] A. V. Tikhonov and V. Y. Arsenin, *Solution of Ill-posed Problems*, Winston & Sons, New York, 1977.

[17] J. F. Traub and H. Wozniakowski, *A General Theory of Optimal Algorithms*, Academic, New York, 1980.

[18] A. Zygmund, *Trigonometric Series*, 2nd ed., Volumes I and II, Cambridge Univ. Press, Cambridge, 1968.

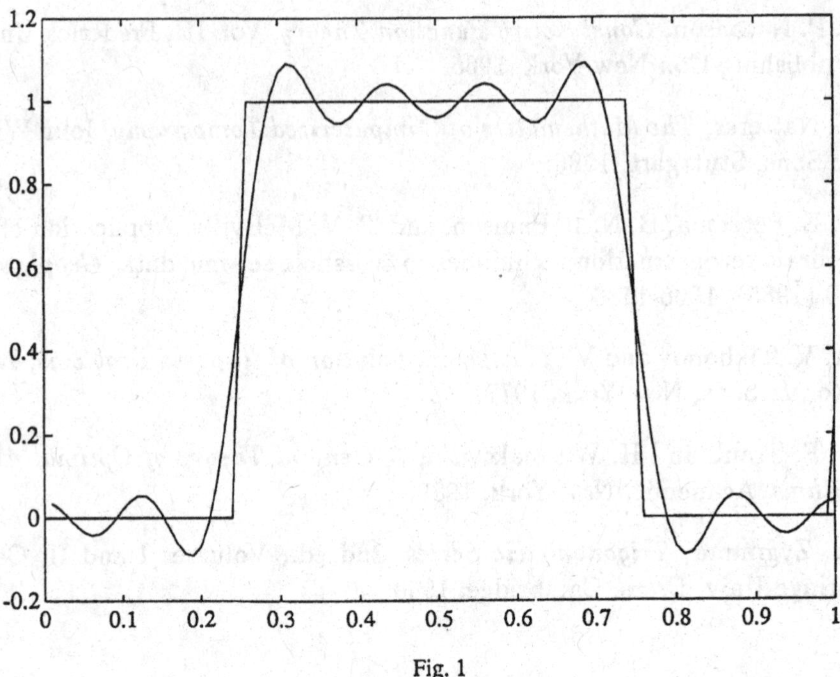
1.2
1
0.8
0.6
0.4
0.2
0
-0.2
0 0.1 0.2 0.3 0.4 0.5 0.6 0.7 0.8 0.9 1

Fig. 1

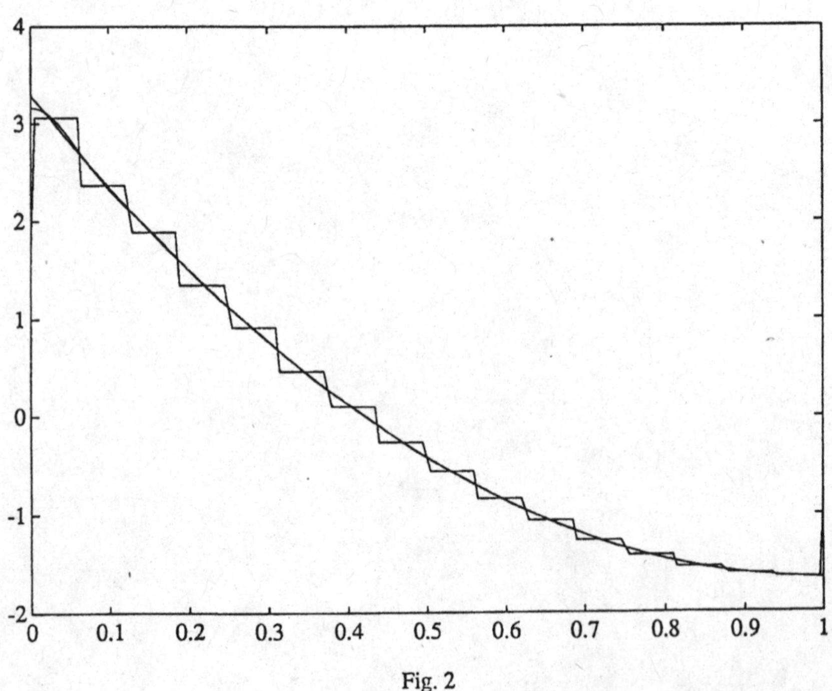
4
3
2
1
0
-1
-2
0 0.1 0.2 0.3 0.4 0.5 0.6 0.7 0.8 0.9 1

Fig. 2

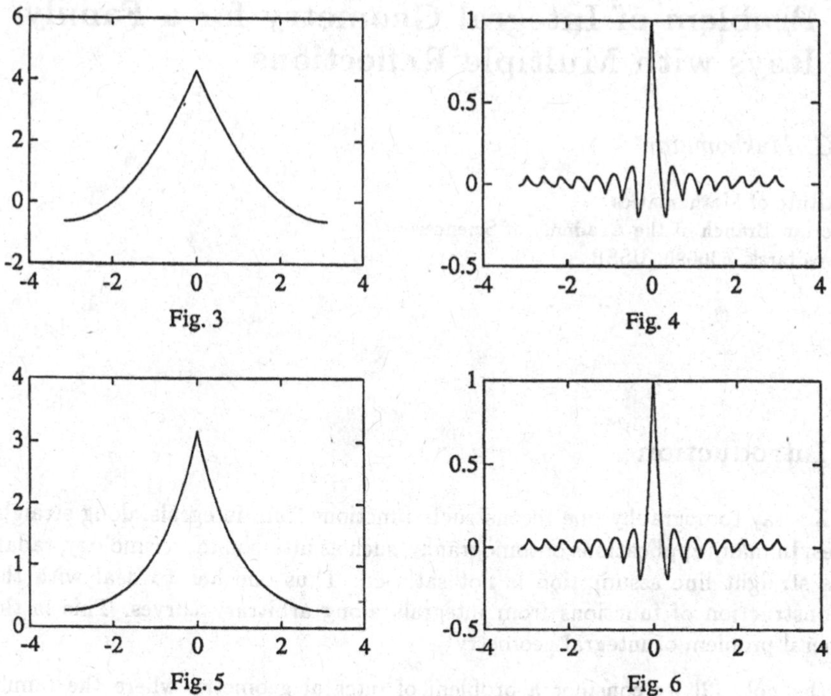

Fig. 3 Fig. 4

Fig. 5 Fig. 6

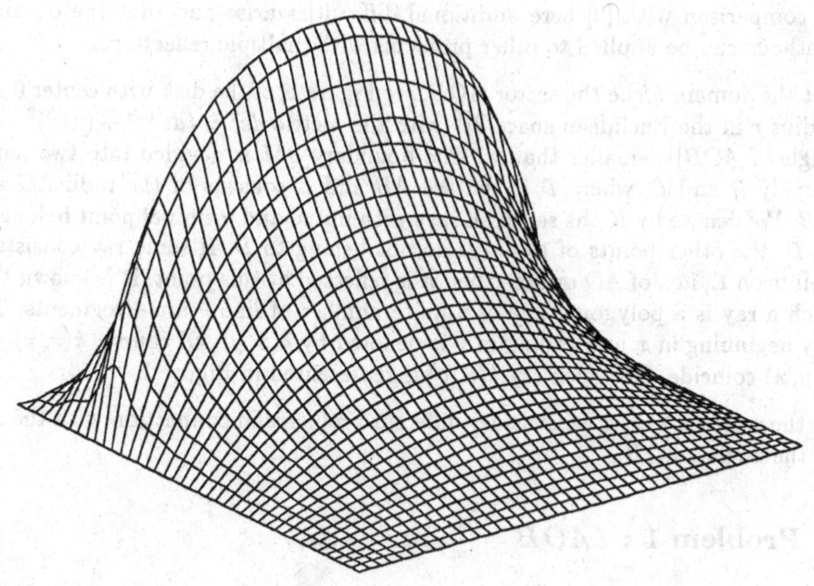

Fig. 7

A Problem of Integral Geometry for a Family of Rays with Multiple Reflections

R.G. Mukhometov

Institute of Mathematics
Siberian Branch of the Academy of Sciences
Novosibirsk, 630090, USSR

1 Introduction

In X - ray tomography one reconstructs functions from integrals along straight lines. In many applications of tomography, such as ultrasound, seismology, radar, this straight line assumption is not satisfied. Thus one has to deal with the reconstruction of functions from integrals along arbitrary curves. This is the general problem of integral geometry.

In the note [2] we consider a problem of integral geometry where the family of rays are reflected once from the boundary of a domain. Of course, there are problems in which the rays are reflected more than one time. In this article we study such problems and obtain stability estimates for their solution. Note that in comparison with [2] here additional difficulties arise and that the obtained methods can be applied to other problems with multiple reflections.

Let the domain M be the sector AOB, see Figure 1, of the disk with center 0 and radius r in the Euclidean space $\mathbb{R}^2$ with the metric $ds^2 = (dx^1)^2 + (dx^2)^2$. The angle of AOB is smaller than π. The boundary ∂M is devided into two parts, namely $\mathcal{D}$ and $\mathcal{L}$, where $\mathcal{D}$ is the arc AB and $\mathcal{L}$ consists of the radii AO and OB. We denote by K the set of all rays with initial and terminal point belonging to $\mathcal{D}$, the other points of the rays do not belong to $\mathcal{D}$. If some ray consists of points on $\mathcal{L}$; i.e., of AO or OB, then it is reflected at this point. It is known that such a ray is a polygonal line of a finite number of line - arc - segments. The ray beginning in x and ending in y is denoted by $k(x, y)$. Of course, $k(x, y)$ and $k(y, x)$ coincide. One such ray $k(x, y)$ is represented in Figure 1.

In the sections 2, 3, 4 we consider different problems in connection with the size of the angle $\angle AOB$.

2 Problem 1 : $\angle AOB = \frac{\pi}{m}, m = 1, 2, \ldots$

We analyze the behaviour of the rays. We shall devide the disk containing the sector AOB into $2m$ sectors each of which is equal to AOB, as shown in Figure

1 for $m = 2$. Associate to each multiply reflected ray $k(x,y)$ the chord xy' so that the ray and the chord have a common direction at the point y. If the ray $k(x,y)$ is reflected the first time from BO then it is convenient to consider, that it passes into the neighboring sector $A'OB$. After the second reflection right from AO the ray passes into the sector $A'OB'$ which is the neighboring sector of $A'OB$ and so on. Thus as domain M we shall consider a multivalent domain, namely consisting of $2m$ domains M which paste together along the radii AO, $B'O, A^{m-1}O, B^2O, A^{m-2}O, \ldots, B^{m-1}O, A'O, BO$. When a ray intersects some of these radii it passes into the neighboring domain. Under such interpretation of the domain M and the rays it is immediately obvious that for any two different points $x, y \in \mathcal{D}$ the different rays $k_i(x,y)$, $i = 0, 1, \ldots, 2m$ exist with the initial point x and terminal point y which are reflected $\lfloor \frac{i+1}{2} \rfloor$ times from the boundary $\mathcal{L}$, where $\lfloor \xi \rfloor$ is the integral part of the number ξ. By $k_i(x,y)$ for $i = 2, 4, \ldots, 2m$ and for $i = 1, 3, \ldots, 2m-1$ we denote the rays which are first reflected from BO respectively from AO. The ray $k_0(x,y)$ is thus the segment connecting the points x and y. So the family K consists of the described rays $k_i(x,y)$, $(x,y) \in \overline{M} \times \overline{M}$. It is clear that for all $x \in M$ and all directions θ the ray $k_i(\cdot,\cdot)$ with some i exists which passes through the point x with the direction θ.

Let for each ray $k_i(x,y)$, $(x,y) \in \mathcal{D} \times \mathcal{D}$, $i = 1, \ldots, 2m$ the integral

$$w_i(x,y) = \int_{k_i(x,y)} u(x_i(s))\rho(x_i(s), \frac{d}{ds}x_i(s))\,ds \tag{1}$$

of the function $u = u(x)$, $x \in \overline{M}$ be given. The known weight function $\rho = \rho(x,a)$ is defined on the tangent bundle TM with $\rho(x, \lambda a) = \rho(x,a)$ for all $\lambda > 0$. By $x_i = x_i(s)$ we denote a parametrization of the ray $k_i(x,y)$ where $x_i = (x_i^1, x_i^2)$. The aim is to determine the function $u = u(x), x \in \overline{M}$.

Because of the homogeneity of the weight function ρ, $\rho(x,\lambda a) = \rho(x,a)$, we restrict the second variable to a unit vector θ which is identified with the direction of the ray, hence $\rho = \rho(x,\theta)$.

For Problem (1) we prove the following theorem.

Theorem 1. *For $u(x) \in C^1(\overline{M})$, $\rho(x,a) \in C^1(\overline{TM})$ we have the estimate*

$$\int\int_M u^2(x)\Big(\int_0^{2\pi}(\rho^2 - \rho_\theta^2)d\theta\Big)dx \le B_m + \sum_{i=0}^{2m-2}(-1)^{q(i)}\int_0^\ell\int_0^\ell \frac{\partial w_i}{\partial z^1}\frac{\partial w_i}{\partial z^2}dz^1dz^2 \tag{2}$$

where $dx = dx^1dx^2$, $q(i) = 1 + \lfloor\frac{i+1}{2}\rfloor$; $w_i = w_i(z^1,z^2)$ is the left part of (1), z^i is the coordinate on $\mathcal{D}$ as the length of the curve, $i = 1,2$; ℓ is the length of $\mathcal{D}$. If m is even then

$$B_m = -\int_0^\ell\Big(\int_0^{\ell-z^1}\frac{\partial w_{2m}}{\partial z^1}\frac{\partial w_{2m}}{\partial z^2}dz^2 + \int_{\ell-z^1}^\ell \frac{\partial w_{2m-1}}{\partial z^1}\frac{\partial w_{2m-1}}{\partial z^2}dz^2\Big)dz^1\,,$$

if m is odd, then

$$B_m = \int_0^\ell\Big(\int_0^{\ell-z^1}\frac{\partial w_{2m-1}}{\partial z^1}\frac{\partial w_{2m-1}}{\partial z^2}dz^2 + \int_{\ell-z^1}^\ell \frac{\partial w_{2m}}{\partial z^1}\frac{\partial w_{2m}}{\partial z^2}dz^2\Big)dz^1\,.$$

Corollary. *If*

$$\int_0^{2\pi} (\rho^2 - \rho_\theta^2) d\theta \geq 0 \ , \tag{3}$$

where equality to zero can hold on a subset of M of measure 0, then (2) is the stability estimate of the solution of Problem 1. The uniqueness of the solution follows from this estimate.

3 Problem 2

In the above analyzed Problem 1 suppose that $\angle AOB = \frac{2\pi}{2m+1}$, $m = 1, 2, \ldots$. In Figure 2 we show $m = 2$ and $2m + 1 = 5$.

We consider the ray which corresponds to the chord xy'. This ray is reflected successively from BO, AO and BO; i.e., the point C is the point B at the closed domain $\overline{M}$. On the other hand, if we consider the chord xy'', then C is the point A at $\overline{M}$. This duality of the point C complicates Problem 2 in the following respect. In Problem 1 for the fixed point $x \in \mathcal{D}$ the parts last reflected from $\mathcal{L}$ of the rays $k_{2m-1}(x, y)$ and $k_{2m}(x, y)$ cover the whole domain M without mutual intersections. In Problem 2, as is obvious from Figure 2, for fixed point $x \in \mathcal{D}$ the domains at M which are covered by the parts of the rays last reflected from L, respectively $k_{2m+1}(x, y)$ and $k_{2m}(x, y)$ for $x \in (0, \ell/2)$ or $k_{2m-1}(x, y)$ and $k_{2m+2}(x, y)$ for $x \in (\ell/2, \ell)$ are intersecting and their intersection is not equal to M. Here $k_{2m+1}(x, y)$ and $k_{2m}(x, y)$ for $x \in (0, \ell/2)$ and $k_{2m-1}(x, y)$ and $k_{2m+2}(x, y)$ for $x \in (\ell/2, \ell)$ are the rays with the largest even and odd indices. This complicates the inequality analoguous to (2), namely the integral term, containing the product of the unknown function $u(x)$ and the known quantity, which has the singularity at the point O, appeared. Of course, provided (3) holds, the uniqueness theorem is correct here too.

For Problem 2 we get the stability estimate of the solution provided that

$$|u(x)| < N \ , \tag{4}$$

where N is an arbitrary constant. We first introduce some notations. In the family K there are the rays consisting of the pairs of the segments xO (the incident part of the ray) and Oy (the reflected part of the ray), $x, y \in D$, but not for all $(x, y) \in D \times D$. Let $y = y(t)$, $t \in [0, \ell]$, be the equation of the arc AB where t is the arc length of the curve. We denote by $k_A(x, y)$ the ray consisting of xO and yO, where $(x, y) \in \{(x(t), y(t)) : t \in [0, \ell]\}$ where $x(t) = y(\ell/2 - t)$ if $t \in [0, \ell/2]$ and $x(t) = y(t - \ell/2)$ if $t \in [\ell/2, \ell]$. Analogously we denote by $k_B(x, y)$ the ray consisting of xO and yO where $(x, y) \in \{(x(t), y(t)) : t \in [0, \ell]\}$ with $x(t) = y(t + \ell/2)$ if $t \in [0, \ell/2]$ and $x(t) = y(3/2\ell - t)$ if $t \in [\ell/2, \ell]$. The set of all rays $k_A(x, y)$ and $k_B(x, y)$ belongs to the family K; i.e., the integrals along these rays are known analogously to (1) and these integrals we denote respectively by $V_A = V_A(z^1)$ and $V_B = V_B(z^1)$, $z^1 \in [0, \ell]$, where $y = y(z^1)$.

Theorem 2. *For $u(x) \in C^1(\overline{M})$ satisfying (4), $\rho(x, a) \in C^1(T\overline{M})$, $|\rho(x, a)| < N_1$ with ρ satisfying condition (3) we have the stability estimate*

$$\int\int_M u^2(x) \int_0^{2\pi} (\rho^2 - \rho_\theta^2) d\theta dx \leq \tag{5}$$

$$\leq \sum_{i=0}^{2m-2} (-1)^{q(i)} \int_0^\ell \int_0^\ell \frac{\partial w_i}{\partial z^1} \frac{\partial w_i}{\partial z^2} dz^1 dz^2 +$$

$$+(-1)^{1+m} \int_0^\ell \Big(\int_0^{\ell/2} \frac{\partial w_{2m-1}}{\partial z^1} \frac{\partial w_{2m-1}}{\partial z^2} dz^1 + \int_{\ell/2}^\ell \frac{\partial w_{2m}}{\partial z^1} \frac{\partial w_{2m}}{\partial z^2} dz^1 \Big) dz^2 +$$

$$+2NN_1 r \int_0^\ell (|\frac{dV_A}{dz^1}| + |\frac{dV_B}{dz^1}|) dz^1 + A_m + B_m \ ,$$

where if m is odd then

$$A_m = -\int_0^{\ell/2} \Big(\int_{\ell/2+z^1}^\ell \frac{\partial w_{2m+1}}{\partial z^1} \frac{\partial w_{2m+1}}{\partial z^2} dz^2 - \int_{\ell/2-z^1}^\ell \frac{\partial w_{2m}}{\partial z^1} \frac{\partial w_{2m}}{\partial z^2} dz^2 \Big) dz^1 \ ,$$

$$B_m = -\int_{\ell/2}^\ell \Big(\int_0^{z^1-\ell/2} \frac{\partial w_{2m+2}}{\partial z^1} \frac{\partial w_{2m+2}}{\partial z^2} dz^2 - \int_0^{3/2\ell - z^1} \frac{\partial w_{2m-1}}{\partial z^1} \frac{\partial w_{2m-1}}{\partial z^2} dz^2 \Big) dz^1 \ ,$$

if m is even then

$$A_m = \int_0^{\ell/2} \Big(\int_0^{\ell/2-z^1} \frac{\partial w_{2m+1}}{\partial z^1} \frac{\partial w_{2m+1}}{\partial z^2} dz^2 - \int_0^{\ell/2+z^1} \frac{\partial w_{2m}}{\partial z^1} \frac{\partial w_{2_,}}{\partial z^2} dz^2 \Big) dz^1 \ ,$$

$$B_m = \int_{\ell/2}^\ell \Big(\int_{3/2\ell - z^1}^\ell \frac{\partial w_{2m+2}}{\partial z^1} \frac{\partial w_{2m+2}}{\partial z^2} dz^2 - \int_{z^1-\ell/2}^\ell \frac{\partial w_{2m-1}}{\partial z^1} \frac{\partial w_{2m-1}}{\partial z^2} dz^2 \Big) dz^1 \ .$$

4 Problem 3

If the angle $\angle AOB = \alpha$ such that $\alpha m + \alpha_1 = 2\pi$, where $m = 2, 3, 4, \ldots$, $0 < \alpha_1 < \alpha$, then we get the stability estimate in the form of (5).

5 Problem 4

Let in Problem 3 the domain M be the intersection of the sector AOB and the ring where the boundaries are the circles with center O and radii r_1 and r with $r_1 < r$. In Figure 3 this domain is the truncated sector $ABCD$. Let the rays with the ends on the arc AB be reflected by the contact with the remaining part of M; i.e., BC, CD, DA. For the problem of integral geometry with this family K of rays we get the stability estimate of the solution without condition (4). This estimate is studied below in Theorem 3. Note that for each ray $k_i(x, y)$, which has no point on CD, there exists a ray $\tilde{k}_i(x, y)$ with the same ends x and y on AB and as much reflections from BC and DA as $k_i(x, y)$, but in contrast to that it has a point of reflection on CD. This follows from the isosceles triangle $xy'd$ in Figure 3. Analogously to (1) the integral along the ray $\tilde{k}_i(x, y)$ we denote by $\tilde{w}_i(x, y)$. Let the angle α satisfy the inequality $0 < \alpha < 2\arccos\frac{r_1}{r} = \beta$. We introduce the notation $p = \lfloor\frac{\beta}{\alpha}\rfloor$,

$$\gamma = \begin{cases} (\alpha + \alpha p - \beta)r & \text{if} \quad \alpha p \neq \beta \\ 0 & \text{if} \quad \alpha p = \beta \end{cases},$$

$$g_i = \frac{\partial w_i}{\partial z^1}\frac{\partial w_i}{\partial z^2} - \frac{\partial \tilde{w}_i}{\partial z^1}\frac{\partial \tilde{w}_i}{\partial z^2} .$$

Theorem 3. *For $u(x) \in C^1(\overline{M})$, $\rho(x, a) \in C^1(T\overline{M})$ where the function $\rho(x, a)$ satisfies condition (3), we have the stability estimate*

$$\int\int_M u^2(x)\Big(\int_0^{2\pi}(\rho^2 - \rho_\theta^2)d\theta\Big)dx \leq$$

$$\leq \sum_{i=0}^{2p-2}(-1)^{q(i)}\int_0^\ell\int_0^\ell g_i dz^1dz^2 +$$

$$+(-1)^{q(2p)}\int_\gamma^\ell\int_0^\ell g_{2p}dz^1dz^2 + (-1)^{2p-1}\int_0^{\ell-\gamma}\int_0^\ell g_{2p-1}dz^1dz^2 +$$

$$+A_p + B_p + C_p + D_p$$

where if p is even then

$$A_p = -\int_0^\gamma\int_0^{\ell-\gamma+z^1} g_{2p}dz^1dz^2 \ ;$$

$$B_p = -\int_{\ell-\gamma}^\ell\int_{z^1-(\ell-\gamma)}^\ell g_{2p-1}dz^1dz^2 \ ;$$

$$C_p = \int_\gamma^\ell\int_{\ell+\gamma-z^1}^\ell g_{2p+2}dz^1dz^2 \ ;$$

$$D_p = \int_0^{\ell-\gamma}\int_0^{\ell-\gamma-z^1} g_{2p+1}dz^1dz^2 \ ;$$

if p is odd, then

$$A_p = \int_0^\ell\int_{\gamma-z^1}^\ell g_{2p}dz^1dz^2 \ ;$$

$$B_p = \int_{\ell-\gamma}^\ell\int_0^{z^1-(\ell-\gamma)} g_{2p-1}dz^1dz^2 \ ;$$

$$C_p = -\int_\gamma^\ell\int_0^{z^1-\gamma} g_{2p+2}dz^1dz^2 \ ;$$

$$D_p = -\int_0^{\ell-\gamma}\int_{z^1+\gamma}^\ell g_{2p+1}dz^1dz^2 .$$

6 Remarks Concerning the Proofs of the Theorems

The proofs of the given theorems are analogous to the proofs of the results in the papers [1], [2].

7 Remark

Note, that the results analogous to the theorems above are also correct for the family K of the geodesics of the Riemannian metric. In that connection we must impose restrictions for the behaviour of the geodesics of this metric so that the family K is analogous to the family K of rays of the Problems 1 - 3.

References

[1] Mukhometov, R.G.: The problem of recovery of a twodimensional Riemannian metric and integral geometry. Dokl. Acad. Nauk SSSR **232** (1977) 32-35; English Transl. : Soviet Math. Dokl. **18** (1977)

[2] Mukhometov, R.G.: On integral geometry in a domain with a reflecting part of the boundary. Dokl. Akad. Nauk SSSR **296** (1987) 279-283; English Transl.: Soviet Math. Dokl. **36** (1988)

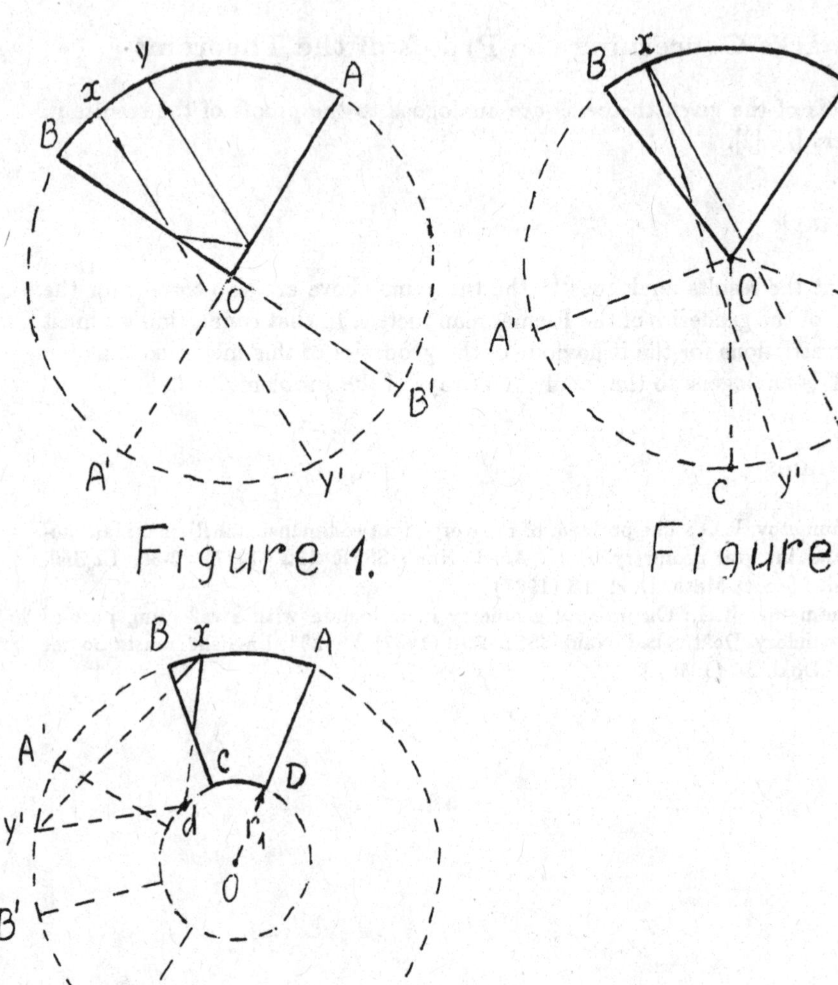

Figure 1.

Figure 2.

Figure 3.

INVERSION FORMULAS FOR THE THREE-DIMENSIONAL RAY TRANSFORM

Victor P.Palamodov
Department of Mathematics and Mechanics
Moscow Lomonosov University
119899 Moscow

§1. Introduction

Consider the problem of reconstruction of a function f on euclidean space $\mathbb{R}^3$ from the knowledge of its integrals over straight lines or rays λ which run over a set Λ. The ray transform of f is the integral

$$R_1 f(\lambda) := \int_\lambda f(x)\, ds, \quad \lambda \in \Gamma,$$

where ds is the Lebesgue measure on λ and Γ is the manifold of all the straight lines or rays in $\mathbb{R}^3$, $\dim \Gamma = 4$ (the symbol R_1 itself means one-dimensional Radon transform). There are a few types of three-dimensional manifolds $\Lambda \subset \Gamma$ for which an explicit formula for the inversion $R_1 f|\Lambda \to f$ is known:

I. Plane by plane inversion of the Radon transform in a family of parallel planes.

II. Let Λ_C be the set of lines λ which meet a fixed curve $C \subset \mathbb{R}P^2$ at infinity such that any plane in $\mathbb{R}^3$ has a non-empty intersection with C. From the data $R_1 f|\Lambda$ one can calculate the (plane) Radon transform $R_2 f$ (Orlov [11]) and then recover this function by the standart method (1). In fact the sampling in the case I is equal to Λ_C, where C is a big circle.

III. Let Λ_C be the set of lines λ which meet a given curve $C \subset \mathbb{R}^3$ or rays starting from points of C. A reconstruction of a function f with a compact support is possible if the following condition (Tuy) is satisfied: any plane H, which has a non-empty intersection with supp f, meets C in a point where H and C are transversal. For such a sampling several methods of reconstruction are known:

i) Kirillov-Tuy's method ([9],[13],[10]): the starting point is the Fourier transform $F_{\vartheta \to \omega}$ of $R_1 f(\lambda(x,\vartheta))$, where $\lambda(x,\vartheta)$ is the ray with the origin x and the direction vector ϑ:

$$f(x) = -i(2\pi)^{-3/2} \int_{S^2} (x'(t),\omega)^{-1}\, \partial/\partial t\, F_{\vartheta\to\omega} R_1 f(\lambda(x,\vartheta))\, d\omega$$

ii) Finch's method [2] is based on a extrapolation of $R_1 f(x,\vartheta)$ to the points (y,ϑ) where y belongs to the convex envelope of C.

iii) A.S.Blagoweshchensky's method [1]: if C is a plane circle ((hence Tuy's condition does not satisfied) function $R_1 f$ is extrapolated by means of an analytic continuation. A similar method in a more general situation was used in [2],[12].

iv) I.M.Gelfand-A.B.Goncharov's approach [4].

v) P.Grangeat's formula [6]. It is equivalent to the following one:

$$\partial/\partial p\, R_2 f(p,\omega) = \int_{\lambda(x,\vartheta)\in H} \partial/\partial\omega\, R_1 f(\lambda(x,\vartheta))\, d\vartheta$$

where the plane H is given by the equation $\langle\omega,x\rangle = p$, the integration on ϑ runs over the unit circle in the plane orthogonal to ω and $\partial/\partial\omega$ means the unit vector field on this circle with the direction ω. This equation is used together with the inversion formula for the Radon transform $R_2 f$:

$$f(x) = -\frac{1}{8\pi^2} \int_{S^2} \partial^2/\partial p^2\, R_2 f(\langle\omega,x\rangle,\omega)\, \sigma(\omega) \tag{1}$$

where $\sigma(\omega)$ is the Lebesgue measure on the sphere.

Remark. All this formulas are not local and are unlike those for inversion of the line transformation in the complex case, where the dimension of line is even.

§2. A necessary condition for a good sampling

Let A be a reconstruction algorithm A: $R_1 f|\Lambda \to f$, defined for functions f, $\operatorname{supp} f \subset\subset U_A$, where U_A is a given open subset of $\mathbb{R}^3$. We call the *error amplifier* of this algorithm the function

$$s_A(N) := \sup_f E/\varepsilon \tag{2}$$

where $\varepsilon = \sup|\delta R_1 f|$, $\delta R_1 f$ is an error of the data $R_1 f|\Lambda$ and $E = \|\delta f\|_\rho$, δf is the error of the reconstruction of f after this algorithm, $N := r\rho$, where r is the diameter of supp f and ρ is the diameter of the spectral sphere $D_\rho \subset \mathbb{R}$ where we measure the error:

$\|g\|_\rho := \sup\{\,|Fg(\xi)|, \xi \in D_\rho\,\}$,

and F is the Fourier transform $x \to \xi$. We call the algorithm A *stable* if the error amplifier is of polynomial growth for big N:

$s_A(N) \le \text{const}.N^k$

For example the standart inversion formula for the Radon transform R_{n-1} in $\mathbb{R}^n$ gives a stable algorithm with $k = n-1$ or n for odd and even n respectively.

In fact the property of stability does not depend in an extent on the choice of the norms for $\delta R_1 f$ and for $\delta f | D_\delta$. In particular we can substitute the sup-norms by the L_p-norm, $p \ge 1$ or by the C^q-norm for arbitrary real q. In the above list of algorithms the items i),ii), iv) and v) are stable but iii) does not. In fact in the case iii) the function $s_A(N)$ is of exponential growth ([12]).

Propostion 1. *If for a sample* Λ *there exists a stable reconstruction algorithm* A: $R_1 f | \Lambda \to f$, *then there is a dense set* Π *of planes in* $\mathbb{R}^3$ *such that any* $H \in \Pi$, *which meets* U_A *contains a line* $\lambda \in \Lambda$. *Hence if* Λ *is compact this condition holds for any* H, $H \cap U_A \ne \Phi$.

We call this condition on Λ the *completeness* condition. In the cases II and III this condition is equivalent to the Orlov's and Tuy's conditions respectively. For an arbitrary compact Λ the completeness property is equivalent to the positivety of the Crofton symbol ([3],[7]). Under this and an additional assumptions Greenleaf and Uhlmann [7] constructed a left pseudodifferential parametrics (cf.[3]). This gives a stable algorithm for reconstruction of only f $\bmod C^\infty$.

§3. A new reconstruction formula

Theorem 2. (V.P.Palamodov, A.S.Denisjuk) *Let* Λ *be the set of all rays tangent to a given smooth surface* $S \subset \mathbb{R}^3$ *and* K *is a compact set in* $\mathbb{R}^3$, H *is a plane such that the intersection* $S \cap H$ *contains an open smooth curve* C_H, *which satisfies the following condition, where* $\tau(x)$ *means a continuous unit tangent field to* C_H:

(*) $\zeta_+^{-1}(K)$ *is a compact set, where* $\zeta_+ : C_H \times \mathbb{R}_+ \to H$ *is defined by* $\zeta_+(x,t) = x + t\tau(x)$, $\mathbb{R}_+ = \{t, t > 0\}$. *Then for any function* $f \in C_0^2(K)$ *the* *equation*

$$\partial/\partial p\, R_2 f(H) = -1/\delta \int_{C_H} (\varkappa\, \partial/\partial q + \langle \nu,\omega\rangle / [\nu,\omega,\tau]\, \partial/\partial s)\, R_1 f(x(s),\vartheta(0))\, ds \quad (3)$$

holds, where

s *is the natural parameter on* C_H *such that* $x'(s) = \tau(x(s))$;

$\varkappa$ *is the curvature:* $x''(s) = \varkappa(\omega\times\tau(s))$, *and* ω *is the unit normal to* H;

ν *is the unit normal field and* $\vartheta(q)$ *is the unit tangent field to* S *at* $x(s)$ *which depends continuously on* $q = \langle\vartheta,\omega\rangle$ *for small* q *and coincides with* τ *for* $q = 0$;

δ *is the degree of the mapping* ζ_+, *where the orientation of* C_H *is defined by* τ *and the orientation of* H *by* ω; *we suppose that* $\delta \neq 0$.

For the line transform $R_1 f$ *the formula* (3) *still holds if the condition* (*) *is valid for the mapping* ζ: $C_H \times \mathbb{R} \to H$, *defined by the same way as* ζ_+.

Remark. We need for accounting of the sign of $\varkappa$ and of δ because of some points of K may be covered by the several rays or lines tangent to S whose number may depend on the point. In the case of the line transform we may change the field τ to $-\tau$. Then we should change in the same way simultaneously the quantities s, $\varkappa$ and δ.

Proof of the theorem. We set $R_1 f(x,q) = R_1 f(\lambda(x,\vartheta(q)))$ and have

$$\partial/\partial s\, R_1 f(x(s),0) = \int \partial/\partial s\, f(x(s)+t\tau)\, dt =$$
$$= \int df(x(s)+t\tau, \tau + t\tau')\, dt = \int t\, df(x(s)+t\tau,\tau')\, dt =$$
$$= \int \varkappa\, t\, df(x(s)+t\tau, \omega\times\tau)\, dt,$$

where $\tau = \tau(x(s))$, because of

$$\int df(x(s)+t\tau),\tau)\, dt = \int \partial/\partial t\, f(x(s)+t\tau)\, dt = 0 \quad (4)$$

The vectors τ and $\nu\times\tau$ form an orthonormal frame in the tangent plane to S at the point $x(s)$, hence for any unit tangent vector $\vartheta = \vartheta(q)$

$$q \equiv \langle\vartheta,\omega\rangle = \langle\vartheta, \nu\times\tau\rangle[\nu,\tau,\omega]$$
$$\vartheta = \langle\vartheta,\tau\rangle\tau + \langle\vartheta,\nu\times\tau\rangle\nu\times\tau = r\tau + q[\nu,\tau,\omega]^{-1}\nu\times\tau,$$

where $r = (1-q^2[\nu,\tau,\omega]^{-2})^{1/2}$. Therefore

$$\partial/\partial q\, \vartheta(q) = q/r\, [\nu,\tau,\omega]^{-2}\tau + [\nu,\tau,\omega]^{-1}\nu\times\tau$$

hence

$$\partial/\partial q\, R_1 F(x,\vartheta(q)) = \int \partial/\partial q\, f(x(s)+t\vartheta(q))\, dt =$$
$$= \int t\, df(x(s)+t\vartheta, [\nu,\tau,\omega]^{-1}\nu\times\tau)\, dt.$$

because of (4), which implies that

$$(x\partial/\partial q + \langle\nu,\omega\rangle/[\nu,\omega,\tau]\partial/\partial s)R_1 f(x(s),\vartheta(0)) =$$

$$= \int x t\, df(x(s)+t\tau,[\nu,\tau,\omega]^{-1}(\nu\times\tau - \langle\nu,\omega\rangle\omega\times\tau)\,dt = \tag{5}$$

$$= \int x t\, df(x(s)+t\tau,\omega)\,dt = \int x t\, g(x(s)+t\tau)\,dt,$$

where $g(x) = \partial/\partial\omega f(x)$ since

$$\nu\times\tau = [\nu,\tau,\omega]\omega + \langle\nu,\omega\rangle\omega\times\tau\ .$$

Integrating over C_H the extreme parts of (5), we get

$$\int (x\partial/\partial q + \langle\nu,\omega\rangle/[\nu,\omega,\tau]\partial/\partial s)R_1 F(x(s),\vartheta(0))\,ds =$$

$$= \int\int x t\, g(x(s)+t\tau)\,dt\,ds.$$

It is easy to check that $x t\,dt\,ds = -\delta\, dH$, where dH is the element of the Lebesgue measure on H. Therefore the right-hand part is equal to

$$-\delta\int_H g(x)\,dH = -\delta\partial/\partial p\int_H f(x)\,dH$$

where δ is the local degree of the map ζ_+ and the theorem follows.

§4. Projective transformations

A projective automorphism L_P of $\mathbb{RP}^n$ is the mapping generated by a nonsingular linear transformation L of $\mathbb{R}^{n+1}$. This transformation defines also an automorphism L_Γ of the manifold Γ of all lines in $\mathbb{RP}^n$ which depends only on L_P. Now we show that any projective automorphism L_P acts on the set of all inversion algorithms in a natural way.

Proposition 3. *Let* ds_x *be the Lebesgue measure on a line* $\lambda\subset\mathbb{R}^n$ *and* ds_y *be the Lebesgue measure on* $L_P(\lambda)$, $\vartheta(\lambda)$ *be a direction vector of* λ. *Then the relation*

$$\|\vartheta(\lambda)\|^{-1} x_0^2\, ds_x = \|\eta(\lambda)\|^{-1} y_0^2\, ds_y \tag{6}$$

holds, where x_0 *be the linear function on* $\mathbb{R}^{n+1}$ *such that* $x_0 \neq 0$ *on* $\mathbb{R}^n$, $y_0 = L_0(x_0,\dots,x_n)$ *is the pull-back of this function under* L *and*

$$\eta(\lambda) = L_0(0,\vartheta(\lambda))L(1,p) - L_0(1,p)L(0,\vartheta(\lambda)),\ p\in\lambda$$

is the direction vector of $L_P(\lambda)$.

A proof can be given by a straightforward computation.

Corollary 4. *If for a set* $\Lambda \subset \Gamma$ *there exists an inversion operator* $I: R_1 f|\Lambda \to f$, *then for any projective transformation* L_P *the set* $L_\Gamma(\Lambda)$ *has the same property.*

In fact the inversion operator $J: R_1 f|L_P(\Lambda) \to f$ can be given in the following way:

$$f(y) = B_0^{-2}(1,y) I(\|\vartheta(\lambda)\|/\|\eta(\lambda)\| \cdot R_1 f(L_P(\lambda)))(x),$$

where $x = B_P(y)$ is the inverse projective transformation whose representation in projective coordinates is $x_i = B_i(y_0, y)$, $i = 0,1,\dots,n$. This relation follows from (6) because of

$$y_0^2 \cdot x_0^{-2} = B_0^{-2}(1,y).$$

Example. Consider the fan-beam transformation in $\mathbb{R}^2$ with sources on a straight line C. A projective transformation L_P of $\mathbb{R}P^2$ which throws C to the infinity, maps the bundle of lines λ which pass through a fixed point $x \in C$ to a family of parallel lines. If there is a gap in sources of beams on C, we get the set of lines $L_P(\lambda)$ with the only restriction on the angle φ, say $|\varphi| \le \alpha < \pi/2$. For a reconstruction of a function $f \in C_0^3(\mathbb{R}\ )$ from this non-complete data one can use the method of consistent extension ([10]) or the method of the interpolation of analytic functions ([12]). Then applying Proposition 2 we get an inversion operator for the fan-beam transform with the non-complete data.

Remark. In the context we see that the classes II and II of §1 can be amalgamated in one projective invariant class **C** : an element of this class is the set Λ_C of all lines which meet a given curve $C \subset \mathbb{R}P^3$. Its projective invariant subclass with plane curves C contains the Orlov's class II. Theorem 2 gives another invariant class **S**: an element of **S** is by definition a sample Λ_S of all lines tangent to a given smooth surface S (the condition of theorem is supposed satisfied for any H which meets a non-empty open set U).

Hypothesis. *The classes* **C** *and* **S** *essentially exhaust the set of all three-manifolds* Λ *for which there is a stable inversion operator* $I: R_1 f|\Lambda \to f$. The word "essentially" means that another examples of Λ's are limit cases for these two classes.

The following arguments are in favour for this hypothesis. According to Proposition 3 the property of Λ to have such kind of inversion operator depends only on projective (but not on euclidean) structure of the space. The following property of a manifold $\Lambda \subset \Gamma$ is projective-invariant as well. This manifold is called *characteristic* if it is tangent at any its point to the subbundle $K \subset T(\Gamma)$. The later may be defined in the following way: for any point $\lambda \in \Gamma$ the fibre K_λ of K is the tangent tangent cone to the variety of all lines μ, which has a common point with λ. This notion in an equivalent form for complex situation is due Gel'fand and Graev [5]. The set of all characteristic three-manifolds Λ essentially coincides with the union of the classes **C** and **S** (a generalization of this result was given by V.Guillemin [8]).

§5. A remark on the integral geometry on a hyperboloid

The starting point for Gel'fand's integral geometry was the problem of reconstruction of a smooth decreasing function defined on the group $Sl(2,\mathbb{C})$ from its integrals over horocycles h. The reconstruction method of [5] was applied for a direct proof of Plancherel formula for the group. The authors considered the group $Sl(2,\mathbb{C})$ was considered as the hyperboloid in $\mathbb{C}^4$ given by the equation:

$$w_0 w_3 - w_1 w_2 = 1$$

Any horocycle h is a complex line in this hyperboloid. Taking the projection onto (w_0, w_1, w_2)- space the authors got the set Λ_C of lines $\lambda = p(h)$ which meet the hyperbola $C = \{w_1 w_2 = -1\}$. Hence the problem was translated into the following one: recover a function f defined on $\mathbb{C}^3$ from its integrals over lines which meet C. According to §4 we attribute this problem to the class **C** in complex situation. (We mention a propos that the real analogue of this problem is more complicated because of Λ_C does not satisfies the completeness condition of §2).

The problem can be dealed in a different way if we choose another direction of projection: rewrite the hyperboloid in the following isometric form:

$$z_1^2 + z_2^2 - z_3^2 - z_4^2 = 2$$

and project it to the (z_1, z_2, z_3)- space. The critical set of this projection mapping q is the two-dimensional hyperboloid

$$S = \{z_1^2 + z_2^2 - z_3^2 = 2\} \tag{7}$$

and for any horocycle h the line $\lambda = q(h)$ is *tangent* to S. The inverse is also true. Hence the method of [5] may be thought as an inversion algorithm for a manifold Λ_S of the class S in the complex situation.

We think now on the real variant to this problem: determine the Radon data $R_2 f$ of a function f with a compact support in $\mathbb{R}^3$ from its integrals on rays or lines tangent to the real (one-sheet) hyperboloid S given by the equation (7). It divides $\mathbb{R}^3$ into two closed sets

$G_{\pm} = \{x: \pm(x_1^2 + x_2^2 - x_3^2) \le 2\}$

We denote by Υ the cone of all time-like lines in the dual space $\mathbb{R}^{*3}$:

$\Upsilon = \{\omega: \omega_3^2 \ge \omega_1^2 + \omega_2^2\}$

For any space-like ω (i.e. for $\omega \in \mathbb{R}^{*3} \setminus \Upsilon$) and for any $p \in \mathbb{R}$ the intersection $C_{\omega,p} = H_{\omega,p} \cap S$ is a hyperbola and $H_{\omega,p} \cap G_+$ is the component between the branches of this hyperbola. This set is twice covered by the tangent lines to $C_{\omega,p}$. Thus we can apply theorem 2 to this curve with $\delta = 2$ and hence reconstruct all the space-like plane wave components of $R_2 f(p,\omega)$ of any function f with a compact support in G_+. For $\omega \in \partial\Upsilon$ the "light" components of $R_2 f$ may be reconstructed as well because of $C_{\omega,p}$ is a parabola whose tangent lines cover twice the set $H_{\omega,p} \cap G_+$.

For any time like $\omega \in \Upsilon$ and any p the set $H_{\omega,p} \cap S$ is an ellipse whose tangent lines cover twice the set $H_{\omega,p} \cap G_-$, hence from the data $R_1 f | \Lambda_S$ we can reconstruct any time-like plane wave component of any function with a compact support in G_-.

§6. Projective invariance for the general Radon transform

Now we consider the k- Radon transform in the euclidean space $\mathbb{R}^n$

$$R_k f(\sigma) = \int_\sigma f(x)dv$$

where dv is the k-dimensional Lebesgue measure on affine k-subspaces σ of $\mathbb{R}^n$. The function $R_k f$ is defined on the manifold $\Sigma = \Sigma_k$ of all k-subspaces. Proposition 3 admits the following generalization:

Proposition 5. *For any projective transformation* L_P *of* $\mathbb{RP}^n$ *and any* $\sigma \in \Sigma_k$ *the following relation between the Lebesgue measures* dv_x *on* σ

and dv_y *on* $L_P(\sigma)$

$$\|L(p_0)\wedge\ldots\wedge L(p_k)\|^{-1} y_0^{k+1}\, dv_y = \|(p_1-p_0)\wedge\ldots\wedge(p_k-p_0)\|^{-1} x_0^{k+1}\, dv_x$$

holds, where $p_0,\ldots,p_k$ *are arbitrary points in* σ *whose affine envelope is equal to* σ, *the product* $(p_1-p_0)\wedge\ldots\wedge(p_k-p_0)$ *is considered as an element of* $\Lambda^k\mathbb{R}^n$.

$$L(p_0)\wedge\ldots\wedge L(p_k) \equiv L_0(p_0)M_0 + \ldots + L_0(p_k)M_k$$

where M_i *is the complement to the element* $L_0(p_i)$ *in the* $n+1\times k$*- matryx* $\|L_i(p_j)\|_{i=0,j=0}^{i=n,j=k}$; M_i *is considered as an element of* $\Lambda^k\mathbb{R}^n$, $\|.\|$ *is the norm in the euclidean algebra* $\Lambda^*\mathbb{R}^n$ *generated by the euclidean structure of* $\mathbb{R}^n$.

Regretfully I do know any reference for this formula and I can only check this formula by a straightforward computation.

It follows that the function $P(x,\lambda) \equiv dv_y/dv_x$ admits a factorization of the form $P(x,\lambda) = p(x)\pi(\lambda)$. In the particular case $k = n-1$ this factorization in an equivalent form was reported independently by J.Boman in his talk on Oberwolfach Conference (August 1990).

Proposition 5 implies an evident generalization of Corollary 4.

REFERENCES

1 BLAGOWESHENSKII, A.S.: *On the reconstruction of functions from the integrals along linear manifolds.* Mathematical Notices **39**, 841-849, (1986) (in Russian).

2 FINCH, D.V.: *Cone beam reconstruction with sources on a curve.* SIAM J. Appl. Math. **45**, 665-673, (1985).

3 GELFAND, I.M. - GINDIKIN, S.G.: *Nonlocal Inversion Formulas in Real Integral Geometry.* Funct. Anal. Appl. **11**, 12-19. (1977) (in Russian).

4 GELFAND, I.M. - GONCHAROV, A.B.: *Reconstruction of finite functions from integrals over straight lines through given points in space.* Dokl. **290**, 1037-1040, (1986) (in Russian).

5 GELFAND, I.M. - GRAEV, M.I. - VILENKIN, N.Ya.: *Generalized Functions*, Vol. **5**. Academic Press 1973.

6 GRANGEAT, P.: *Analyse d'un systeme d'imagerie 3D par reconstruction à partir de radiographies X en gèomètrie conique.* These de doctorat, Grenoble (1987).

7 GREENLEAF, A. - UHLMANN, G.: *Nonlocal inversion formulas for the X-ray transform.* Duke Math. J. **58**, 205-240, (1989).

8 GUILLEMIN, V.: *On some results of Gelfand in integral geometry.* Proc. Symp. Pure Math. **43**, 149-155, (1985).

9 KIRILLOV, A.A.: *On a problem of I.M. Gel'fand.* Soviet Math. Dokl. **2**, 268-269, (1961).

10 NATTERER, F.: *The mathematics of computerized tomography.* Wiley-Teubner (1986).

11 ORLOV, S.S.: *Theory of three-dimensional reconstruction. II. The recovery operator.* Kristallographiya **20**, 701-709, (1975).

12 PALAMODOV, V.P.: *Some Singular Problems in Tomography*, in: GELFAND, I.M. - GINDIKIN, S.G.: *Mathematical Problems of Tomography*, p. 123-140. Translations of Mathematical Monographs, Vol. **81**, AMS 1990.

13 TUY, H.K.: *An inversion formula for cone-beam reconstruction.* SIAM J. Appl. Math. **43**, 546-552, (1983).

BACKSCATTERED PHOTONS — ARE THEY USEFUL FOR A SURFACE-NEAR TOMOGRAPHY?

Volkmar Friedrich
Sektion Mathematik, Technische Universität Chemnitz
PSF 964, 9010 Chemnitz

1. The problem

Can backscattered photons be used to determine inhomogeneities in surface-near tissue? This problem was stated by physisists for medical purposes where X-rays should not be used.

Which mathematical formulation is the most appropriate to this problem? A beam of optical rays can be thought as a collection of photons with the velocity $v = c\Omega_Q$, which enter to a body G at a certain position $x_Q \in \partial G$. The further interaction of each of these photons with the tissue in G will be determined by scattering and absorption events. The mean free way between two scattering events is denoted by $m_s(x)$, $m_a(x)$ characterizes the mean way of a photon up to its absorption. The dependence of these physical parameters on the space variable $x \in G$ is emphasized by these notations. After a random number of scattering events a photon either will die by absorption or will emerge from the region G at a point x_E in the direction Ω_E. The flux $F(x_E, \Omega_E)$ of photons leaving the region G contains some information about the interesting parameters $m_s(x)$ and $m_a(x)$.

2. The simplest model and its physical limitations

The simplest model takes into account only the first scattering event of each photon. After a possible second scattering the photon will not be followed up.
For the outcoming flux $F(x_E, \Omega_E; x_Q, \Omega_Q)$ of photons scattered only once near x_P we have the relation

$$F(x_E, \Omega_E; x_Q, \Omega_Q) \approx \frac{I_o}{m_s(x_P)} \exp(-\int_{x_Q x_P x_E} \mu(x) ds) \qquad (1)$$

x_P, Ω_Q, Ω_E, x_Q, x_E

with

$$\mu(x) = \frac{1}{m_s(x)} + \frac{1}{m_a(x)}.$$

This proportionality can also take into account certain assumptions how the scattering depends on the angle between the two directions Ω_Q and Ω_E. For this model we could try to determine the parameters m_s and μ from a set of at least two different measurements for each point x_P.

Unfortunately this model seems not to be appropriate for most of the medical situations in view of the physical limitations: Multiple scattered photons form a neglegtible part ($\leq$ 5-10%) of the whole flux of backscattered photons, only if the distances $x_Q x_P$ and $x_P x_E$ are not larger then about 0.75 m_s, as we have learned from a numerical simulation of the behaviour of a large number of photons. (The mathematical investigation of this first model instead would be much more easy then of the following ones, because we get linear relations by taking the logarithm of (1) for which a singular-value-approach for selecting the useful information would be possible.)

3. Boltzmann- versus Helmholtz-equation

The distribution of photons $p(x,\Omega)$, $(x,\Omega) \in G \times S^2$ (S^2 denotes the surface of the unit ball in R^3) and the measurable flux F of backscattered photons at x_E into the direction Ω_E can be modelled by the Boltzmann-equation

$$(\text{grad}_x p, c\Omega) + (\lambda + \alpha)p = \frac{\lambda}{4\pi} \int_{S^2} p(x,\Omega')d\Omega' + \text{source term} \tag{2}$$

(this source term depends on x_Q and Ω_Q!) and the relation

$$F(x_E,\Omega_E) = cp(x_E,\Omega_E)\cos(n_E,\Omega_E),$$

where $\frac{c}{\lambda} = m_s$, $\frac{c}{\alpha} = m_a$ and n denotes the outer normal to G at $x \in \partial G$. For this model we have got a very good correspondence with the result of the simulation of the large sample of photons mentioned above.

In some papers the densitiy of photons

$$p_0(x) = \frac{1}{4\pi} \int_{S^2} p(x,\Omega)d\Omega$$

is used instead of the distribution $p(x,\Omega)$, where the density is governd by the Helmholtz-equation

$$-\text{div}(D(x)\text{grad}p_0) + A(x)p_0 = \text{source term} \tag{3}$$

with the following relations to the parameters of the model (2):

$$D = \frac{c}{3(\lambda+\alpha)}, \quad A = \frac{\alpha}{c}.$$

The arguments under which a simplification of the Boltzmann-equation to a Helmholtz-equation is admissible will not fit our situation: The obvious boundary condition

$$p(x,\Omega) = 0 \quad \text{for} \quad x \in \partial G \quad \text{and} \quad \cos(\Omega, n) < 0 \tag{4}$$

does not have an exact equivalent for the density p_0. (4) usually is approximated by the relation

$$\int_{\cos(\Omega,n)<0} \Omega p(x,\Omega)d\Omega = 0$$

for the 'amount of motion' of incoming photons. This relation together with the assumption

$$p(x, \Omega) = p_o(x) + 3(q(x), \Omega) \tag{5}$$

gives us the boundary condition

$$p_0 = -2D\frac{\partial p_0}{\partial n}$$

for the Helmholtz-equation.

When comparing this model with the simulation of a large number of photons mentioned above we did not found a sufficient accordance with the result of the simulation experiment. The reason for this difference we found in the essential violation of the assumption (5), especially for points x which are near to the boundary ∂G.

4. The correct mathematical formulation

The correct formulation of the analysis of backscattered photons is the following: Find parameters $m_s(x)$ and $m_a(x)$ such that the measurements $z(x_E, \Omega_E; x_E, \Omega_E)$ are in good correspondence to the flux values F for the Boltzmann-equation (2).

A complete analysis of the sensitivity of the solution of this problem to measurement errors has not been done up to now. Some difficulties of our problem comes to light even if we solve the direct problem (2). The outcoming flux F shows only a rather small dependence on the parameters m_s and m_a in a depth which is greater then four - five times the mean free way m_s. Therefore we must expect large errors in the reconstruction of details in the depth of the tissue (similar to the limited-angle-problem). Furthermore the accuracy of the calculated flux F is rather sensitive to the discretization of the Boltzmann-equation in the direct neighbourhood of the surface ∂G.

Similar considerations on models for the transport of light in biological tissue see also [1].

[1] G.A.Navarro and A.E.Profio, "Contrast in diaphanography of the breast", Medical Physics 15,181-187 (1988)

MATHEMATICAL FRAMEWORK OF CONE BEAM 3D RECONSTRUCTION VIA THE FIRST DERIVATIVE OF THE RADON TRANSFORM

Pierre Grangeat

LETI - Département Systèmes - SETIA, Centre d'Etudes Nucléaires de Grenoble
85 X - 38041 GRENOBLE CEDEX - FRANCE

Abstract

Either for medical imaging or for non destructive testing, X-ray provides a very accurate mean to investigate internal structures. The object is described by a 3D map f of the local density. The use of a 2D X-ray detector like an image intensifier in front of the ponctual X-ray source defines a cone beam geometry. When the source moves along a curve, the acquisition measurements are modelized by the cone beam X-ray transform of the function f. This same model can be applied to emission tomography when cone beam collimators are used.

The aim of the 3D reconstruction is to recover the original function f. We have established an exact formula between the cone beam X-ray transform and the first derivative of the 3D Radon transform. We propose to use the planes as information vectors to achieve the rebinning from the coordinates system linked to the cone beam geometry, to the spherical coordinates system of the Radon domain. Then the reconstruction diagram is to compute and to invert the first derivative of the 3D Radon transform.

In this publication, we describe the mathematical framework of this reconstruction diagram. We emphasize the special case of the circular acquisition trajectory.

Key-words : Cone beam. Three-dimensional reconstruction. Radon transform. X-ray. Transmission tomography. Gamma-ray. Emission tomography.

1. INTRODUCTION

In 3D image reconstruction, the object to investigate is characterized by the 3D map f of a physical parameter, the local density in transmission tomography or the local activity in emission tomography. For a given curve Γ, the cone beam X-ray transform Xf does associate to each half line starting of one point on the curve, the integral of the function f over this half line. The cone beam X-ray transform does modelize the acquisition system for tomographic imaging devices where a focal point S moves along the acquisition trajectory Γ and a 2D detector on the opposite side provides a parametrization of the half-lines starting from S, crossing the object, and intersecting the detector. For X-ray transmission acquisitions, the X-ray source defines the focal point S and an image intensifier can be used as 2D detector. For gamma-ray emission acquisitions, the point S is the focal point of a cone beam collimator and the 2D detector is a gamma camera. The main technological interests are to speed the acquisition by the use of a 2D detector and to improve the spatial resolution by the magnification effect induced by the cone beam geometry.

The cone beam X-ray transform describes a new generation of 3D tomographic imaging devices using 2D detectors. Some examples in X-ray medical imaging are the Dynamic Spatial Reconstructor [ROBB (1985)] to investigate the beating heart and lungs, or the TRIDIMOS project developped at the LETI for the CNES to measure the bone mineral content of lumbar vertebrae [GRANGEAT (1989)], or the MORPHOMETRE project of GE-CGR, with the LETI as partner, to image vessel trees and bone structures [SAINT-FELIX et al. (1990), GRANGEAT (1990c)] or a 3D X-ray microtomograph to investigate small objects like biopsies [MORTON et al. (1990)]. In nuclear medicine, cone beam collimators are used with large gamma cameras to focalize the acquisition on small region of interest like the brain [JASZCZAK et al. (1988)] or the heart [GULLBERG et al. (1989)]. Moreover, it enables to put a X-ray source at the focal point in order to reconstruct the attenuation map from cone beam transmission measurements [MANGLOS et al. (1990)], to correct the auto-attenuation effect of the gamma-rays. Finally, in X-ray Non Destructive Testing, cone beam 3D tomographs are developped to control small pieces like ceramic materials [FELDKAMP et al. (1984), VICKERS et al. (1989)]. The LETI is one partner of the Evaluation of Voludensitometric Analysis (EVA) project of the EEC [RIZO and GRANGEAT (1989), SIRE et al. (1990)].

The reconstruction algorithm has to recover the original function f from its cone beam X-ray transform Xf. We will only review the transform methods. This inverse problem has been studied in the following publications [KIRILLOV (1961), HAMAKER et al. (1980), FINCH and SOLMON (1980, 1983), TUY (1983), FINCH (1985)]. TUY has proposed a first inversion formula using the homogeneous extension of functions. All these studies have given mathematical results but could not lead directly to a numerical implementation.

So the first approach has been to generalize to the 3D cone beam geometry the 2D fan beam reconstruction algorithm. This direct processing is based on a convolution cone beam backprojection algorithm. This has first been suggested by FELDKAMP [FELDKAMP et al. (1984)]. This idea has induced large developments [WEBB et al. (1987), JACQUET (1988)]. BRUCE SMITH has expressed the mathematical steps to reach this convolution cone beam backprojection formula [SMITH B. (1985)]. He gives a survey on cone beam tomography in [SMITH B. (1990)]. But the hypothesis the trajectory has to fullfill are too restrictive. The only general framework which can deal with the largest class of trajectories is to use the Radon transform. The first attempts have been formulated in [MINERBO (1979), GRANGEAT (1985, 1986a, 1986b)]. But an approximation was used. To get an exact relation, the solution is to work either with the first derivative R'f of the Radon transform [GRANGEAT (1987b)] or with the Hilbert transform HDRf of the first derivative of the Radon transform. This second solution can be derived from [SMITH B. (1985, 1987, 1990), KUDO and SAITO (1990a, 1990b)]. The main advantage of our first solution is that it involves only partial differentiation which means local filtering, whereas the second needs a global filtering to achieve the Hilbert transform.

In our oral communication at Oberwolfach [GRANGEAT et al. (1990b)], we have presented and compared reconstructions with both FELDKAMP's algorithm and ours. In this written publication, we describe the mathematical framework of our reconstruction algorithm via the first derivative R'f of the Radon transform.

After some preliminary definitions in chapter 2, we describe how to compute the first derivative R'f of the 3D Radon transform. We first introduce in chapter 3 the fundamental relation between the cone beam X-ray transform Xf and the first derivative R'f of the Radon transform. Then we give in chapter 4 the expression of this fundamental relation in the coordinates system of the detection plane, in order to prepare the numerical implementation. In the chapter 5, we give the necessary and sufficient condition on the trajectory to describe all the Radon domain of the object support and we introduce a geometrical description of set of planes. Finally, we emphasize the special case of the circular trajectory in the chapter 6. We depict the shadow zone in the Radon domain and its processing by interpolation. We introduce the rebinning equation.

Then we describe in the chapter 7 the inversion of the first derivative R'f of the Radon transform using two steps, a first convolution backprojection step to compute the filtered rebinned X-ray transform and a second backprojection step to recover the original object function f.

2. PRELIMINARY DEFINITIONS

2.1. The cone beam X-ray transform Xf

Let us take a curve Γ in $\mathbb{R}^3$. For a given point S on Γ and for a unit vector $\vec{u}$ in S^2, we use $(S,\vec{u})$ to characterize the half-line of direction $\vec{u}$, with S as origin point. For a given function f on $\mathbb{R}^3$, the cone beam X-ray transform Xf associates to each half-line $(S,\vec{u})$ with S moving along Γ, the integral of f over this half line :

$$Xf\left(S,\vec{u}\right) = \int_{a=0}^{+\infty} f\left(S + a.\vec{u}\right) da \tag{2.1}$$

for $S \in \Gamma$ and $\vec{u} \in S^2$.

It is supposed throughout that the support Ω of f is a compact convex subset of $\mathbb{R}^3$ and that the function f is an element of $C^2(\Omega)$ the space of two times differentiable functions, with continuous second differential functions, vanishing outside Ω. The discussion over more general functions spaces is not in the scope of this paper.

For the curve Γ, we don't need strong regularity conditions. For mechanical feasibility, we will assume that Γ is a piecewise C^1 curve, which means that Γ is the image in $\mathbb{R}^3$ of the union of a finite number of intervals in $\mathbb{R}$, under a map C^1 on each interval. We suppose the curve Γ lies outside the support Ω.

On a physical device, we will have the X-ray source S on one side of the object and the two-dimensional X-ray detector on the opposite side, as it is represented on the figure 1. This acquisition geometry will move around the object. We choose an origin point 0 for the object. If the motion of the acquisition geometry as a fixed point, for instance a center of rotation, this will be selected as origin point 0. We will assume that the front side of the detector is a plane P_dX. Each point A_d of this plane P_dX defines an unique half-line issued from S. So these points can be used to parametrize the cone beam X-ray transform for each unit vector directed toward this plane.

To simplify, we assume that this plane is perpendicular to the line (S,O). To avoid the use of scaling factor, we will consider the detection plane PX which we define as the plane crossing the origin O and perpendicular to the line (S,O). Thus this detection plane PX is parallel to the detector front side P_dX.

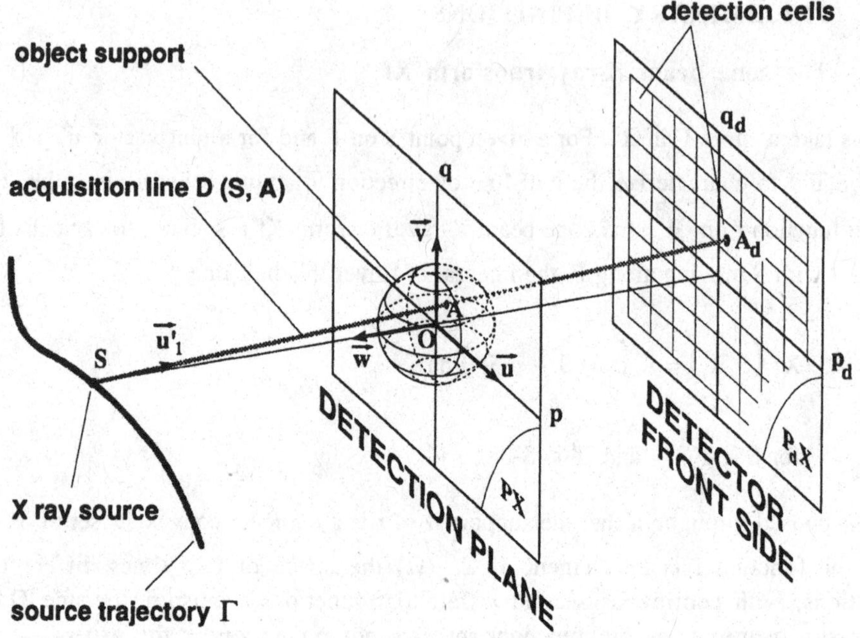

Figure 1 : The cone beam X-ray transform

To describe more precisely the acquisition procedure, we give now a new definition of the cone beam X-ray transform Xf :

$$Xf\,(S,A) = \int_{a=0}^{+\infty} f\left(S + a.\vec{u'_1}\right) da \qquad (2.2)$$

for $S \in \Gamma$, $A \in PX$ and with $\vec{u'_1} = \dfrac{\vec{SA}}{\|\vec{SA}\|}$.

In this definition, we assume that the support Ω of f belongs to the half-space described by the half-lines (S,A) when A moves within the detection plane PX, for each position of the source S on the curve Γ.

2.2. The first derivative R'f of the Radon transform

Let us set $(O,\vec{i},\vec{j},\vec{k})$ the orthonormal object reference system in $\mathbb{R}^3$ and (x,y,z) the cartesian coordinates system to parametrize the object points M.

Each plane P is characterized by one of its orthogonal unit vector $\vec{n}$ and by its algebraic distance to the origin O (cf figure 2) :

$$M \in P(\rho,\vec{n}) \quad \Leftrightarrow \quad \overrightarrow{OM}.\vec{n} = \rho \qquad\qquad (\rho,\vec{n}) \in \mathbb{R} \times S^2 \qquad (2.3)$$

We use the spherical coordinates system (θ,φ) to parametrize the unit vector $\vec{n}$. The colatitude angle θ is the angle between the axis $(O,\vec{z})$ and the vector $\vec{n}$. The longitude angle φ is the angle between the axis (O,x) and the orthogonal projection of $\vec{n}$ on the $(\vec{i},\vec{j})$ vectorial plane.

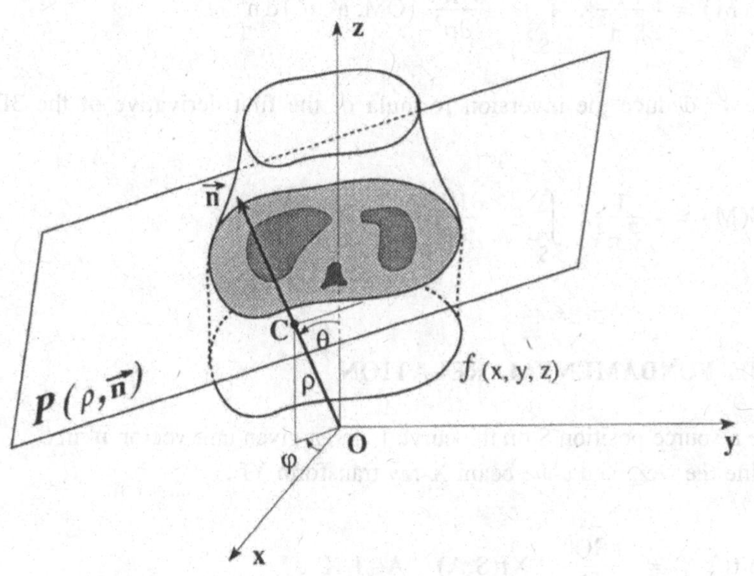

Figure 2 : The 3D Radon transform parameters

For a given object function f on $\mathbb{R}^3$, its 3D Radon transform Rf is defined as the set of its integrals over the planes of $\mathbb{R}^3$ [NATTERER (1986)] :

$$Rf\left(\rho,\vec{n}\right) = \iint_{M \in P(\rho,\vec{n})} f(M)\ dM \tag{2.4}$$

We define the first derivative R'f of the Radon transform as the partial derivative of Rf with respect to the algebraic distance ρ :

$$R'f\left(\rho,\vec{n}\right) = \frac{\partial Rf}{\partial \rho}\left(\rho,\vec{n}\right) \tag{2.5}$$

We shall remark that the definition set of the planes can be restricted to the planes which do intersect the function support Ω, because Rf and R'f are null on the others.

Let us now write the inversion formula of the 3D Radon transform [NATTERER (1986)] :

$$f(M) = -\frac{1}{8\pi^2} \cdot \int_{S^2} \frac{\partial^2 Rf}{\partial \rho^2}\left(\vec{OM}.\vec{n},\vec{n}\right) d\vec{n} \tag{2.6}$$

From this, we deduce the inversion formula of the first derivative of the 3D Radon transform :

$$f(M) = -\frac{1}{8\pi^2} \cdot \int_{S^2} \frac{\partial R'f}{\partial \rho}\left(\vec{OM}.\vec{n},\vec{n}\right) d\vec{n} \tag{2.7}$$

3. THE FUNDAMENTAL RELATION

Let us take a source position S on the curve Γ and a given unit vector $\vec{n}$ in S^2.
Let us define the weighted cone beam X-ray transform Yf :

$$Yf(S,A) = \frac{\|\vec{SO}\|}{\|\vec{SA}\|} \cdot Xf(S,A) \quad A \in PX \tag{3.1}$$

We define the integration plane $P\left(\vec{OS}.\vec{n},\vec{n}\right)$ as the uniq· · plane perpendicular to the vector $\vec{n}$ and crossing S. The point C orthogonal projection of the origin O on this integration plane is called its characteristic point.

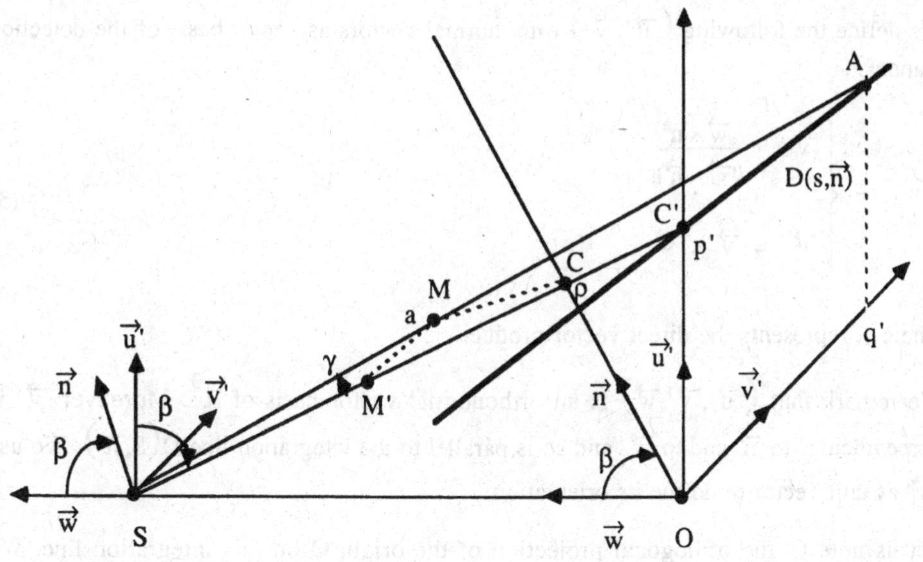

Figure 3 : Parameters of the fundamental relation

We note $\vec{w}$ the unit vector which gives the direction of the source point S from the origin O :

$$\vec{w} = \frac{\overrightarrow{OS}}{\|\overrightarrow{OS}\|}$$

If the vectors $\vec{n}$ and $\vec{w}$ are not parallel, the integration plane $P\left(\overrightarrow{OS}.\vec{n},\vec{n}\right)$ does intersect the detection plane PX along a straight line $D\left(S,\vec{n}\right)$ that we call the integration line.

We define the following $(\vec{u}\,',\vec{v}\,')$ orthonormal vectors as vector basis of the detection plane :

$$\begin{cases} \vec{v}\,' = \dfrac{\vec{w}\wedge\vec{n}}{\|\vec{w}\wedge\vec{n}\|} \\ \\ \vec{u}\,' = \vec{v}\,'\wedge\vec{w} \end{cases} \tag{3.2}$$

where $\wedge$ represents the direct vector product.

We remark that $(\vec{u}\,',\vec{v}\,',\vec{w})$ is an orthonormal vector basis of $\mathbb{R}^3$. Moreover $\vec{v}\,'$ is perpendicular to $\vec{n}$ and to $\vec{w}$ and so is parallel to the integration line $D(S,\vec{n})$. We use $\vec{v}\,'$ as unit vector to define its orientation.

Let us note C' the orthogonal projection of the origin O on this integration line. We define $SYf(S,\vec{n})$ as the integration of the weighted cone beam X-ray transform Yf over the integration line $D(S,\vec{n})$:

$$SYf(S,\vec{n}) = \int_{A\in D(S,\vec{n})} Yf(S,A)\ dA \tag{3.3}$$

$$= \int_{q_1=-\infty}^{+\infty} Yf\left(S,\ C' + q'.\vec{v}\,'\right) dq'$$

Let us write (p', q') the coordinates system in the $(O,\vec{u}\,',\ \vec{v}\,')$ reference system of the detection plane. If we consider all the integration lines parallel to $\vec{v}\,'$, we can use p' as a parameter of $SYf(S,\vec{n})$.

Then we can introduce **the fundamental relation between the cone beam X-ray transform Xf and the first derivative R'f of the Radon transform** :

$$\frac{\|\vec{OS}\|^2}{\|\vec{OS}\wedge\vec{n}\|^2}\cdot\frac{\partial SYf}{\partial p'}\left(S,\vec{n}\right) = R'f\left(\vec{OS}.\vec{n}\,,\ \vec{n}\right) \tag{3.4}$$

This formula and its proof has been published in 1987 in our thesis [GRANGEAT (1987)] which we consider as the reference publication. This formula has been introduced first in our talk [GRANGEAT (1986)] in the last meeting at Oberwolfach :

Theory and Application of Radon Transforms. In 1984, we have proved a first relation equivalent to this, using the homogeneous extension of Xf, as it is defined in Tuy's paper [TUY (1983)]. It was written in a private communication with D. FINCH and D. SOLMON [GRANGEAT (1984)] which is reproduced in our thesis [GRANGEAT (1987)].

We will give here the proof of this Grangeat's formula. The reader should refer to the figure 3 to follow the presentation.

Let us define two coordinates systems to parametrize the points M in $\mathbb{R}^3$.

The first is the acquisition cartesian coordinates system (x',y',z') associated to the $(S, \vec{u}', \vec{v}', \vec{w})$ reference system with the origin at the source point S.

The second is a spherical coordinates system to parametrize the cone beam geometry. The origin is at S and $\vec{v}'$ is the polar axis. Let us note M' the orthogonal projection of M on the $(S, \vec{w}, \vec{u}')$ plane.

We define the longitude parameter β as the angle between $\vec{SM'}$ and $\vec{u}'$ and the latitude parameter γ as the angle between $\vec{SM}$ and $\vec{SM'}$. The parameter a describes the distance between the point M and the source point S.

We remind that we have assumed the points M are restricted to the subspace $\mathbb{R}^2 \times \mathbb{R}^-$ in the acquisition cartesian coordinates system, which corresponds to :

$$(a, \beta, \gamma) \in \mathbb{R}^+ \times [0,\pi] \times \left[-\frac{\pi}{2}, \frac{\pi}{2}\right]$$

The cone beam coordinate system is related to the acquisition cartesian coordinate system by the following equations :

$$\begin{cases} x' = a.\cos\gamma.\cos\beta \\ y' = a.\sin\gamma \\ z' = -a.\cos\gamma.\sin\beta \end{cases} \tag{3.5}$$

The angular parameter β can be used to describe the integration lines instead of p'. We have :

$$p' = \|\vec{OS}\|.\operatorname{cotg}\beta \tag{3.6}$$

and so : $\dfrac{d\beta}{dp'} = -\dfrac{\sin^2\beta}{\|\vec{OS}\|}$

But on the integration plane, we have :

$$\sin^2 \beta = \frac{\|\overrightarrow{OS} \wedge \vec{n}\|^2}{\|\overrightarrow{OS}\|^2}$$

So we get :

$$\frac{\|\overrightarrow{OS}\|^2}{\|\overrightarrow{OS} \wedge \vec{n}\|^2} \cdot \frac{\partial SYf(S,\vec{n})}{\partial p'} = - \frac{1}{\|\overrightarrow{OS}\|} \cdot \frac{\partial SYf}{\partial \beta}(S,\vec{n}) \qquad (3.7)$$

Let us express the function $SYf(S,\vec{n})$ in the cone beam coordinates system.

For a given half-line starting from S and crossing the detection plane at the point A of coordinates (p',q'), we have :

$$q' = \|\overrightarrow{SC'}\| \cdot \operatorname{tg} \gamma \qquad (3.8)$$

If we use the angular parameters (β,γ) to parametrize the half-lines issued from S, we get :

$$SYf(S,\vec{n}) = \int_{\gamma=-\frac{\pi}{2}}^{+\frac{\pi}{2}} Yf(S,\beta,\gamma) \cdot \frac{\|\overrightarrow{SC'}\|}{\cos^2\gamma} \cdot d\gamma \qquad (3.9)$$

But :

$$\frac{\|\overrightarrow{SO}\|}{\|\overrightarrow{SA}\|} = \frac{\|\overrightarrow{SO}\|}{\|\overrightarrow{SC'}\|} \cdot \frac{\|\overrightarrow{SC'}\|}{\|\overrightarrow{SA}\|}$$

$$= \frac{\|\overrightarrow{SO}\|}{\|\overrightarrow{SC'}\|} \cdot \cos \gamma$$

So :

$$Yf \cdot \frac{\|\overrightarrow{SC'}\|}{\cos^2\gamma} = Xf \cdot \frac{\|\overrightarrow{SO}\|}{\cos\gamma}$$

As :

$$Xf(S,\beta,\gamma) = \int_{a=0}^{+\infty} f(a,\beta,\gamma)\, da$$

We get the following relation :

$$SYf(S,\vec{n}) = \int_{\gamma=-\frac{\pi}{2}}^{+\frac{\pi}{2}} \int_{a=0}^{+\infty} f(a,\beta,\gamma) \cdot \frac{\|\vec{SO}\|}{\cos\gamma} \, da \, d\gamma \tag{3.10}$$

Now we introduce the basic relation, induced by the moment effect if we derive f with respect to the angular variable β. For all the points M of the integration plane, we have :

$$\frac{\partial f(M)}{\partial \beta} = - \frac{\partial f(M)}{\partial \rho} \cdot a \cdot \cos\gamma \qquad M \in P\left(\vec{OS}.\vec{n},\vec{n}\right) \tag{3.11}$$

It can be stated with reference to the cartesian coordinates system :

$$\frac{\partial f}{\partial \beta} = - \, a.\cos\gamma.\sin\beta. \frac{\partial f}{\partial x'} \;\; - \, a.\cos\gamma.\cos\beta. \frac{\partial f}{\partial z'}$$

If β is the longitude of the integration plane, the coordinates of its orthogonal unit vector $\vec{n}$ in the $\left(\vec{u}',\vec{v}',\vec{w}\right)$ basis are :

$$\vec{n} \;\; \begin{vmatrix} \sin\beta \\ 0 \\ \cos\beta \end{vmatrix}$$

And so the partial derivative in the direction of $\vec{n}$ is given by :

$$\frac{\partial f}{\partial \rho} = \sin\beta. \frac{\partial f}{\partial x} + \cos\beta. \frac{\partial f}{\partial z}$$

So we get the moment formula (3.11). We can now conclude the demonstration. We differentiate the relation (3.10) and we apply the differentiation operation before the integration. We get :

$$\frac{1}{\|\vec{SO}\|} \cdot \frac{\partial SYf}{\partial \beta} \left(S,\vec{n}\right) = - \int_{\gamma=-\frac{\pi}{2}}^{+\frac{\pi}{2}} \int_{a=0}^{+\infty} \frac{\partial f}{\partial \beta} (a,\beta,\gamma) \cdot \frac{1}{\cos\gamma} \; da \;\; d\gamma$$

We apply the moment formula (3.11) :

$$\frac{1}{\|\overrightarrow{SO}\|} \cdot \frac{\partial SYf}{\partial \beta}\left(S, \vec{n}\right) = - \int_{\gamma=-\frac{\pi}{2}}^{+\frac{\pi}{2}} \int_{a=0}^{+\infty} \frac{\partial f}{\partial \rho}(a, \beta, \gamma) \, . \, a \, da \, d\gamma$$

The second member of this equation is the integration in polar coordinates of the partial derivative of f in the direction of the unit vector $\vec{n}$. If we apply the differentiation operator after the integration, we get the first derivative of the Radon transform :

$$\frac{\partial Rf}{\partial \rho}\left(\overrightarrow{OS}.\vec{n}, \vec{n}\right) = \frac{\partial}{\partial \rho}\left[\iint_{M \in P(\overrightarrow{OS}.\vec{n}, \vec{n})} f(M) \, dM\right]$$

$$= \int_{\gamma=-\frac{\pi}{2}}^{+\frac{\pi}{2}} \int_{a=0}^{+\infty} \frac{\partial f}{\partial \rho}(a, \beta, \gamma) \, . \, a \, da \, d\gamma \qquad (3.12)$$

And so :

$$\frac{1}{\|\overrightarrow{SO}\|} \cdot \frac{\partial SYf}{\partial \beta}\left(S, \vec{n}\right) = - \frac{\partial Rf}{\partial \rho}\left(\overrightarrow{OS}.\vec{n}, \vec{n}\right)$$

If we use now the relation (3.7), we get the fundamental relation (3.4).

4. EXPRESSIONS OF THE FUNDAMENTAL RELATION IN THE COORDINATES SYSTEM OF THE DETECTION PLANE

We want now to prepare the numerical computation of the fundamental relation.

We refer to the schematic representations of the figures 1 and 4. We consider that the acquisition system provides a sampling of the function Xf on a regular rectangular grid. Then we define the $(O, \vec{u}, \vec{v})$ orthonormal reference system such that the vector $\vec{u}$ is parallel to the rows of the grid, the vector $\vec{v}$ to the columns, and such that $\left(\vec{u}, \vec{v}, \vec{w}\right)$ represents a direct orthonormal basis, with :

$$\vec{w} = \frac{\overrightarrow{OS}}{\|\overrightarrow{OS}\|}$$

We note (p,q) the coordinates of the points A on the detection plane.

For a given unit vector $\vec{n}$, we have defined in the last paragraph the $(O,\vec{u}',\vec{v}')$ orthonormal reference system of the detection plane, such that the integration line $D(S,\vec{n})$ is parallel to the axis $(O,\vec{v}')$.

We call α the rotation angle around $\vec{w}$ to go from the $(\vec{u},\vec{v})$ basis to the $(\vec{u}',\vec{v}')$ basis.

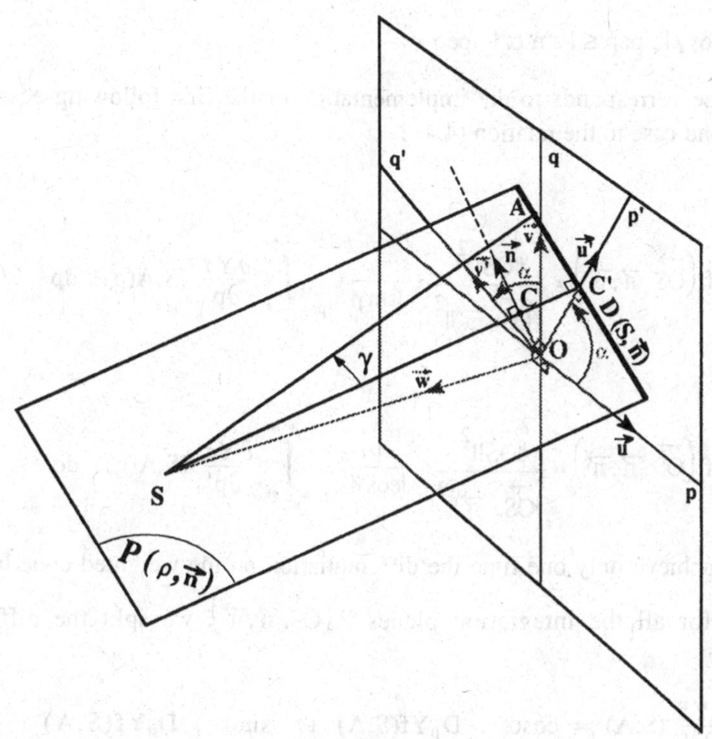

Figure 4 : Coordinates systems on the detection plane

In the (p',q') coordinates system associated to $(O,\vec{u}',\vec{v}')$, we can express the fundamental relation (3.4) in the following way, writting the differentiation operator inside the integration operator :

$$R'f\,(\vec{OS}.\vec{n},\vec{n})) = \frac{\|\vec{OS}\|^2}{\|\vec{OS}\wedge\vec{n}\|^2} \int_{q'=-\infty}^{+\infty} \frac{\partial Yf}{\partial p'}\,(S,A(q'))\;dq' \qquad (4.1)$$

The computation of the integration operator is equivalent to the computation of the X-ray transform Xf of a function f in two-dimensions from its representation on a rectangular sampling grid. This operation is called the reprojection. In our case we call it the integration processing. To get an efficient implementation, we use the algorithm described by JOSEPH [JOSEPH (1982)]. The principle is to sample the integration line either using the intersection points A(p) with the columns of the projection grid or using the intersection points A(q) with the rows of the projection grid. Let us describe as pep, respectively peq, the sampling distances between the columns, respectively the rows, of the grid. In order to get the sampling points as near as possible, we will choose either the first solution, if the following condition is fullfilled, or the second :

$$| \cos\gamma | \,.\, pep \leq | \sin \alpha | \,.\, peq \tag{4.2}$$

The first case corresponds to the implementation of the first following equation (4.3), and the second case to the relation (4.4) :

case 1 :

$$R'f\left(\overrightarrow{OS}.\vec{n},\vec{n}\right) = \frac{\|\overrightarrow{OS}\|^2}{\|\overrightarrow{OS}\wedge\vec{n}\|^2} \cdot \frac{1}{|\sin\gamma|} \cdot \int_{p=-\infty}^{+\infty} \frac{\partial Yf}{\partial p'}(S,A(p))\, dp \tag{4.3}$$

case 2 :

$$R'f\left(\overrightarrow{OS}.\vec{n},\vec{n}\right) = \frac{\|\overrightarrow{OS}\|^2}{\|\overrightarrow{OS}\wedge\vec{n}\|^2} \cdot \frac{1}{|\cos\gamma|} \cdot \int_{q=-\infty}^{+\infty} \frac{\partial Yf}{\partial p'}(S,A(q))\, dq \tag{4.4}$$

In order to achieve only one time the differentiation on the weighted cone beam X-ray transform, for all the integration planes $P\left(\overrightarrow{OS}.\vec{n},\vec{n}\right)$, we split the differentiation operator :

$$\frac{\partial Yf}{\partial p'}(S,A) = \cos\alpha \,.\, D_pYf(S,A) + \sin\alpha \,.\, D_qYf(S,A)$$

where D_p and D_q are the differentiation operators along the rows and the columns of the grid :

$$D_pYf = \frac{\partial Yf}{\partial p}$$

$$D_qYf = \frac{\partial Yf}{\partial q}$$

Finally, we get the expressions of the fundamental relation which are used to achieve the numerical implementation :

case 1 :

$$R'f\left(\vec{OS}.\vec{n},\vec{n}\right) = C_1.\left[\cos\alpha\,.\int_{p=-\infty}^{+\infty} D_pYf(S,A(p))\,dp + \sin\alpha\,.\int_{p=-\infty}^{+\infty} D_qYf(S,A(p))\,dp\right]$$

$$\text{with}\quad C_1 = \frac{\|\vec{OS}\|^2}{\|\vec{OS}\wedge\vec{n}\|^2}\cdot\frac{1}{|\sin\alpha|} \tag{4.5}$$

case 2 :

$$R'f\left(\vec{OS}.\vec{n},\vec{n}\right) = C_2.\left[\cos\alpha\,.\int_{q=-\infty}^{+\infty} D_pYf(S,A(q))\,dq + \sin\alpha\,.\int_{q=-\infty}^{+\infty} D_qYf(S,A(q))\,dq\right]$$

$$\text{with}\quad C_2 = \frac{\|\vec{OS}\|^2}{\|\vec{OS}\wedge\vec{n}\|^2}\cdot\frac{1}{|\cos\alpha|} \tag{4.6}$$

5. FROM THE CONE BEAM X-RAY TRANSFORM Xf TO THE FIRST DERIVATIVE R'f OF THE RADON TRANSFORM.

For a given source position S and a given unit vector $\vec{n}$, the fundamental relation (3.4) allows to compute the first derivative R'f of the Radon transform on the integration plane $P\left(\vec{OS}.\vec{n},\vec{n}\right)$. This can be applied to every unit vector $\vec{n}$ in S^2. It means that we can assign its value R'f for every plane crossing S. The case of the unit vector $\vec{n}$ parallel to the source vector $\vec{SO}$ is a singularity only because we use the detection plane to parametrize the cone beam X-ray transform.

The basic idea to design the reconstruction algorithm is to achieve a rebinning operation. But in the three-dimensional space $\mathbb{R}^3$, the set of straight lines intersecting the object support is a four-dimensional space and the set of straight lines intersecting a curve is a three-dimensional space. So there is no change of parameters possible. Whereas the set of planes intersecting the object support and the set of planes intersecting the curve are both three-dimensional spaces. So it becomes possible to achieve a rebinning operation, if we use the planes as information vectors.

We assign to each plane its integral value R'f. Thanks to the fundamental relation (3.4), this value R'f can be computed from the cone beam X-ray transform Xf for the planes which cross the trajectory Γ at least at one source position S. The condition on the trajectory to apply the rebinning is to describe all the first derivative R'f of the Radon transform. As the function f is null out of its support Ω, the definition set of R'f can be restricted to the planes which cross the object support Ω, because R'f is null for the others.

Now we can express **the necessary and sufficient condition on the curve** Γ : the curve Γ, which defines the cone beam X-ray transform Xf, allows to compute the first derivative R'f of the Radon transform if and only if every plane which does intersect the object support Ω does intersect the curve Γ at least at one point.

This condition is quiet equivalent to the KIRILLOV-TUY condition [KIRILLOV (1961), TUY (1983)], but is more general because we don't need that the planes should not be tangent to the curve at their intersection points. Such a condition have been proposed in [SMITH B. (1985)] using the reconstruction diagram via the Hilbert transform of R'f.

We have defined the cone beam X-ray transform for a source point moving on a curve Γ. But it can be generalized to a source S moving on a surface Σ. Then the same necessary and sufficient condition on the surface Σ can be stated : the surface Σ allows to compute the R'f transform if and only if every plane which does intersect the object support Ω does intersect the curve Γ at least at one point.

Let us introduce now a geometrical description of the planes. The reader should refer to the figures 2 and 5.

We define as the characteristic point C of a plane P, the orthogonal projection of the origin O on P. This description is one-one for the planes which don't cross the origin O. The parameters (ρ,θ,φ) of the Radon transform correspond to the spherical coordinates of the characteristic points C. We have the following relations :

$$\begin{cases} \overrightarrow{OC} = \rho \,.\, \vec{n} \\ M \in P\left(\rho, \vec{n}\right) \Leftrightarrow \overrightarrow{OM} \,.\, \vec{n} = \rho \end{cases} \tag{5.1}$$

Let us take a point M different from the origin O. We note $\mathcal{A}(M)$ the set of the characteristic points C of the planes crossing the point M. This set $\mathcal{A}(M)$ is defined by the following equation :

$$C \in \mathcal{A}(M) \quad \Leftrightarrow \quad \overrightarrow{CM} \,.\, \overrightarrow{CO} = 0 \tag{5.2}$$

It is equivalent to define $\mathcal{A}(M)$ as the set of the points C such that MCO is a right angle. So $\mathcal{A}(M)$ is the spherical surface of diameter (O,M).

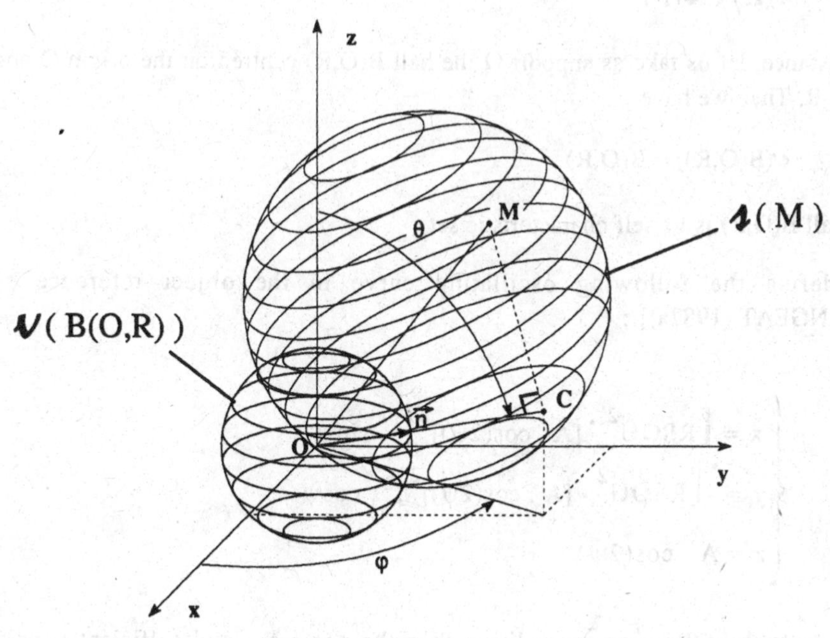

Figure 5 : Characteristic sets $\mathcal{A}(M)$ for the point M and $\mathcal{V}(B(O,R))$ for the ball B(O,R).

For the curve Γ, and respectively for the support Ω, we define the characteristic set $\mathcal{V}(\Gamma)$, and respectively $\mathcal{V}(\Omega)$, as the set of the characteristic points of the planes which intersect the curve Γ, and respectively the support Ω. This sets are defined by the following relations :

$$\mathcal{V}(\Gamma) = \bigcup_{S \in \Gamma} \mathcal{A}(S) \tag{5.3}$$

$$\mathcal{V}(\Omega) = \bigcup_{M \in \Omega} \mathcal{A}(M) \tag{5.4}$$

Then we give a geometrical description of the necessary and sufficient condition on the curve Γ. Every plane which does intersect the object support Ω does intersect the curve Γ at least at one point if and only if :

$$\mathcal{V}(\Omega) \subset \mathcal{V}(\Gamma)$$

For instance, let us take as support Ω the ball B(O,R) centred on the origin O and with radius R. Then we have :

$$\mathcal{V}(B(O,R)) = B(O,R) \tag{5.5}$$

The ball B(O,R) is its self characteristic set.

We define the following oscillating curve in the object reference system [GRANGEAT (1987a)] :

$$\begin{cases} x = \left[RSOU^2 - [A \cdot \cos(2\psi)]^2\right]^{\frac{1}{2}} \cdot \sin\psi \\ y = -\left[RSOU^2 - [A \cdot \cos(2\psi)]^2\right]^{\frac{1}{2}} \cdot \cos\psi \\ z = A \cdot \cos(2\psi) \end{cases} \tag{5.6}$$

If we have the following inequalities, then the necessary and sufficient condition is fullfilled [GRANGEAT (1987b)] :

$$R \leq A \quad \text{and} \quad \sqrt{3} \cdot A \leq RSOU$$

6. THE SPECIAL CASE OF THE CIRCULAR TRAJECTORY

The circular trajectory is the most convenient to design. Moreover it has a revolution symetry which induces simplifications and efficiency in the reconstruction processing. But it is a special case because it doesn't fullfill the necessary and sufficient condition on the acquisition curves.

Indeed, if Γ is a circular trajectory, the characteristic set $\mathcal{V}(\Gamma)$ is a torus (cf. figure 6). It is the hull of the set of spheres $\mathcal{S}(S)$ of diameter (O,S), for S moving along the circular trajectory Γ. If the support Ω is the ball B(O,R), we see on the figure 6 that the necessary and sufficient condition is not fullfilled : $\mathcal{V}(\Omega)$ is not included within $\mathcal{V}(\Gamma)$. There exists a shadow zone in the characteristic set $\mathcal{V}(\Omega)$, which corresponds to the planes almost parallel to the trajectory plane and which don't cross the circular trajectory Γ.

Then, from the cone beam X-ray transform Xf we get an incomplete description of the first derivative R'f of the Radon transform. As in 2D for a limited angular acquisition, it does induce artefacts on the reconstructed function. To lower these artefacts, it is necessary to fill R'f by interpolation on this shadow zone. This ability to process the shadow zone is the main difference between the FELDKAMP'S algorithm [FELDKAMP et al. (1984)] and ours [GRANGEAT (1987b)].

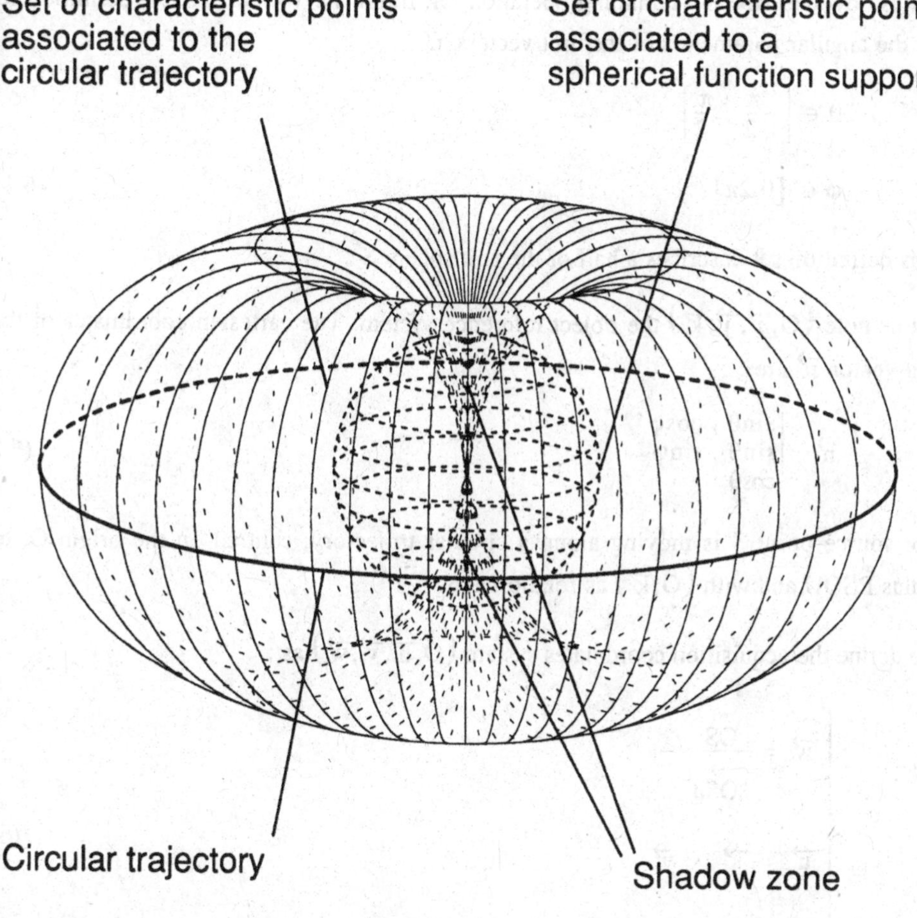

Figure 6 : Shadow zone in the Radon domain associated to a circular trajectory

The easiest way to achieve the interpolation on the shadow zone is to consider on each meridian plane, specified by a longitude angle φ, and on each circle, specified by a given distance ρ to the origin, the two upper and respectively the two lower limit points of the shadow zone. Then, on these circles we proceed either to a nearest neighbour interpolation or to a more sophisticated one like a linear interpolation or a B-spline interpolation.

In the inversion formula (7.1) of R'f, the values on this shadow zone are weighted by $\sin\theta$ and the colatitude angle θ is small. So a high precision on the interpolated data is not necessary.

Let us now describe the rebinning operation (cf. figure 7). We consider as definition set for the angular parameters of the unit vectors $\vec{n}$:

$$\theta \in \left[-\frac{\pi}{2}, \frac{\pi}{2}\right]$$

$$\varphi \in [0,2\pi] \tag{6.1}$$

This definition set describes a half of the unit sphere S^2.

Let us note $(O,\vec{i},\vec{j},\vec{k})$ the object reference system. The cartesian coordinates of the unit vector $\vec{n}$ are :

$$\vec{n} \left| \begin{array}{l} \sin\theta \,.\, \cos\varphi \\ \sin\theta \,.\, \sin\varphi \\ \cos\theta \end{array} \right. \tag{6.2}$$

The source point S is moving along a circular trajectory, centred on the origin O, of radius RSOU and with $(O,\vec{k})$ as rotation axis.

We define the acquisition coordinates system $(O,\vec{u},\vec{v},\vec{w})$ as :

$$\begin{cases} \vec{w} = \dfrac{\vec{OS}}{\|\vec{OS}\|} \\ \vec{u} = \vec{k} \wedge \vec{w} \\ \vec{v} = \vec{k} \end{cases} \tag{6.3}$$

$(O,\vec{u},\vec{v})$ is an orthonormal reference system for the detection plane.

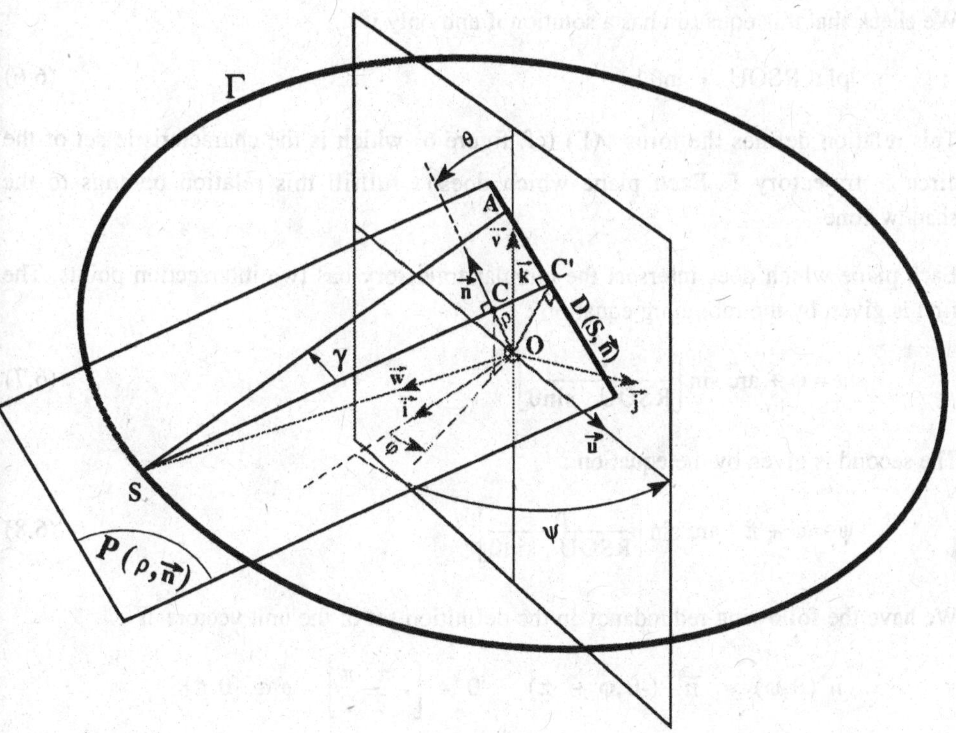

Figure 7 : Reference systems for the circular trajectory

The vector $\vec{u}$ belongs to the vectorial plane associated to the $(\vec{i}, \vec{j})$ vectorial basis. We use as angular parameter ψ to describe the source position S, the angle between the vectors $\vec{u}$ and $\vec{i}$. The cartesian coordinates of the source position S within the object reference system are :

$$S \left| \begin{array}{l} RSOU \,.\, \sin\psi \\ -RSOU \,.\, \cos\psi \\ 0 \end{array} \right. \tag{6.4}$$

The principle of our algorithm is to fill the Radon domain. For each plane $P(\rho, \vec{n})$,we must find one source position S which belongs to that plane, such that we can apply the fundamental relation (3.4). This source position S is given by the following equation :

$$\vec{OS} . \vec{n} = \rho \quad \Leftrightarrow \quad RSOU \,.\, \sin\theta \,.\, \sin(\psi - \varphi) = \rho \tag{6.5}$$

We check that this equation has a solution if and only if :

$$|\rho| \leq RSOU \,.\, |\sin\theta| \tag{6.6}$$

This relation defines the torus $\mathcal{V}(\Gamma)$ (cf. figure 6) which is the characteristic set of the circular trajectory Γ. Each plane which doesn't fullfill this relation belongs to the shadow zone.

Each plane which does intersect the circular trajectory has two intersection points. The first is given by the rebinning equation :

$$\psi = \varphi + \text{arc sin}\left[\frac{\rho}{RSOU \,.\, \sin\theta}\right] \tag{6.7}$$

The second is given by the equation :

$$\psi = \varphi + \pi - \text{arc sin}\left[\frac{\rho}{RSOU \,.\, \sin\theta}\right] \tag{6.8}$$

We have the following redundancy in the definition set of the unit vectors $\vec{n}$:

$$\vec{n}\,(\theta,\varphi) = \vec{n}\,(-\theta,\varphi + \pi) \qquad \theta \in \left[-\frac{\pi}{2}, \frac{\pi}{2}\right], \ \varphi \in [0,\pi]$$

So we don't loose any solution if we consider only the first equation (6.7) that we have called the rebinning equation.

For a given (ρ,θ) couple of parameters, the rebinning from the source coordinate system to the Radon coordinate system is a rotation with the constant angle :

$$-\text{ arc sin}\left[\frac{\rho}{RSOU \,.\, \sin\theta}\right]$$

So the rebinning algorithm is very efficient for a circular trajectory [GRANGEAT (1986b), GRANGEAT (1987b)].

Finally, we remark that if the distance RSOU between the source S and the origin O increases to infinity, the cone beam X-ray transform becomes the parallel beam X-ray transform. We can check that there is no more shadow zone. Moreover, no rebinning is necessary, as it is described by the limit of the rebinning equation (6.7) :

$$\psi = \varphi$$

7. FROM THE FIRST DERIVATIVE R'f OF THE RADON TRANSFORM TO THE OBJECT FUNCTION f.

The reconstruction of the object function f from the first derivative R'f of its Radon transform is given by the inversion formula (2.7). If we use the definition set

$\left[-\frac{\pi}{2},\frac{\pi}{2}\right]$ x $[0,2\pi]$ for the angular parameters (θ,φ) of the unit vector $\vec{n}$, we get :

$$f(M) = -\frac{1}{8\pi^2} \cdot \int_{\theta=-\frac{\pi}{2}}^{\frac{\pi}{2}} \int_{\varphi=0}^{2\pi} \frac{\partial R'f}{\partial \rho}\left(\vec{OM}.\vec{n},\vec{n}\right).\, |\sin\theta| \quad d\theta\, d\varphi \qquad (7.1)$$

To achieve an efficient implementation of this inversion formula [MARR and al. (1980)], we must split the computation of this double integral in two steps, first an integration over θ for all the meridian planes and second an integration over φ for all the axial planes. For the numerical aspects, we refer to [LOUIS (1983), GRANGEAT (1987b)].

Let us introduce the rebinned X-ray transform $\tilde{X}f$ as the acquisition in parallel geometry along straight lines perpendicular to the axis $(O,\vec{k})$. We note $D(\varphi,B)$ the straight line perpendicular to the meridian plane of longitude φ, with B as intersection point (cf. figure 8). Then the rebinned X-ray transform $\tilde{X}f$ is defined by :

$$\tilde{X}f(\varphi,B) = \int_{M\in D(\varphi,B)} f(M)\ dM \qquad (7.2)$$

Let us define the filtered rebinned X-ray transform $HD\tilde{X}f$ as the convolution of the rebinned X-ray transform $\tilde{X}f$ with the classical ramp filter HD along all the lines perpendicular to the axis $(O,\vec{k})$. The two-dimensional Fourier transform F_2 [HD] of this filter HD is given by :

$$F_2\,[HD]\ (\nu_r,\nu_z) = |\nu_r| \qquad (7.3)$$

if (ν_r,ν_z) are the frequential coordinates in the directions respectively perpendicular and parallel to the axis $(O,\vec{k})$.

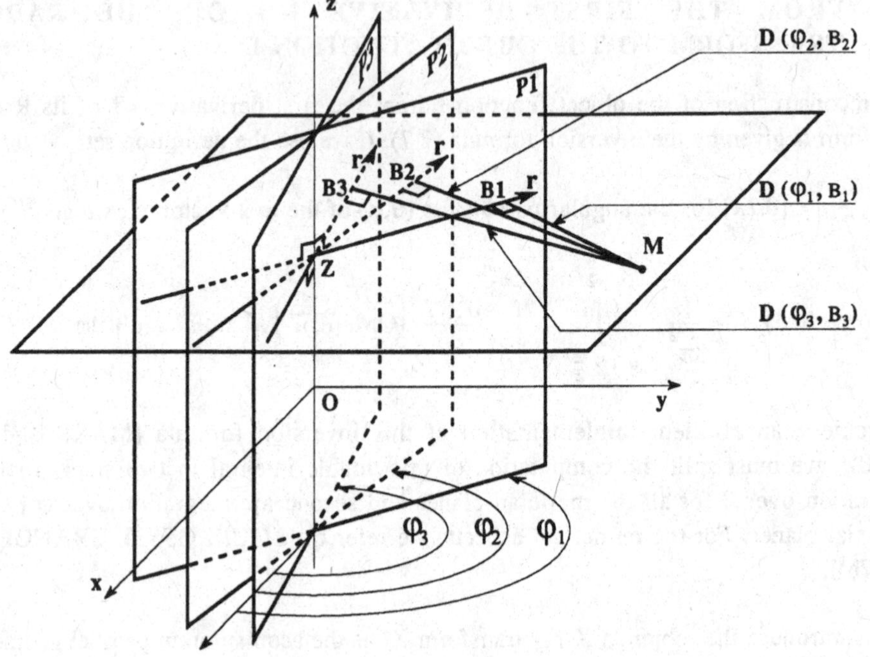

Figure 8 : The rebinned X-ray transform $\tilde{X}f$

The same relation can be defined if this frequential plane is parametrized with the polar coordinates (ν,θ) :

$$F_2\,[HD]\,(\nu,\theta) = |\,\nu\,|\,.\,|\,\sin\theta\,| \tag{7.4}$$

On each meridian plane of longitude φ, we get the following relation for the first convolution backprojection step :

$$HD\tilde{X}f\,(\varphi,B) = -\frac{1}{4\pi^2}\cdot\int_{\theta=-\frac{\pi}{2}}^{\frac{\pi}{2}} \frac{\partial R'f}{\partial\rho}\left(\overrightarrow{OB}.\vec{n},\vec{n}\right).\,|\,\sin\theta\,|\quad d\theta \tag{7.5}$$

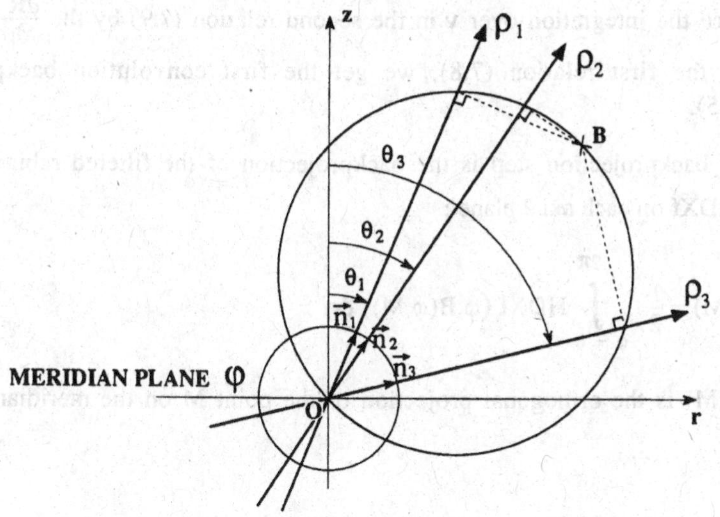

Figure 9 : The first convolution backprojection step on each meridian plane

The relation (7.5) can be proved from the central silice theorems. If $\hat{f}$ is the three-dimensional Fourier transform of the function f, we have the folloving relations :

$$Rf\left(\rho,\vec{n}\right) = \int_{\nu=-\infty}^{+\infty} \hat{f}\left(\nu,\vec{n}\right) . e^{2i\pi\nu\rho} \, d\nu \tag{7.6}$$

$$\tilde{X}f\,(\varphi,B) = \int_{\theta=-\frac{\pi}{2}}^{\frac{\pi}{2}} \int_{\nu=-\infty}^{+\infty} \hat{f}\left(\nu,\vec{n}\right) . e^{2i\pi\nu\overrightarrow{OB}.\vec{n}} . |\nu| \; d\theta \; d\nu \tag{7.7}$$

After the filtering, we get :

$$\frac{\partial R'f}{\partial\rho}\left(\rho,\vec{n}\right) = -4\pi^2 . \int_{\nu=-\infty}^{+\infty} \hat{f}\left(\nu\;,\vec{n}\right) . e^{2i\pi\nu\rho} . \nu^2 \; d\nu \tag{7.8}$$

$$HD\tilde{X}f\,(\varphi,B) = \int_{\theta=-\frac{\pi}{2}}^{\frac{\pi}{2}} \int_{\nu=-\infty}^{+\infty} \hat{f}\left(\nu,\vec{n}\right) . e^{2i\pi\nu\overrightarrow{OB}.\vec{n}} . \nu^2 \cdot |\sin\theta| \;\; d\theta \; d\nu \tag{7.9}$$

If we replace the integration over ν in the second relation (7.9) by the $\frac{\partial R'f}{\partial \rho}$ function defined by the first relation (7.8), we get the first convolution backprojection formula (7.5).

The second backprojection step is the backprojection of the filtered rebinned X-ray transform $HD\tilde{X}f$ on each axial plane :

$$f(M) = \frac{1}{2} \cdot \int_{\varphi=0}^{2\pi} HD\tilde{X}f\,(\varphi, B(\varphi,M))\, d\varphi \tag{7.10}$$

where B(φ,M) is the orthogonal projection of the point M on the meridian plane of longitude φ.

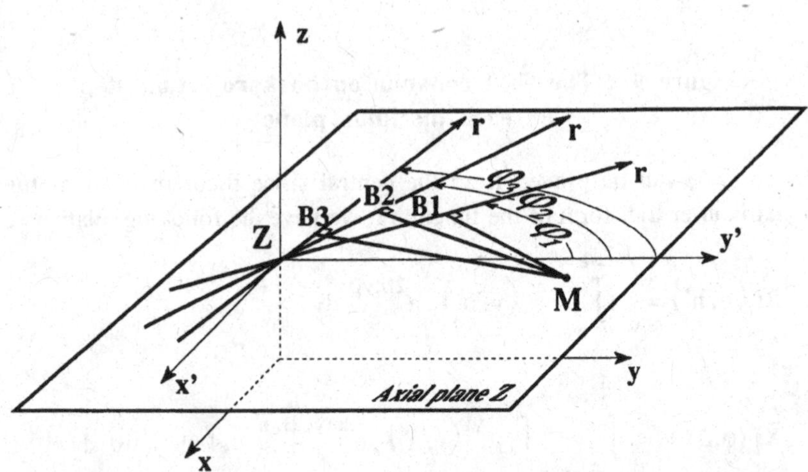

Figure 10 : The second backprojection step on each axial plane

This relation is the classical inversion formula of the X-ray transform in parallel geometry.

For the implementation of these formulas, we consider a given number NPHI of meridian angles φ, which is equal to the number NPSI of source positions for a circular trajectory. If this number is even, we have a redundancy in the description of the Radon domain because :

$$\vec{n}\,(\theta,\varphi) = \vec{n}\,(-\theta, \varphi + \pi) \quad (\theta,\varphi) \in \left[-\frac{\pi}{2}, \frac{\pi}{2}\right] \mathrm{x}\, [0,\pi] \tag{7.11}$$

To reduce by a factor 2 the number of backprojections, we first compute the average value AR'f (θ,φ) for opposite meridians :

$$A'Rf(\theta,\varphi) = \frac{1}{2}\left[R'f(\theta,\varphi) + R'f(-\theta,\varphi+\pi)\right] \tag{7.12}$$

$$\text{For } (\theta,\varphi) \in \left[-\frac{\pi}{2}, \frac{\pi}{2}\right] \times [0,\pi]$$

Then the first convolution backprojection step can be restricted to the longitude angles φ between 0 and π, and the second backprojection step becomes :

$$f(M) = \int_{\varphi=0}^{\pi} HD\tilde{X}f\left(\varphi, B(\varphi,M)\right) d\varphi \tag{7.13}$$

8. CONCLUSION

In this publication, we have described the mathematical framework of our cone beam 3D reconstruction algorithm via the first derivative of the Radon transform. It is based first on the fundamental relation (3.4) between the cone beam X-ray transform Xf and the first derivative R'f of the Radon transform, second on the rebinning operation on planes from the acquisition coordinates system to the Radon spherical coordinates system, third on the inversion of the first derivative R'f of the Radon transform to recover the original function f. This inversion diagram gives a direct reconstruction algorithm for a large class of acquisition trajectories. The induced large family of cone beam 3D tomographic devices associated to this reconstruction process have been patented [GRANGEAT (1987a)]. The description of the mathematical theory and of the numerical processing is presented in our thesis [GRANGEAT (1987b)].

The numerical implementation of the algorithm does proceed in three steps : first the differentiation integration operations on each projection and the rebinning,to compute the first derivative R'f of the Radon transform from the cone beam X-ray transform Xf, second the parallel backprojection step on each meridian to get the filtered rebinned X-ray transform $HD\tilde{X}f$, from R'f, third the parallel backprojection step on each axial plane to compute the function f from $HD\tilde{X}f$. Each step is a sequential processing of elementary 2D files. So this algorithm is well suited for parallelization and vectorization. It uses only the four fondamental operations of reconstruction algorithms that are convolution, rebinning, backprojection, reprojection. So it can be implemented on reconstruction processors [CAQUINEAU and AMANS (1990a), CAQUINEAU (1990b)]. Today, at the LETI, we have developped a software for the cone beam 3D reconstruction via the first derivative of the Radon transform, that we call RADON [GRANGEAT et al. (1990a), SIRE et al. (1990)]. For the moment, it does process the cone beam acquisitions only for a circular trajectory. We have take care to the vectorization of the algorithm. The experimental comparison between the FELDKAMP'S reconstruction software and this RADON software is under study [RIZO and ELLINGSON (1990a), RIZO et al. (1990b)]. The next extension of the RADON software will be to process the acquisitions with a double circular trajectory [RIZO et al. (1990c)]. So we conclude that all this mathematical framework has lead at the LETI to large algorithmical and technological developments.

REFERENCES

CAQUINEAU C., AMANS J.L. (1990a). “A processor architecture for the image and volume reconstruction”. ICASSP 1990, Session M1, M1.3, 1849 - 1852.

CAQUINEAU C. (1990b). Architecture de processeurs pour la reconstruction d'images et de volumes à partir de projections. Thèse de doctorat. Université de Technologie de Compiègne.

FELDKAMP L.A., DAVIS L.C., KRESS J.W. (1984). “Practical cone-beam algorithm”. J. Opt. Soc. Am., 1 (6), 612 - 619.

FINCH D.V., SOLMON D.C. (1980). “Stability and consistency for the divergent beam X-ray transform” in HERMAN G.T., NATTERER F., Mathematical Aspects of Computerized Tomography, 100 - 111, Springer - Verlag.

FINCH D.V., SOLMON D.C. (1983). “A characterization of the range of the divergent beam X-ray transform”. SIAM J. Math. Anal., 14 (4), 767 - 771.

FINCH D.V. (1985). “Cone beam reconstruction with sources on a curve”. SIAM J. Appl. Math., 45 (4), 665 - 673.

GRANGEAT P. (1984). “Theoretical background of the cone-beam reconstruction algorithm”. Private communication with D. FINCH and D. SOLMON, published in GRANGEAT P. (1987). Analyse d'un Système d'Imagerie 3D par Reconstruction à partir de Radiographies X en Géométrie Conique. Thèse de doctorat. Ecole Nationale Supérieure des Télécommunications.

GRANGEAT P. (1985). “3D reconstruction for diverging X-ray beams”. Computer Assisted Radiology (Berlin), CAR'85, 59 - 64, Springer - Verlag.

GRANGEAT P. (1986a). “Description of a 3D reconstruction algorithm for diverging X-ray beams”. Biostereometrics 85, A.M. Coblentz, R.E. Heron ed, proc. SPIE-602, 92 - 108.

GRANGEAT P. (1986b). “Voludensitométrie : optimisation du calcul de la transformée de Radon 3D à partir de radiographies X en géométrie conique”, Deuxième Colloque Image (Nice), CESTA, 512 - 516.

GRANGEAT P. (1986c). "An analysis of the divergent beam X-ray transform based on the 3D Radon transform". Communication at the siminar organized by HERMAN G.T. and NATTERER F. at the Mathematisches Forschungsinstitut Oberwolfach : Theory and Application of Radon transforms.

GRANGEAT P. (1987a). "Procédé et dispositif d'imagerie tridimensionnelle à partir de mesures bidimensionnelles de l'atténuation". French patent n° 8777 07134. European patent (1988) n° 88 401234.5, publication n° EP 0292 402 A1.

GRANGEAT P. (1987b). Analyse d'un Système d'Imagerie 3D par Reconstruction à partir de Radiographies X en Géométrie Conique. Thèse de doctorat. Ecole Nationale Supérieure des Télécommunications.

GRANGEAT P. (1989). TRIDIMOS : Imagerie 3D de la minéralisation des vertèbres lombaires. Rapport final contrat CNES-LETI n° 853/CNES/89/5849/00 (référence CEA : n° GR 771.576).

GRANGEAT P., HATCHADOURIAN G., LE MASSON P., SIRE P. (1990a). Logiciel Radon : Notice descriptive des algorithmes et des programmes. Note technique LETI n° 1546.

GRANGEAT P., LE MASSON P., MELENNEC P., SIRE P. (1990b). "3D cone beam reconstruction". Communication at the seminar organized by HERMAN G.T., LOUIS A.K., NATTERER F., at the Matematisches Forschungsinstitut Oberwolfach : Mathematical Methods in Tomography.

GRANGEAT P. (1990c). "Reconstruire les structures tridimensionnelles internes de l'organisme humain". Submitted to Le Courrier du CNRS.

GULLBERG G.T., ZENG G.L., CHRISTIAN P.E., TSUI B.M.W., MORGAN H.T. (1989). "Single photon emission computed tomography of the heart using cone beam geometry and non circular detector rotation". In Information Processing in Medical Imaging, XI th IPMI International conference, Berkeley, CA.

HAMAKER C., SMITH K.T., SOLMON D.C., WAGNER S.L. (1980). "The divergent beam X-ray transform". Rocky Mount. J. of Math., 10 (1), 253 - 283.

JACQUET I. (1988). Reconstruction d'Image 3D par l'Algorithme Eventail Généralisé. Mémoire de Diplôme d'Ingénieur. Conservatoire National des Arts et Métiers.

JASZCZAK R.J., GREER K.L., COLEMAN R.E. (1988). "SPECT using a specially designed cone beam collimator". J. Nucl. Med., 29, 1398 - 1405.

JOSEPH P.M. (1982). "An improved algorithm for reprojecting rays through pixel images". IEEE Trans. on Med. Imag., MI - 1 (3), 192 - 196.

KIRILLOV A.A. (1961). "On a problem of I.M. Gel' fand". Soviet Math. Dokl., 2, 268 - 269.

KUDO H., SAITO T. (1989a). "3-D tomographic image reconstruction from incomplete cone beam projections". In Proc. Topical Meeting OSA, Signal Recovery and Synthesis, Cape Code, USA, 170 - 173.

KUDO H., SAITO T. (1989b). "Feasible cone beam scanning methods for exact 3-D tomographic image reconstruction". In Proc. Topical Meeting OSA, Signal Recovery and Synthesis, Cape Code, USA, 174 - 177.

LOUIS A.K. (1983). "Approximate inversion of the 3D Radon transform". Math. Meth. in the Appl. Sci., 5, 176 - 185.

MANGLOS S.H., BASSANO D.A., DUXBURY C.E., CAPONE R.B. (1990). "Attenuation maps for SPECT determined using cone beam transmission computed tomography". IEEE Trans. on Nucl. Sci., NS-37 (2), 600 - 608.

MARR R.B., CHEN C., LAUTERBUR P.C. (1980). "On two approaches to 3D reconstruction in NMR zeugmatography" in HERMAN G.T. and NATTERER F., Mathematical Aspects of Computerized Tomography, 225 - 240, Springer - Verlag.

MINERBO G.N. (1979). "Convolution reconstruction from cone-beam projection data". IEEE Trans. Nucl. Sci., NS - 26 (2), 2682 - 2684.

MORTON E.J., WEBB S., BATEMAN J.E., CLARKE L.J., SHELTON C.G. (1990). "Three-dimensional X-ray microtomography for medical and biological applications". Phys. Med. Biol., 35 (7), 805 - 820.

NATTERER F. (1986). The Mathematics of Computerized Tomography. Wiley/Teubner.

RIZO Ph., GRANGEAT P. (1989). "Development of a 3D cone beam tomographic system for NDT of ceramics". In Topical Proceedings of the ASNT : Industrial Computerized Tomography, Seattle, July 25-27, 24 - 28.

RIZO Ph., ELLINGSON W.A. (1990a). "An initial comparison between two 3D X-ray CT algorithms for characterizing ceramic materials". Proc. of the conference on Non Destructive Evaluation of Modern Ceramics, Columbus, Ohio, July 9 - 12.

RIZO Ph., GRANGEAT P., SIRE P., LE MASSON P., MELENNEC P. (1990b). "Comparison of two 3D cone beam reconstruction algorithm with a circular source trajectory". Submitted to J. Opt. Soc. Am.

RIZO Ph., GRANGEAT P., SIRE P., LE MASSON P., DELAGENIERE S. (1990c). "Cone beam 3D reconstruction with a double circular trajectory". Communication at the 1990 Fall Meeting of the Material Research Society, Boston.

ROBB R.A. (1985). "X-ray Computed Tomography : Advanced Systems in Biomedical Research" in ROBB R.A. (1985), Three Dimensional Biomedical Imaging, CRC Press, Volume I, Chapter 5, 107 - 164.

SAINT-FELIX D., TROUSSET Y., PICARD C., ROUGEE A. (1990). "3D reconstruction of high contrast objects using a multi-scale detection/estimation scheme" in HÖHNE K.H., FUCHS H., PIZER S., 3D Imaging in Medicine : Algorithms, Systems, Applications, NATO ASI Series, Springer - Verlag, Series F, Vol. 60, 147 - 158.

SIRE P., GRANGEAT P., LE MASSON P., MELENNEC P., RIZO Ph. (1990). "NDT applications of the 3D Radon transform algorithm for cone beam reconstruction". Communication at the 1990 Fall Meeting of the Material Research Society, Boston.

SMITH B.D. (1985). "Image reconstruction from cone-beam projections : necessary and sufficient conditions and reconstruction methods". IEEE Trans. on Med. Imag., MI - 4 (1) 14 - 25

SMITH B.D. (1987). Computer-aided tomographic imaging from cone-beam data. Ph. D. dissertation. University of Rhode Island.

SMITH B.D. (1990). "Cone-beam tomography : recent advances and a tutorial review". Optical Engineering, 29 (5), 524 - 534.

TUY H.K. (1983). "An inversion formula for cone-beam reconstruction". SIAM J. Appl. Math., 43 (3), 546 - 552.

VICKERS D., COX W., Mc CROSKEY W., KOHRS B., ZAHN R., CARLSON R. (1989). "A revolutionary approach to industrial CT using cone-beam reconstruction". In Topical Proceedings of the ASNT : Industrial Computerized Tomography, Seattle, July 25-27, 39 - 45.

WEBB S., SUTCLIFFE J., BURKINSHAWL, HORSMAN A. (1987). "Tomographic reconstruction from experimentaly obtained cone-beam projections". IEEE Trans. on Med. Imag., MI - 6 (1), 67 - 73.

DIFFRACTION TOMOGRAPHY
SOME APPLICATIONS AND EXTENSION TO 3-D ULTRASOUND IMAGING

Patricia GRASSIN, Bernard DUCHENE, Walid TABBARA
Laboratoire des Signaux et Systèmes
(CNRS-ESE) Plateau de Moulon - 91192 Gif-sur-Yvette Cedex, France

ABSTRACT

Diffraction tomography is investigated in our laboratory since the beginning of the eighties. We first present an overview of the results obtained at microwave and ultrasound frequencies. Next, since the authors are mainly involved in acoustical imaging, we emphasize the extension of this technique to 3D imaging using ultrasound waves.

1. OVERVIEW OF APPLICATIONS

In some sense, Diffraction Tomography (DT) is an extension of the well known Computerized Tomography (CT). Unlike the latter, DT does not require any assumption on the way energy propagates from the emitter to the receiver (propagation along straight rays in CT).

They share the facts that both are multiview imaging techniques and they lead to experimental set up similar in their basic principles. While CT provides an image which is a map of a physical parameter of the medium inside the object (attenuation, speed of sound,...), DT which takes into account all diffraction phenomena, reconstructs a map of the density of the induced sources (or Huygens sources) inside the object. This density is a function of the physical parameters whose retrieval requires more processing, and until now this final step is still an open problem.

Diffraction Tomography has been introduced in 1979 [1] and since then is the subject of numerous investigations using mainly synthesized data [2, 3]. Applications in various fields [4, 5] has been considered and evaluated by means of simulations or through experimentation.

The contribution of our group to the understanding and application of DT in acoustics and electromagnetics includes both theoretical and experimental results, a large part of them being reported in [4, 6, 7].

We have dealt with biomedical applications along with others in the field of nondestructive testing in civil engineering and control of faults in metallic structures. The main conclusions of these investigations can be stated as follow :

- DT has a large spectrum of potential applications.

- It is well suited for objects whose dimensions are of the order of few wavelengths. Few views (usually between 30 and 60) are necessary to produce an acceptable (in terms of contrast and sharpness of the boundaries) image of a horizontal cross-section of the object. For vertical cross-sections (this is 3D imaging) one view is enough.

- DT provides in most cases a qualitative image, this means that the basic processing of the measured data does not provide information about the physical parameters of the object (permittivity, speed of sound, conductivity,...). The retrieval of the latter requires additional analysis of the development of new approaches [8, 9, 10].

- It has been shown that first-order approximations such as Born's and Rytov's usually fail when applied to real world problems.

- Biomedical applications involve highly inhomogeneous media whose physical parameters are not known with enough accuracy. In vitro experimental results in DT led us to the conclusion that this technique reproduces accurately the contours of each homogeneous region in an inhomogeneous cross-section of a biological medium. Combining DT with differential imaging shows an interesting ability to monitor small variation in the values of these parameters. These conclusions are expected to help in monitoring temperature in hyperthermia treatment of cancers.

- In civil engineering, DT has been used to image metallic bars in concrete blocks. For a block with a low humidity rate, multifrequency DT provides images of bars deeply buried in the concrete. On the opposite for high humidity rates the quality of the image decreases very rapidly. In this experiment a view is related to the data at one frequency since the emitter and the receiver do not move with respect to the object.

- The detection of flaws or changes in the conductivity of metallic structures is within the reach of eddy currents DT. Numerical results have shown that small cracks can be imaged when present near the surface of a metallic block. Accuracy decreases with the burial depth.

Actual work in our group is mainly in the development on one hand of quantitative imaging algorithms for 2D and 3D problems, and on the other hand of a new generation of devices that are able to use these algorithms to provide images in various fields of application.

2. 3-D ULTRASOUND IMAGING

2.1 Basic formulation

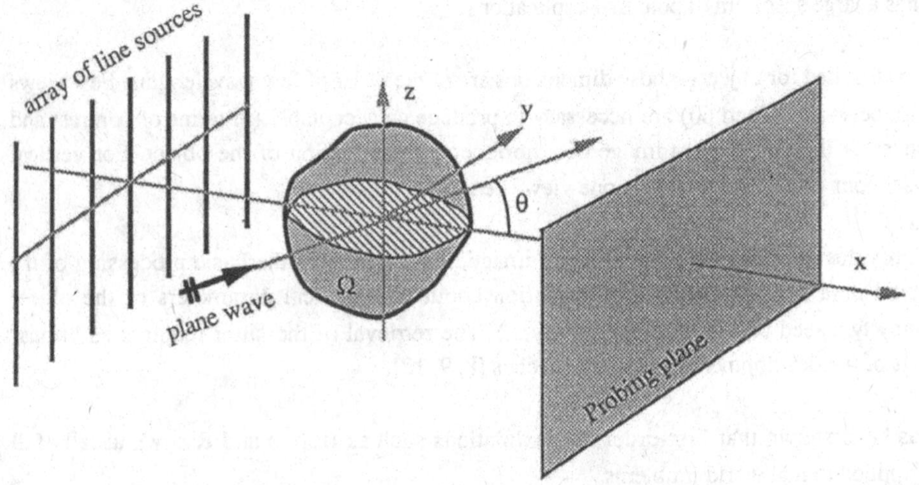

Figure 1 : *Geometry of the scattering problem*

As shown on figure 1, a 3-D object is defined by the speed of sound $C(\vec{x})$ inside its volume Ω where $\vec{x} = (x, y, z)$ is the coordinate vector. The surrounding medium is made of water where a source, operating at frequency f_0, illuminates the object. Density is constant and equal to that of water throughout space. The scattered field is measured on a 2-D planar array located opposite to the source with respect to the object and perpendicular to the x-axis. We note k_0 the wave number in water and $k(\vec{x})$ the one within the object. The source is either a plane wave propagating in the (x, y) plane along a direction defined by its angle θ, or an array of line sources parallel to the z-axis and separated by a distance equal to $\lambda_0/2$ (λ_0 : wavelength in water). In this latter case the arrays of emitters and receivers are at equal distances from the center of the object. The incident pressure field is given by :

$$p_0(\vec{x}) = e^{j\vec{k}_0.\vec{x}} \qquad \text{plane wave}$$

$$p_0(\vec{x}) = \frac{j}{4} H_0^1(k_0|\vec{x} - \vec{x}_s|) \qquad \text{line source located at } \vec{x}_s = (x_s, y_s)$$

The position of a receiver in the array is specified by its coordinate vector $\vec{x}_r = (x_r, y_r, z_r)$.

Proceeding as in the 2-D case [6], it is easy to show that the total pressure $p(\vec{x})$ everywhere in space is given by :

$$p(\vec{x}) = p_0(\vec{x}) + \int_{\Omega} J(\vec{x}')\, G(\vec{x} - \vec{x}')\, d\vec{x}'$$

$$J(\vec{x}') = (k^2(\vec{x}') - k_0^2)\, p(\vec{x}') \quad \text{density of induced sources} \tag{1}$$

$$G(\vec{x}-\vec{x}') = \frac{e^{j k_0 |\vec{x} - \vec{x}'|}}{4\pi |\vec{x} - \vec{x}'|} \quad \text{Green's function}$$

We introduce the normalized functions :

$$\Psi(\vec{x}) = (p(\vec{x}) - p_0(\vec{x})) / p_0(\vec{x})$$
$$\varphi(\vec{x}) = J(\vec{x}) / p_0(\vec{x}) \tag{2}$$

the Fourier transform of the normalized scattered field :

$$\hat{\Psi}(\alpha_{y_r}, \alpha_{z_r}) = \iint_{-\infty}^{+\infty} \Psi(y_r, z_r)\, e^{-j(\alpha_{y_r} y_r + \alpha_{z_r} z_r)}\, dy_r\, dz_r \quad \text{plane wave}$$

$$\hat{\Psi}(\alpha_{y_r}, \alpha_{z_r}, \alpha_{y_s}) = \iiint_{-\infty}^{+\infty} \Psi(y_r, z_r, y_s)\, e^{-j(\alpha_{y_r} y_r + \alpha_{z_r} z_r + \alpha_{y_s} y_s)}\, dy_r\, dz_r\, dy_s \quad \text{line sources} \tag{3}$$

and the Fourier transform of the normalized induced sources :

$$\hat{\varphi}(\mu, \nu, \gamma) = \iiint_{-\infty}^{+\infty} \varphi(x', y', z')\, e^{-j(\mu x' + \nu y' + \gamma z')}\, dx'\, dy'\, dz'$$

Applying the Fourier transform to both sides of (1) leads to :

$$\hat{\varphi}(\mu, \nu, \gamma) = -2j\beta\,\widehat{\Psi}(\alpha_{y_r}, \alpha_{z_r})\, e^{-j(\beta - k_0)x_r}$$

$$\begin{aligned}
\beta &= \sqrt{k_0^2 - (\alpha_{y_r}^2 + \alpha_{z_r}^2)} \\
\mu &= (\beta - k_0)\cos\theta - \alpha_{y_r}\sin\theta \\
\nu &= (\beta - k_0)\sin\theta + \alpha_{y_r}\cos\theta \\
\gamma &= \alpha_{z_r}
\end{aligned} \tag{4.a}$$

for a plane wave illumination and to :

$$\begin{aligned}
&\hat{\varphi}(\mu, \nu, \gamma) = -4\beta_s\beta_r\,\widehat{\Psi}(\alpha_{y_r}, \alpha_{z_r}, \alpha_{y_s})\, e^{-j(\beta_r x_r - \beta_s x_s)} \\
&\beta_r = \sqrt{k_0^2 - (\alpha_{y_r}^2 + \alpha_{z_r}^2)} \;,\quad \beta_s = \sqrt{k_0^2 - \alpha_{y_s}^2} \\
&\mu = \beta_r - \beta_s \;,\quad \nu = \alpha_{y_r} + \alpha_{y_s} \;,\quad \gamma = \alpha_{z_r}
\end{aligned} \tag{4.b}$$

in the case of an array of line sources. Equations (4.a, 4.b) are satisfied in the spectral space over restricted domains :

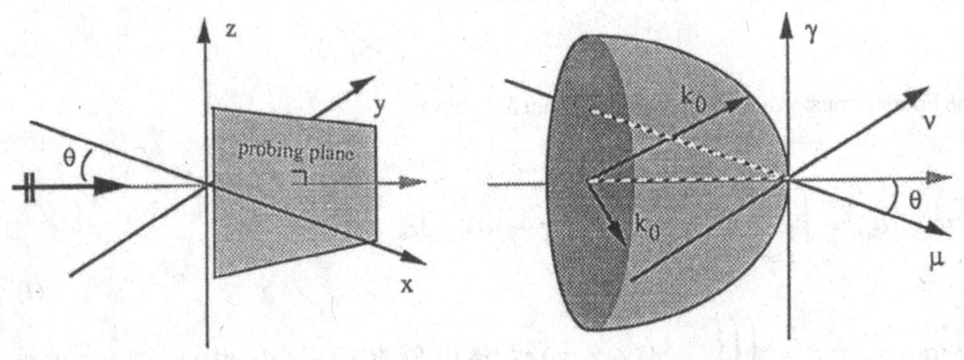

Figure 2 : *Geometry in the (x, y, z) space and in the (μ, ν, γ) spectral space*

in the case of a plane wave illumination, for each view (each direction of incidence) the spectral data are located on a hemisphere (radius k_0, center $(-k_0\cos\theta, -k_0\sin\theta, 0)$ shown in Figure 2 (in the case where the receiving array is perpendicular to the direction of illumination). Multiview data are collected as described in [6] and the spectral data located on a set of hemispheres. In the case of a line source no displacement of the source or of the receivers occurs.

A regular cubic grid is built in the spectral space by interpolating the data (nearest neighbor interpolation) from the set of hemispheres. Finally an inverse Fourier transform is applied in order to retrieve $\varphi(x, y, z)$ and the map of its modulus is displayed as the image of a cross-section of the object lying in the xy - and yz - planes.

2.2. Results

We have considered the case of sources operating at a frequency of 2 MHz and of an array of 33 x 33 receivers located at a distance equal to $3\lambda_0$ from the center of the object. For a plane wave source 17 views have been used, and in the second type of illumination 17 lines sources have been considered. The objects were : 1) a spherical shell : inner radius λ_0, thickness $\lambda_0/2$, $C(\vec{x})$ = 1560 m/s in the shell and 1470 m/s (water) inside the sphere; 2) a $3\lambda_0$-sided T shaped object with $C(\vec{x})$ = 1 560 m/s. The results are shown on the coloured plate.

2.2.1 Plane wave illumination

Figure 3 shows the reconstruction of a spherical shell built up from one view. It can be seen that the transverse cross-section, (parallel to the plane of the receiver : left) is much better described than the longitudinal one (in the xy-plane : right). However the latter is greatly improved when several views are used for the reconstruction, as shown in Figure 4 which depicts longitudinal cross-sections of a spherical shell (left) and of a T-shaped object (right) built-up from 12 views (incident wave and probing plane being rotated all around the object).

In all figures the continuous lines represent the true boundaries of the objects. As shown here and in other reconstructed images the boundaries are accurately determined and thus one can expect the frontiers of each of the homogeneous region of an inhomogeneous object to be well reconstructed. These examples and others we have obtained show that for plane wave illumination the behavior of 3-D diffraction tomography is similar to the 2-D case, except for the reconstruction of vertical cross-sections.

2.2.2 Line source illumination

Figure 5 shows longitudinal cross-sections built-up from 17 views of a spherical shell (same as in 2.2.1) illuminated either by line-sources (left) or by a plane wave (right). Remember that here the probing plane do not move as previously, and remains perpendicular to the x-axis. The set of 17 line sources are seen from the center of the sphere within a sector of 80°, whereas the 17 plane waves ly in the same sector with equal angular separation. This comparison shows that there is significant differences between the two set-ups of sources. In the case of line-source illumination, due to the dispersion of energy, the front face of the object (the part facing the

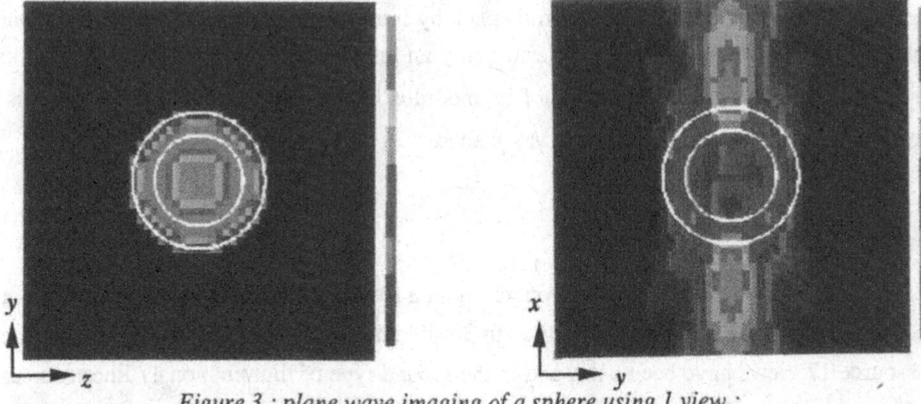

Figure 3 : plane wave imaging of a sphere using 1 view :
left = transverse plane, right = longitudinal plane

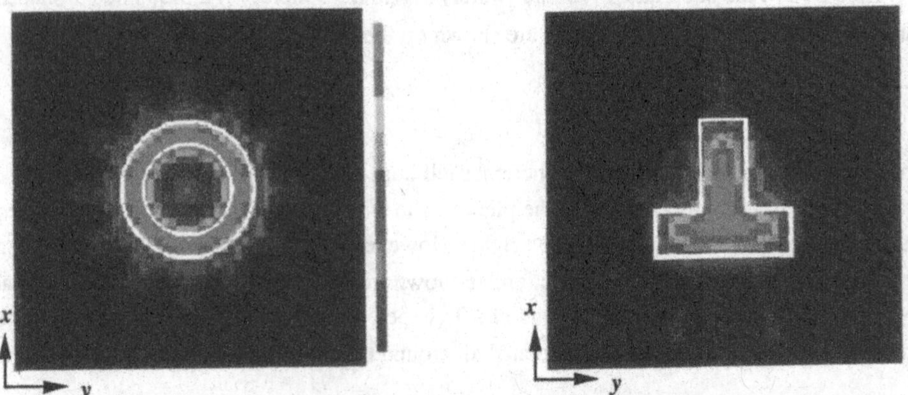

Figure 4 : Plane wave imaging using 12 views :
left = case of a sphere, right = case of a T

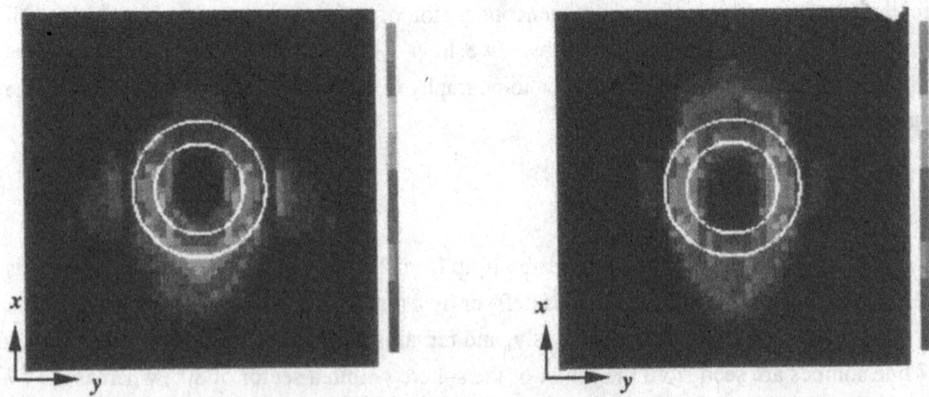

Figure 5 : 17-view images of a sphere :
left = line source illumination, right = plane wave illumination

source) is enhanced compared to the plane wave illumination case, whereas the rear face becomes almost invisible.

Thus, one cannot expect to reduce the number of views (or of mechanical rotations) by using still line sources. On the other hand vertical cross sections are accurately reconstructed.

CONCLUSION

After reviewing the main results we have obtained from the evaluation of DT through various applications to real world problems, we have presented some preliminary results in 3-D ultrasonics DT. As a general conclusion one can notice that DT is an efficient imaging technique usefull in many applications. It does not require complex and expensive experimental setups and in most cases provides accurate qualitative images. Its main limitation lies in its inability to reconstruct the intrinsic physical parameters of the object at least by means of the present formulation of DT. In spite of this handicap, there remains many applications where DT, in its present state of development, is an efficient tool of investigation.

REFERENCES

[1] R.K. Mueller et al., Proc. IEEE, vol. 67, n° 4, pp. 567-587, 1979.
[2] A.J. Devaney, Ultrasonic Imaging, vol. 4, pp. 336-350, 1982.
[3] A.J. Devaney et al., Ultrasonic Imaging, vol. 6, pp. 181-193, 1984.
[4] J.Ch. Bolomey et al., IEEE Trans. Microwave Theory Tech., vol. MTT-30, n° 11, pp. 1998-2000, 1982.
[5] A.J. Witten et al., IEEE Trans. Geosci. Remote Sensing, Vol. GE-24, n° 5, pp. 655-662, 1986.
[6] W. Tabbara et al., Inverse Problems, vol. 4, pp. 305-331, 1988.
[7] B. Duchêne et al., J. Opt. Soc. Am., A, vol. 2, pp. 1937-1953, 1985.
[8] N. Joachimowicz, Thesis, Univ. of Paris-Sud, March 1990 (available from the authors).
[9] A. Franchois, in Inverse Methods in Inverse Methods in Action, Edit. P.C. Sabatier, pp. 62-68, Springer, 1990.
[10] R. Zorgati, Thesis, Univ. of Paris-7, June 1990 (available from the authors).

Diffuse Tomography: A Refined Model

F. ALBERTO GRÜNBAUM
DEPARTMENT OF MATHEMATICS
UNIVERSITY OF CALIFORNIA
BERKELEY, CA 94720

Table of Contents

1. Introduction
2. The original model
3. The forward problem
4. Refining the model

1. Introduction.

In [1] we presented a model of "diffuse tomography" that considers the problem of reconstruction local characteristics of tissue from radiation that undergoes attenuation and scattering as it travels through the medium. Some aspects of the problem have also been discussed in [2,3,4,5,6].

In the limiting case when scattering effects can be ignored this model reduces to the well studied problem of "X-ray tomography". However, as long as scattering (or diffusion) is a part of the problem to be solved for, we have a considerable harder problem. In fact a proper treatment of the problem requires an ab-initio three dimensional formulation, since low energy photons that are unwilling to stay on a straight line are equaly unwilling to stay on a given plane, and they will scatter out of the plane of the source.

The discussion in [1] addresses the three dimensional situation, and presents the results of some numerical simulations based on this model. One also finds in [1] some numerical simulations based on a (somewhat less physically correct) two dimensional model. All these results make it worth while to study the simpler two dimensional case a bit further: the three dimensional problem is in some sense easier (see the remark at the end of Section 3), although the computational issues make the two dimensional model a preferable one.

The main limitations of the model discussed in [1,2,3,4,5] consists in having discretized positions and velocities in a rather primitive fashion. This, as well as other possible pitfalls inherent to any discretization process, has led us and some of our friends to look for a more refined model. I want to acknowledge the remarks from L. Shepp in this connection, [7]. He bears no responsibility for the model discussed here, but his (and mine) unhappiness with discretized models have spurned me in the search for a more refined model.

Research partially supported by NSF DMS-87-20007 and AFOSR-88-0250.

2. The original model.

Subdivide the object (thought of as a square, or a cube if we were dealing with the three dimensional version) into an array of $n \times n$ pixels, each pixel being labeled by a pair of indices (i,j).

Each pixel is characterized by four parameters (three of which are independent), namely the attenuation coefficient v_{ij}, and the forward, sidewise, and backward scattering coefficients f_{ij}, s_{ij}, b_{ij}. The first one, v_{ij}, gives the probability that a photon that enters pixel (i,j) will die there, while the other three parameters give the conditional probability that a photon that does not die will either preserve its incoming direction (forward scattering), turn ninety degrees either to the left or the right (sidewise scattering) or reverse its direction (backward scattering).

These parameters are connected by one relation, namely

$$b_{ij} = 1 - f_{ij} - 2s_{ij}$$

expressing the fact that, conditional on the photon not being absorbed at pixel (i,j), it has to get out of it in one of four different ways.

Notice that the transition from one pixel to any of its adjacent pixels is made by means of one of four possible directions: the state of a photon at any instant of time is given by its pixel indices (i,j) plus the direction with which the photon came into this pixel.

The description of the local characteristics in the model is now complete.

The problem that we consider is that of determining the values of the parameters $v_{ij}, f_{ij}, s_{ij}, b_{ij}$ for each one of the $n \times n$ pixels from the data consisting of the following "measurements": for each "exposed pixel" (i,j) with i or j equal to 1 or n, consider the probability that a photon that is "pushed in" in a direction orthogonal to the edge of pixel (i,j) will emerge at one of the "exposed pixels" after meandering its way through the object.

Since we have $4n$ edges corresponding to "exposed pixels", and we have placed (at consecutive times) a source at each one of them we get a total of $4n \times 4n$ measurements. A moment's thought shows that our assumption that right and left scattering have a common value, implies that reversing sources and detectors results in the same measurements (this assumption is not crucial, and can be disposed of). Therefore the total number of (hopefully independent) measurements is

$$4n + (4n \times 4n - 4n)/2 = 8n^2 + 2n$$

The number of unknowns is $3n^2$, so that in principle we have a chance to invert the NONLINEAR equations relating the unknowns to the data.

3. The forward problem.

The first step in handling this problem consists in solving the "forward problem", namely writing down a set of expressions for the data in terms of the unknowns. This is described, for the problem at hand, in [2,4]. The possibility of writing down in a closed form the solution to the forward problem constitutes the main result of the papers mentioned earlier. It rests entirely on the invertibility of the matrix A described in [2,4]. A sufficient condition for the invertibility of A is, for instance, $0 \leq s_{ij} + b_{ij} < 1$. An example of non-invertible A is given by $b_{ij} \equiv 1$, $s_{11} = 0$, $s_{22} = 1$.

We give below a general derivation of the solution to the forward problem from scratch. This formulation will apply to the refined model given in the next section.

The set of "states" is divided into four disjoint sets: incoming, outgoing, hidden, and absorbing states. Denote by $P_{\alpha\beta}$ the (one step) transition probabilities among states α,β and by $Q_{\alpha,\beta}$ the probability of ever reaching state β from state α.

The transition probabilities from hidden to incoming variables are zero; those among incoming states or among outgoing states also vanish identically. Finally, the transition probability out of an absorbing state is zero.

If the incoming states are labelled a_i, the outgoing states b_j and the hidden ones c_k, we've for a fixed outgoing state b_r the following equations for each i and each k

$$Q_{a_i b_r} = P_{a_i b_r} + \sum_k P_{a_i c_k} Q_{c_k b_r}$$

$$Q_{c_k b_r} = P_{c_k b_r} + \sum_l P_{c_k c_l} Q_{c_l b_r}.$$

The last set of equations can be solved for the vector $Q_{c_k b_r}$ and we get

$$Q_{c_k b_r} = \sum_\mu ((I-P)^{-1})_{k,\mu} P_{c_\mu b_r}$$

where P denotes the matrix of transition probabilities restricted to hidden states. Of course, this expression holds only when $I - P$ is invertible.

Plugging this into the first set of equations, we get

$$\begin{aligned} Q_{a_i b_r} &= P_{a_i b_r} + \sum\sum P_{a_i c_k}((I-P)^{-1})_{k\mu} P_{c_\mu b_r} \\ &= P_{a_i b_r} + \sum P_{a_i c_k} P_{c_k b_r} + \sum P_{a_i c_k} P_{c_k c_l} P_{c_l b_r} + \dots \end{aligned}$$

One can see clearly the relation between these expressions and those given in [2,4]. In these references the "input-output" matrix takes the form

$$D - CA^{-1}B$$

where: D is the transition matrix between incoming and outgoing states, C the transition matrix between incoming and hidden states, B the transition matrix between hidden and outgoing states and finally A denotes the difference between the transition matrix among hidden states and the identity matrix. The explicit matrices A, B, C, D

given in [4] are written with respect to a basis (resulting from a peculiar ordering of the hidden states) which is not too fortunate. For this reason we give these matrices anew for the simple two-by-two case in the original model.

$$A = \begin{matrix} -1 & b12 & 0 & s12 & 0 & 0 & 0 & 0 \\ b11 & -1 & 0 & 0 & 0 & 0 & s11 & 0 \\ 0 & s12 & -1 & b12 & 0 & 0 & 0 & 0 \\ 0 & 0 & b22 & -1 & 0 & s22 & 0 & 0 \\ 0 & 0 & s22 & 0 & -1 & b22 & 0 & 0 \\ 0 & 0 & 0 & 0 & b21 & -1 & 0 & s21 \\ 0 & 0 & 0 & 0 & s21 & 0 & -1 & b21 \\ s11 & 0 & 0 & 0 & 0 & 0 & b11 & -1 \end{matrix} \qquad B = \begin{matrix} 0 & s12 & f12 & 0 & 0 & 0 & 0 & 0 \\ s11 & 0 & 0 & 0 & 0 & 0 & 0 & f11 \\ 0 & f12 & s12 & 0 & 0 & 0 & 0 & 0 \\ 0 & 0 & 0 & s22 & f22 & 0 & 0 & 0 \\ 0 & 0 & 0 & f22 & s22 & 0 & 0 & 0 \\ 0 & 0 & 0 & 0 & 0 & s21 & f21 & 0 \\ 0 & 0 & 0 & 0 & 0 & f21 & s21 & 0 \\ f11 & 0 & 0 & 0 & 0 & 0 & 0 & s11 \end{matrix}$$

$$C = \begin{matrix} s11 & 0 & 0 & 0 & 0 & 0 & f11 & 0 \\ 0 & s12 & 0 & f12 & 0 & 0 & 0 & 0 \\ 0 & f12 & 0 & s12 & 0 & 0 & 0 & 0 \\ 0 & 0 & s22 & 0 & 0 & f22 & 0 & 0 \\ 0 & 0 & f22 & 0 & 0 & s22 & 0 & 0 \\ 0 & 0 & 0 & 0 & s21 & 0 & 0 & f21 \\ 0 & 0 & 0 & 0 & f21 & 0 & 0 & s21 \\ f11 & 0 & 0 & 0 & 0 & 0 & s11 & 0 \end{matrix} \qquad D = \begin{matrix} b11 & 0 & 0 & 0 & 0 & 0 & 0 & s11 \\ 0 & b12 & s12 & 0 & 0 & 0 & 0 & 0 \\ 0 & s12 & b12 & 0 & 0 & 0 & 0 & 0 \\ 0 & 0 & 0 & b22 & s22 & 0 & 0 & 0 \\ 0 & 0 & 0 & s22 & b22 & 0 & 0 & 0 \\ 0 & 0 & 0 & 0 & 0 & b21 & s21 & 0 \\ 0 & 0 & 0 & 0 & 0 & s21 & b21 & 0 \\ s11 & 0 & 0 & 0 & 0 & 0 & 0 & b11 \end{matrix}$$

We close this section with the observation, alluded to in the introduction given above, that the three dimensional (and more correct) version of this problem is in some sense "easier" except for the computational demands. This comes about by observing that the number of unknowns grows now like the cube of the number n of pixels on each side of the object, while the amount of data grows like the fourth power of n. In the two-dimensional case both quantities grow like the square of n.

4. Refining the model.

It would be desirable to have a continuous version of our problem, and then proceed to some discretization of it. This is not the route we take.

Instead consider the same spatial discretization of section 2 into $n \times n$ pixels labelled by indices (i,j) and strive for a more sophisticated discretization of the velocities.

A photon can only arrive at a pixel (i,j) through one of its four neighbourhs, $(i-1,j),(i+1,j),(i,j+1),(i,j-1)$. However, in contrast to the original model, we now allow for many directions into each pixel. More explicitely: the state of a photon is given by its present pixel position (i,j) and the knowledge of the previous pixel it occupied plus the direction that was used in making this transition (in the previous model this last piece of information is not needed).

If the directions are attached to the edges of the pixels then it is clear that the "states" of our system are exactly the sets of all arrows in the figure given below: each arrow tells you which pixel you are in, what pixel you came from and furthermore what direction was used in this transition. Absorbing states are added to account for the attenuation at each pixel. Finally, each detector adjacent to an "exposed pixel" contributes a number of "outgoing states" or arrows.

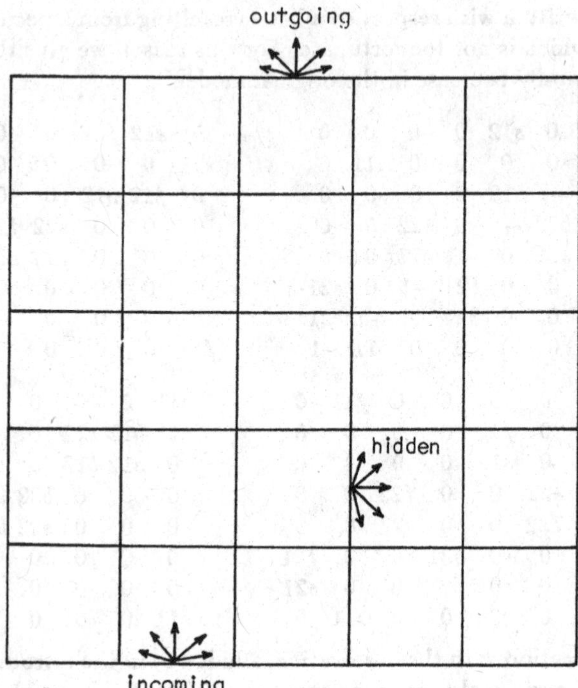

On this enlarged state space we have a Markov transition mechanism just as in the case of the original model.

Another way of formulating the model is to say that for each edge of a pixel we have a "fan" of directions that can be considered the directions into the pixel in question. If a photon does not die at a given pixel, then it chooses one of its four adjacent pixels to migrate to, once this decision is made it has to decide how to change the direction that it used to get into its present pixel to a new direction that will be considered its direction into the previously chosen new pixel.

Once again, notice that if the "fan" is replaced by a single direction, orthogonal to the edge in question and pointing into the pixel, then this refined model reduces to the original one.

At the level of the parameters that describe the model, notice that the refined model is obtained from the old one by replacing each of the quantities f_{ij}, s_{ij}, b_{ij} by a matrix which gives the probability of changing what had been a direction into pixel (i,j) into a direction chosen from four "fans" of directions: if we have a forward transition like

$i-1,j) \to (i,j)$ followed by $(i,j) \to (i+1,j)$ then the change in direction is governed by the matrix f_{ij}, etc.

Most of the arrows become "hidden states". Some of the arrows corresponding to "exposed pixels" become the "incoming states". The detectors adjacent to these pixels provide the "outgoing states" and finally the center of each pixel can be thought of as an "absorbing state". We are thus in the framework of the model described in Section 2 and the solution of the forward problem given there applies in this refined model.

We intend to pursue the "inverse problem" in a future publication.

References

1. J. Singer, F. A. Grünbaum, P. Kohn and J. Zubelli, *Image reconstruction of the interior of bodies that diffuse radiation*, Science **248** (1990), 990–993.
2. F. A. Grünbaum, *Tomography with diffusion*, in "Inverse Methods in Action", Proceedings of the Multicentennials Meeting on Inverse Problems, Montpellier, November 27–December 1, 1989, (ed. P. C. Sabatier) Springer-Verlag (1990), 16–21.
3. F. A. Grünbaum, *Backscattering comes to the rescue*, AMS Conference on the Radon Transform, Arcata, 1989, to appear in Contemporary Mathematics, T. Quinto, editor.
4. F. A. Grünbaum, *An inverse problem in transport theory: diffuse tomography*, SIAM Volume in Honor of Robert Krueger, to appear (1991).
5. F. A. Grünbaum, P. Kohn, J. Singer and J. Zubelli, *Imaging of media that diffuse and scatter radiation*, IMA Volume II in Radar and Sonar, Workshop June 1990, Minneapolis, Minn.
6. F. A. Grunbaum, G. Latham and J. Zubelli, *An inverse problem for a model of scattered and diffused radiation, to appear.*
7. L. Shepp, Private communication.

Three Dimensional Reconstructions in Inverse Obstacle Scattering

Rainer Kress and Axel Zinn

Institut für Numerische und Angewandte Mathematik, Universität Göttingen, Lotzestr. 16–18, D3400 Göttingen, Germany

1 Introduction

The inverse problem we consider is to reconstruct the shape of an obstacle from the knowledge of the far-field pattern for the scattering of incident time-harmonic acoustic or electromagnetic waves. It occurs in a variety of applications such as remote sensing, ultrasound tomography and seismic imaging and is difficult to solve since it is nonlinear and improperly posed. We desribe a method for the approximate solution which belongs to a new group of schemes and stabilizes the inverse scattering problem by reformulating it as a nonlinear optimization problem. A guideline of this survey will be to consider in detail only inverse scattering from an impenetrable acoustically sound-soft obstacle. But we note that the analysis can be extended to impenetrable scatterers with other boundary conditions and also to penetrable obstacles and to electromagnetic waves. We will desribe the numerical implementation of the method and also include some three dimensional examples for reconstructions, whereas most of the numerical reconstructions published so far in the literature are in two dimensions. Only Colton and Monk [9] have given three dimensional reconstructions for the full nonlinear problem in the resonance region.

2 The inverse scattering problem

The scattering of time-harmonic acoustic waves by an impenetrable sound-soft obstacle D imbedded in a homogeneous isotropic medium in $\mathbb{R}^3$ leads to an exterior Dirichlet boundary value problem for the *Helmholtz equation*

$$\Delta u + k^2 u = 0 \quad \text{in } \mathbb{R}^3 \setminus \overline{D}. \tag{1}$$

Here u denotes the space dependent part of the velocity potential $u(x)e^{-i\omega t}$ with frequency ω and the wave number k is given by $k = \omega/c$ with c denoting the speed of sound. Consider the scattering of an incident plane wave $u^i(x) = e^{ik\, d\cdot x}$ where d is a unit vector giving the direction of propagation of the incident wave. Since prescribing the values of u on the boundary ∂D of the obstacle physically corresponds to prescribing the pressure of the acoustic wave on the boundary, the *direct acoustic scattering problem* consists in determining the total field $u = u^i + u^s$ as a solution to (1) with vanishing total pressure

$$u = 0 \quad \text{on } \partial D. \tag{2}$$

The scattered wave u^s is required to satisfy the *Sommerfeld radiation condition*

$$\frac{\partial u^s}{\partial r} - iku^s = o\left(\frac{1}{r}\right), \quad r = |x| \to \infty, \tag{3}$$

uniformly in all directions $\hat{x} = x/|x|$. This radiation condition ensures the uniqueness for the exterior boundary value problem by Rellich's lemma (see [6]).

As in classical potential theory, for smooth boundaries, for example ∂D of class C^2, existence of a solution for the exterior Dirichlet problem (1) to (3) can be based on boundary integral equations. For details we refer to [6]. The continuous dependence of the solution on the boundary in a $C^{1,\beta}$–Hölder norm setting can be shown either by integral equation methods as in [1] or by weak solution techniques as in [22].

From the Sommerfeld radiation condition (3) it follows that the scattered wave u^s has an asymptotic behaviour of the form

$$u^s(x) = \frac{e^{ik|x|}}{|x|}\left\{u_\infty(\hat{x}) + O\left(\frac{1}{|x|}\right)\right\}, \quad |x| \to \infty, \tag{4}$$

uniformly in all directions $\hat{x} = x/|x|$. The function u_∞, defined on the unit sphere Ω in $\mathbb{R}^3$, is known as *far-field pattern* or *scattering amplitude* of the radiating wave u^s. A vanishing far-field pattern $u_\infty = 0$ on the unit sphere implies

$$\lim_{r\to\infty} \int_{|x|=r} |u^s(x)|^2 ds = 0$$

whence $u^s = 0$ follows by Rellich's lemma (see [6]). On occasion, in order to indicate the dependence of the far-field pattern on the direction d of the incoming wave we will write $u_\infty(\hat{x}; d)$

The *inverse problem* we want to consider now is, given the far-field pattern u_∞ of the scattered wave u^s for one incoming plane wave u^i with one single incident direction d and one single wave number k or possibly several incoming plane waves u^i with different incident directions d and wave numbers k, determine the shape of the scatterer D. As opposed to the direct problem the inverse problem is ill-posed. The solution - if it exists at all - does not depend continuously on the given far-field pattern in any reasonable norm. Therefore the numerical solution requires the incorporation of some regularization technique. In addition, the inverse scattering problem is nonlinear since the far-field pattern depends nonlinearly on the boundary surface.

Based on a result due to Schiffer, the question of uniqueness has been addressed by Colton and Sleeman [10] and by Jones [11]. The obstacle D is uniquely determined by the far-field pattern for a countable set of plane waves *either* with one fixed incident direction and (a bounded set of) different wave numbers *or* with one fixed wave number and different incident directions. Given an a-priori information on the size of the obstacle, for example on the diameter of D, then a finite number of incident plane waves suffices for uniquely determining D. Note that due to analyticity it suffices to know the far-field pattern for all observation directions $\hat{x}$ in an open subset of the unit sphere Ω. As a challenging open problem we wish to point out that so far it is not known if one incoming plane wave for one single direction and one single wave number completely determines the scatterer.

For this survey we are interested in the approximate solution of the inverse problem for wave numbers k in the *resonance region*, that is, the wave length is of the same magnitude as the diameter of the unknown object. In this case linearizations by high frequency asymptotics like geometric and physical optics do not lead to valid approximations and it is necessary to treat the full nonlinear problem.

3 Numerical methods

An obvious concept for an approximate solution of the inverse obstacle scattering problem is to try solving the ill-posed nonlinear operator equation

$$A(\partial D) = u_\infty \tag{5}$$

by standard inversion methods. Here $A : X \to L^2(\Omega)$ stands for the forward operator mapping the boundary ∂D into the far-field pattern u_∞ of the scattered wave and X is a suitably chosen subset of a some Banach space representing the possible boundary surfaces.

Newton type methods for the approximate solution of (5) have been implemented by Roger [23], by Murch, Tan and Wall [19], by Wang and Chen [24] and by Onishi [21]. The ill-posedness of the inverse scattering problem requires appropriate measures to stabilize the Newton iteration, for example by a Tikhonov regularization or a singular value cut-off in each Newton step.

The method of quasi-solutions has been investigated by Angell, Colton and Kirsch [1]. Here the inverse scattering problem is replaced by minimizing the defect functional

$$\|A(\Lambda) - u_\infty\|_{L^2(\Omega)} \tag{6}$$

over all surfaces Λ in a suitable admissible set U. To restore stability U is assumed to be a compact subset of the space X of all starlike closed $C^{1,\beta}$–surfaces Λ. A Tikhonov type regularization of the defect minimization (6) has been employed by Kristensson and Vogel [18]. Here the constraint for the admissible subset U to be compact is replaced by minimizing a penalized defect functional of the form

$$\|A(\Lambda) - u_\infty\|_{L^2(\Omega)} + p(\Lambda) \tag{7}$$

with a suitable penalty term p.

A common feature of all the above methods is that they are of an iterative nature and require the numerical solution of the forward scattering problem for different domains at each iteration step. The method which we describe in the sequel and which was proposed by Kirsch and Kress[13,14,15] does not need the solution of the direct problem at all. The principal idea is to stabilize the inverse scattering problem by reformulating it as a nonlinear optimization problem. Of course, the numerical solution of the optimization problem again relies on iteration techniques. However, the actual performance of these iterations will be less costly due to a simple structure of the cost functional. The motivation of the method is divided into two parts: the first part deals with the ill-posedness and the second part with the nonlinearity of the inverse scattering problem.

We choose an auxiliary closed surface Γ contained in the unknown scatterer D. The knowledge of such an internal surface Γ requires a weak a-priori information about D. Without loss of generality we may assume that the wave number k is not a Dirichlet eigenvalue for the interior G of Γ, that is, the Helmholtz equation $\Delta u + k^2 u = 0$ in G with homogeneous boundary condition $u = 0$ on Γ admits only the trivial solution $u = 0$. We try to represent the scattered field $u^s = S\varphi$ as an acoustic single-layer potential

$$(S\varphi)(x) := \int_\Gamma \frac{e^{ik|x-y|}}{|x-y|} \varphi(y)\, ds(y) \tag{8}$$

with an unknown density $\varphi \in L^2(\Gamma)$. Simple asymptotics shows that the far-field pattern of the single-layer potential is described through the integral operator $F : L^2(\Gamma) \to L^2(\Omega)$ defined by

$$(F\varphi)(\hat{x}) := \int_\Gamma \varphi(y) e^{-ik\,\hat{x}\cdot y}\, ds(y), \quad \hat{x} \in \Omega. \tag{9}$$

Hence, given the far-field pattern u_∞, we have to solve the integral equation of the first kind

$$F\varphi = u_\infty \tag{10}$$

for the density φ. The integral operator F has a smooth kernel and therefore equation (10) is severely ill-posed. Its solvability can be related to the analytic continuation of the scattered field u^s across the boundary ∂D. The integral equation (10) can be shown to have at most one solution and it is solvable if and only if u_∞ is the far-field of a solution to the Helmholtz equation in the exterior of Γ with boundary data in the Sobolev space $H^1(\Gamma)$. Whether such an analytic continuation is possible can be decided only in special cases of boundary surfaces like spheres and ellipsoids.

Provided a solution of (10) exists we can apply the Tikhonov regularization technique (see [17]) for a stable numerical treatment and obtain an approximation $u^s_{\text{approx}} = S\varphi_{\text{approx}}$ for the scattered field by the single-layer potential. Then we seek the boundary of the scatterer D as the location of the zeros of $u^i + u^s_{\text{approx}}$ in a minumum norm sense, i.e., we approximate ∂D by minimizing the defect

$$\|u^i + u^s_{\text{approx}}\|_{L^2(\Lambda)} \tag{11}$$

over some suitable class U of admissible surfaces Λ. For example we may choose U to be a compact subset of the set V of all starlike closed $C^{1,\beta}$-surfaces Λ satisfying some a-priori information of the form $\Gamma < \Lambda_1 \leq \Lambda \leq \Lambda_2$. Here, by $\Gamma < \Lambda$ or $\Gamma \leq \Lambda$ we mean that Γ is contained in the interior of Λ or the closure of the interior of Λ, respectively.

Since, however, in general we do not have existence of a solution to the integral equation (10) we combine its Tikhonov regularization and the defect minimization (11) into one cost functional. Given u^i and u_∞, we minimize the sum

$$\mu(\varphi, \Lambda; \alpha, \gamma) := \|F\varphi - u_\infty\|^2_{L^2(\Omega)} + \alpha\|\varphi\|^2_{L^2(\Gamma)} + \gamma\|u^i + S\varphi\|^2_{L^2(\Lambda)} \tag{12}$$

simultaneously over all $\varphi \in L^2(\Gamma)$ and $\Lambda \in U$. Here, $\alpha > 0$ denotes the regularization parameter for the Tikhonov regularization of (10) represented by the first two terms in (12) and $\gamma > 0$ denotes a coupling parameter which has to be chosen appropriately for the numerical implementation. For this reformulation of the inverse scattering problem we can state the following existence and convergence results due to Kirsch and Kress [15].

Theorem 1. *The optimization formulation of the inverse scattering problem has a solution.*

Proof. The proof follows from the compactness of U, the weak compactness of bounded subsets of $L^2(\Gamma)$ and the fact that the cost functional in (12) is weakly sequentially closed with respect to φ due to the compactness of the integral operators $F : L^2(\Gamma) \to L^2(\Omega)$ and $S : L^2(\Gamma) \to L^2(\Lambda)$. For the details we refer to [17].

Theorem 2. *If u_∞ is the exact far-field pattern of a domain D with $\partial D \in U$, then for the cost functional there holds convergence*

$$\inf_{\varphi \in L^2(\Gamma),\, \Lambda \in U} \mu(\varphi, \Lambda; \alpha, \gamma) \to 0, \quad \alpha \to 0,$$

and for any sequence (φ_n, Λ_n) of solutions with parameters $\alpha_n \to 0$, $n \to \infty$, there exists a convergent subsequence of (Λ_n) and on each limit surface Λ the exact total field $u^i + u^s$ vanishes.

Proof. The zero limit of the cost functional is a consequence of the fact that the operator $S : L^2(\Gamma) \to L^2(\partial D)$ has dense range and the continuous dependence of the far-field pattern on the boundary data. The existence of the limit surface Λ follows from the compactness of V. As mentioned above the solution to the forward problem depends continuously on the boundary in the $C^{1,\beta}$–Hölder norm. This together with the vanishing limit of the cost functional implies that the scattered wave u^s_Λ for the boundary Λ has the same far-field pattern u_∞ as the scattered wave u^s for the true boundary ∂D whence $u^s_\Lambda = u^s$ follows. Again we refer to [17] for the details of the proof.

Since we do not have uniqueness either for the inverse scattering problem or for the optimization problem, in general, we cannot expect more than convergent subsequences. In addition, due to the lack of a uniqueness result for one wave number and one incident plane wave, we cannot assure that we always have convergence towards the boundary of the unknown scatterer. The latter insufficiency can be remedied by using more incident waves $u_1^i, \ldots, u_n^i$ with different directions $d_1, \ldots, d_n$ with corresponding far-field patterns $u_{\infty,1}, \ldots, u_{\infty,n}$ with the total number n depending on the size of the a-priori known surfaces Λ_1 and Λ_2. Then we have to minimize the sum

$$\sum_{j=1}^{n} \left\{ \|F\varphi_j - u_{\infty,j}\|^2_{L^2(\Omega)} + \alpha\|\varphi_j\|^2_{L^2(\Gamma)} + \gamma\|u_j^i + S\varphi_j\|^2_{L^2(\Lambda)} \right\} \tag{13}$$

over all $\varphi_1, \ldots, \varphi_n \in L^2(\Gamma)$ and all $\Lambda \in U$. Of course, we also can expect more accurate reconstructions by using more than one incoming directions.

The basic idea of the above method is to suitably approximate the scattered wave u^s. In principle, the approximation through the single-layer potential can be replaced by any other convenient approximation. For example Angell, Kleinman and Roach [4] have suggested to use an expansion with respect to spherical wave functions. Numerical implementations of this approach in two dimensions are given in [2], [3] and [12]. Using a single-layer potential approximation on an auxiliary internal surface Γ has the advantage of allowing the incorporation of a-priori information on the unknown scatterer by a suitable choice of Γ whereas from the validity of expansions with respect to spherical wave functions one can expect satisfactory reconstructions only for scatterers not too much deviating from a spherical shape.

We briefly sketch the main idea of the method introduced by Colton and Monk [7,8], which in contrast to our approach may be considered as an approximation of an incoming field yielding the simplest possible far-field pattern, namely a constant far-field belonging to an acoustic monopol

$$v^s(x) := \frac{e^{ik|x|}}{|x|}, \quad x \neq 0, \tag{14}$$

at the origin as corresponding scattered wave. We try to represent the corresponding incident field $v^i = H\psi$ as a *Herglotz wave function*, that is, a superposition of incident plane waves

$$(H\psi)(x) := \int_{\Omega} \psi(d) e^{ik\, x \cdot d}\, ds(d) \tag{15}$$

with density $\psi \in L^2(\Omega)$. Then clearly the corresponding far-field pattern is obtained by superposing the far-field patterns $u_\infty(\cdot\,; d)$ for the incoming directions d and in order to achieve (14) as the scattered wave we have to solve the integral equation of the first kind

$$\mathcal{F}\psi = 1 \tag{16}$$

where the integral operator $\mathcal{F} : L^2(\Omega) \to L^2(\Omega)$ is defined by

$$(\mathcal{F}\psi)(\hat{x}) := \int_{\Omega} \psi(d) u_\infty(\hat{x}; d)\, ds(d), \quad \hat{x} \in \Omega. \tag{17}$$

The integral operator $\mathcal{F}$ has a smooth kernel and therefore equation (16) again is severely ill-posed. Its solvability can be related to the interior Dirichlet problem

$$\triangle v^i + k^2 v^i = 0 \quad \text{in } D \tag{18}$$

with boundary condition

$$v^i + v^s = 0 \quad \text{on } \partial D. \tag{19}$$

If we assume that the homogeneous Dirichlet problem for the Helmholtz equation in D admits only the trivial solution, then the integral equation (16) turns out to have at most one solution and to be solvable if and only if the solution to (18) and (19) possesses an analytic continuation across the boundary ∂D in the form of a Herglotz wave function.

As in the previous method we combine a Tikhonov regularization for the integral equation (16) with the minimum norm search over surfaces Λ in U for the location of the zeros of the total field $v^i + v^s$ in the minimization of the sum

$$\nu(\psi, \Lambda; \alpha, \gamma) := \|\mathcal{F}\psi - 1\|^2_{L^2(\Omega)} + \alpha\|\psi\|^2_{L^2(\Omega)} + \gamma\|H\psi + v^s\|^2_{L^2(\Lambda)} \tag{20}$$

simultaneously over all $\psi \in L^2(\Omega)$ and $\Lambda \in U$. For this optimization problem now results similar to those given through Theorems 1 and 2 can be proven (see [8]).

For a description of the numerical implementation of the latter method and for numerical examples in two and three dimensions we refer to [8,9]. A detailed comparison of the Kirsch–Kress and the Colton–Monk method in the two dimensional case is carried out in [16].

The extension of the Kirsch–Kress and the Colton–Monk method for the inverse problem for electromagnetic waves scattering from a perfect conductor has been studied by Blöhbaum [5].

In both methods, so far we have assumed the far-field pattern to be known for all observation directions $\hat{x}$. Theoretical and numerical extensions to the *limited-aperture problem*, that is, to the case where the far-field pattern is known only on a part of the unit sphere have been given by Ochs [20] and Zinn [26].

4 Numerical results

We briefly describe some details on the numerical implementation of the Kirsch–Kress method. For the data we have to rely on synthetic far-field data obtained through the numerical solution of the forward scattering problem. Here we wish to emphasize that in order to avoid trivial inversion of finite dimensional problems for reliably testing the performance of the approximation method for the inverse problem it is crucial that the synthetic data are delivered through a forward solver which has no connection to the inverse solver under consideration.

Unfortunately some of the numerical experiments in inverse obstacle problems which appeared in the literature do not meet with this obvious requirement. In our numerical examples the far-field data were obtained through the classical boundary integral equations via the combined double- and single-layer approach (see [6]). For its numerical solution we employed a Nyström type method using numerical quadratures based on approximations through spherical harmonics. This method is exponentially convergent for smooth boundaries and has been recently developed by Wienert [25].

For the numerical method for the inverse problem the evaluation of the cost functional (12) including the integral operators S and F requires the numerical evaluation of integrals with integrands over the smooth surfaces Ω, Γ and Λ. We approximate integrals over the unit sphere by the Gauss trapezoidal product rule. By $-1 < t_1 < t_2 < \cdots < t_m < 1$ we denote the zeros of the Legendre polynomial P_m and by

$$\alpha_j := \frac{2}{(1-t_j^2)\,[P_m'(t_j)]^2}, \quad j = 1,\ldots,m,$$

the weights of the Gauss–Legendre quadrature rule for the interval $[-1, 1]$. Then the Gauss trapezoidal rule reads

$$\int_\Omega f\,ds \approx \frac{\pi}{m}\sum_{j=1}^{m}\sum_{k=0}^{2m-1} \alpha_j f(x_{jk}) \tag{21}$$

where the knots x_{jk} are given in polar coordinates by

$$x_{jk} := (\sin\theta_j\cos\varphi_k, \sin\theta_j\sin\varphi_k, \cos\theta_j)$$

for $j = 1,\ldots,m$ and $k = 0,\ldots,2m-1$ with $\theta_j := \arccos t_j$ and $\varphi_k = \pi k/m$. Integrals over the surfaces Γ and Λ are transformed into integrals over Ω through appropriate substitutions.

For the numerical solution, of course, we also must discretize the optimization problem. This is achieved through replacing $L^2(\Gamma)$ and U by finite dimensional subspaces. Denote by Z_n the linear space of all spherical harmonics of order less than or equal to n. Let $q : \Gamma \to \Omega$ be bijective and and define $X_n \subset L^2(\Gamma)$ by

$$X_n := \{\varphi = Y \circ q : Y \in Z_n\}.$$

Further we denote by U_n the set of all starlike surfaces described by

$$x(a) := r(a)a, \quad a \in \Omega, \quad r \in Z_n,$$

satisfying some a-priori information

$$0 < r_1(a) \le r(a) \le r_2(a)$$

with given functions r_1 and r_2 representing Λ_1 and Λ_2. Then we replace (12) by the finite dimensional problem where we minimize over the finite dimensional set $X_n \times U_n$ instead of $L^2(\Gamma) \times U$. Denote by (φ_n, Λ_n) for $n \in \mathbb{N}$ a solution to this finite dimensional minimization problem. Then it can be shown (see Zinn [27]) that there exists a subsequence $(\varphi_{n(j)}, \Lambda_{n(j)})$ which converges to a solution of (12) as $j \to \infty$. The finite dimensional minimization problem is a nonlinear least squares problem with $2(n+1)^2$ unknowns. For its numerical solution we used a Levenberg-Marquard algorithm as one of the most efficient nonlinear least squares routines. It does not allow the imposition of constraints, but we found in practice that the constraints are unnecessary due to the increase in the cost functional as Λ approaches Γ or tends to infinity.

The Figures 1 to 3 show some examples of our numerical experiments. For these the regularization parameter α and the coupling parameter γ were selected by trial and error, the actual numerical values were $\alpha = 10^{-8}$ and $\gamma = 10^{-6}$. For the internal surface Γ we choose ellipsoids with centre at the origin and axes coinciding with the axes of the cartesian coordinates. As starting surface Λ for the Levenberg–Marquardt algorithm we used an ellipsoid parallel and with distance 0.2 from Γ, and as starting density we choose $\varphi = 0$. In all examples we worked with only one incident plane wave with the wave number $k = 1$. In the figures the arrow marks the direction of the incident wave. The parameter for the numerical quadrature is $m = 12$ and the dimension of the approximating subspace is $n = 6$.

The examples show that our method yields reasonable reconstructions even in the case of non-convex scatterers. Of course, the approximations are less accurate in the shadow region and somewhat poorer for perturbed data. The numerical experiments also indicate that the appropriate choice of Γ, that is, the available a-priori information has an impact on the quality of the reconstruction.

Figure 1 shows the reconstruction of the oblate ellipsoid

$$x_1^2 + x_2^2 + \left(\frac{2}{3}\,x_3\right)^2 = 1$$

for data with 5% random noise. The internal ellipsoid is a sphere with radius 0.6.

Figure 2 shows the reconstruction of a peanut given through its radial distance in terms of the polar angle θ by

$$r(\theta) = \frac{3}{2}\left(\cos^2\theta + \frac{1}{4}\sin^2\theta\right)^{1/2}.$$

The internal ellipsoid again is a sphere with radius 0.6.

Figure 3 finally shows the reconstruction of an acorn given by

$$r(\theta) = \frac{3}{5}\left(\frac{17}{4} + 2\cos 3\theta\right)^{1/2}.$$

Here the internal ellipsoid has major axis 0.6, 0.6 and 1.2.

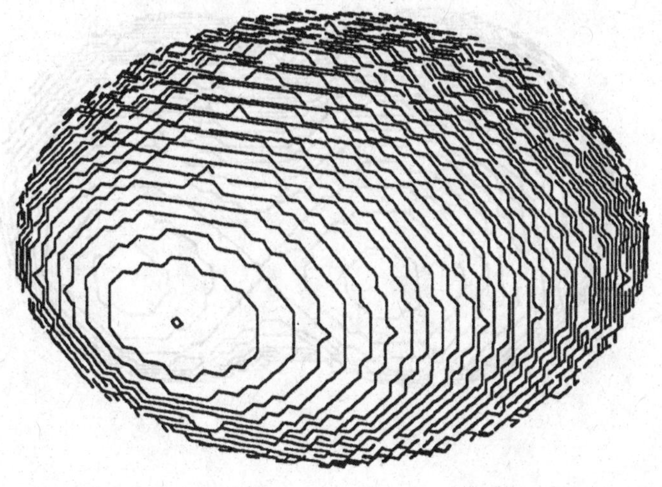

(a) Original

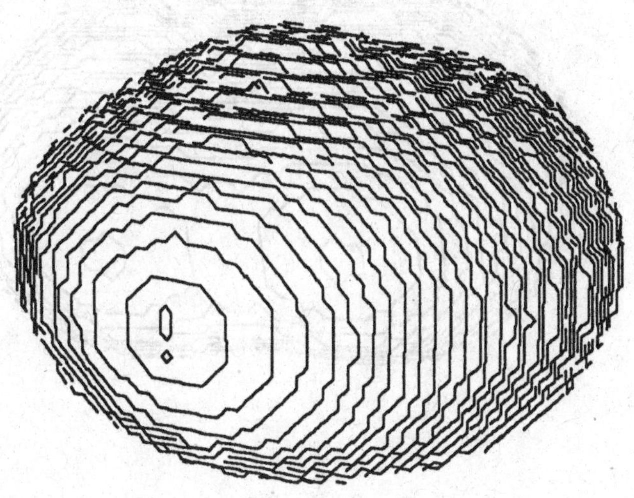

(b) Reconstruction

Fig. 1. The oblate ellipsoid and its reconstruction

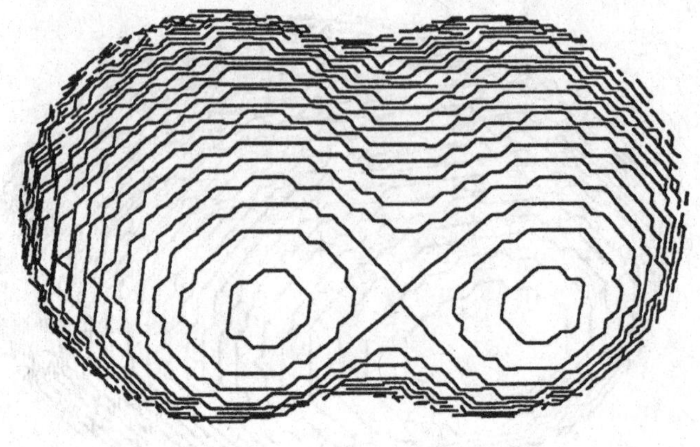

(a) Original

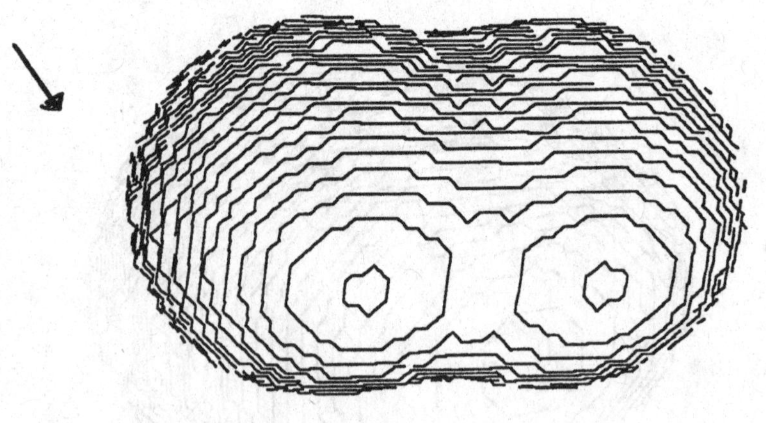

(b) Reconstruction

Fig. 2. The peanut and its reconstruction (turned by 90°)

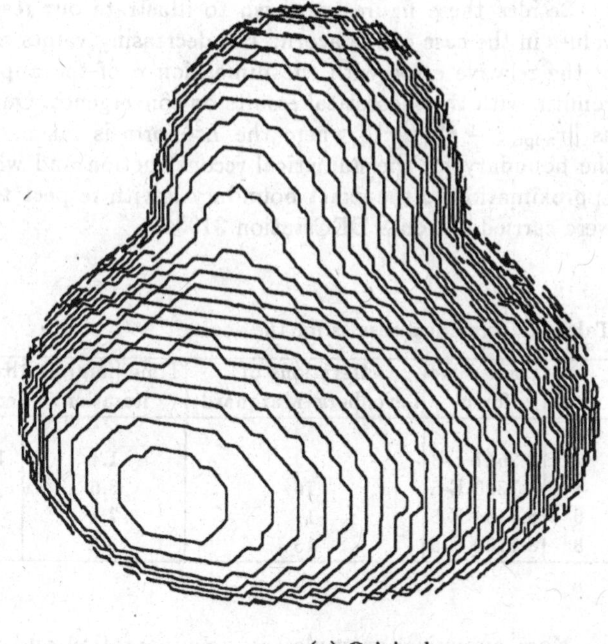

(a) Original

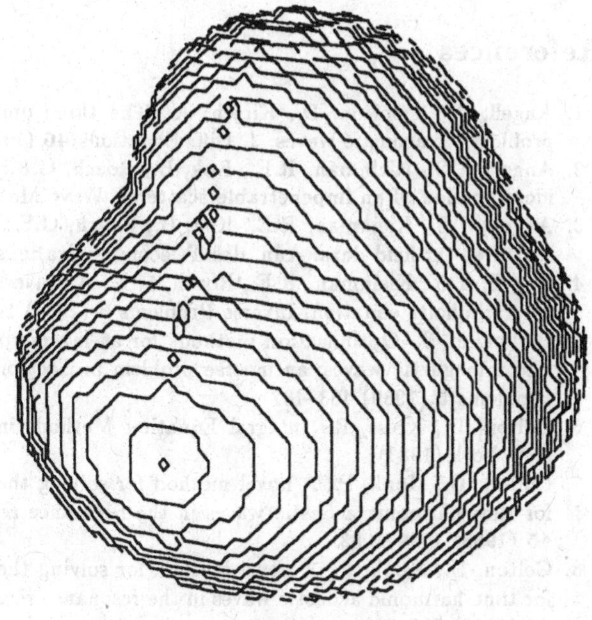

(b) Reconstruction

Fig. 3. The acorn and its reconstruction

Besides these figures we wish to illustrate our results by a few numerical values in the case of the acorn. The decreasing values of the cost functional and of the relative error with the dimension n of the approximating subspace Z_n confirm with the theoretical results on convergence. Our relative error is defined as $\|r_{\text{approx}} - r^*\|/\|r^*\|$ where the L^2-norm is taken, where r_{approx} represents the boundary for the numerical reconstruction and where r^* denotes the best approximation to the exact boundary r with respect to Z_n. The computations were carried out on a DECstation 3100.

Table 1. Numerical results for the acorn

n	Final value for μ	Iterations of Levenberg–Marquardt	Time [min] per iteration	Relative error %
2	8.2617 E-3	9	1.4	10.59
4	8.1200 E-5	16	3.6	8.45
6	8.1184 E-5	11	7.4	8.23
8	8.1181 E-5	13	13.2	8.09

More numerical examples are in preparation and will be published in due course.

References

1. Angell, T.S., Colton, D., Kirsch, A.: The three dimensional inverse scattering problem for acoustic waves. J. Diff. Equations **46** (1982) 46–58
2. Angell, T.S., Kleinman, R.E., Kok, B., Roach, G.F.: A constructive method for identification of an impenetrable scatterer. Wave Motion **11** (1989) 185–200
3. Angell, T.S., Kleinman, R.E., Kok, B., Roach, G.F.: Target reconstruction from scattered far field data. Ann. des Télécommunications **44** (1989) 456–463
4. Angell, T.S., Kleinman, R.E., Roach, G.F.: An inverse transmission problem for the Helmholtz equation. Inverse Problems **3** (1987) 149–180
5. Blöhbaum, J.: Optimisation methods for an inverse problem with time-harmonic electromagnetic waves: an inverse problem in electromagnetic scattering. Inverse Problems **5** (1989) 463–482
6. Colton, D., Kress, R.: Integral Equation Methods in Scattering Theory. Wiley, New York (1983)
7. Colton, D., Monk, P.: A novel method for solving the inverse scattering problem for time-harmonic acoustic waves in the resonance region. SIAM J. Appl. Math. **45** (1985) 1039–1053
8. Colton, D., Monk, P.: A novel method for solving the inverse scattering problem for time-harmonic acoustic waves in the resonance region II. SIAM J. Appl. Math. **46** (1986) 506–523
9. Colton, D., Monk, P.: The numerical solution of the three dimensional inverse scattering problem for time-harmonic acoustic waves. SIAM J. Sci. Stat. Comp. **8** (1987) 278–291

10. Colton, D., Sleeman, B.D.: Uniqueness theorems for the inverse problem of acoustic scattering. IMA J. Appl. Math. **31** (1983) 253–259
11. Jones, D.S.: Note on a uniqueness theorem of Schiffer. Applicable Analysis **19** (1985) 181–188
12. Jones, D.S., Mao, X.Q.: The inverse problem in hard acoustic scattering. Inverse Problems **5** (1989) 731–748
13. Kirsch, A., Kress, R.: On an integral equation the first kind in inverse acoustic scattering. In: Inverse Problems. (Cannon, Hornung eds.) ISNM **77** (1986) 93–102
14. Kirsch, A., Kress, R.: A numerical method for an inverse scattering problem. In: Inverse Problems (Engl, Groetsch eds.), Academic Press, (1987) 279–290
15. Kirsch, A., Kress, R.: An optimization method in inverse acoustic scattering. In: Boundary elements IX, Vol 3. Fluid Flow and Potential Applications (Brebbia, Wendland and Kuhn, eds). Springer-Verlag, Heidelberg, (1987) 3–18
16. Kirsch, A., Kress, R., Monk, P., Zinn, A.: Two methods for solving the inverse acoustic scattering problem. Inverse Problems **4** (1988) 749–770
17. Kress, R.: Linear Integral Equations. Springer-Verlag, New York (1989)
18. Kristensson, G., Vogel, C.R.: Inverse problems for acoustic waves using the penalised likelihood method. Inverse Problems **2** (1986) 461–479
19. Murch, R.D., Tan, D.G.H., Wall, D.J.N.: Newton–Kantorovich method applied to two-dimensional inverse scattering for an exterior Helmholtz problem. Inverse Problems **4** (1988) 1117–1128
20. Ochs, R.L.: The limited aperture problem of inverse scattering: Dirichlet boundary conditions. SIAM J. Appl. Math. **6** (1987) 1320–1341
21. Onishi, K.: Numerical methods for inverse scattering problems in two-dimensional scalar field. (to appear)
22. Pironneau, O.: Optimal shape design for elliptic systems. Springer-Verlag, New York (1984)
23. Roger, A.: Newton Kantorovitch algorithm applied to an electromagnetic inverse problem. IEEE Trans. Ant. Prop. **AP-29** (1981) 232–238
24. Wang, S.L., Chen, Y.M.: An efficient numerical method for exterior and interior inverse problems of Helmholtz equation. (to appear)
25. Wienert, L.: Die numerische Approximation von Randintegraloperatoren für die Helmholtzgleichung im $\mathbb{R}^3$. Dissertation, Göttingen (1990)
26. Zinn, A.: On an optimisation method for the full- and limited-aperture problem in inverse acoustic scattering for a sound-soft obstacle. Inverse Problems **5** (1989) 239–253
27. Zinn, A.: Ein Rekonstruktionsverfahren für ein inverses Streuproblem bei der zeitharmonischen Wellengleichung. Dissertation, Göttingen (1990)

Mathematical Questions of a Biomagnetic Imaging Problem

Alfred K. Louis

Universität des Saarlandes
Fachbereich Mathematik
D-6600 Saarbrücken

Abstract A simple mathematical model used in the first commercial scanners for the biomagnetic imaging problem is considered. We discuss the restrictions in the resolution inherent in the mathematical model. It is shown that only the position of the dipole is computable not its strength. An approximate inversion formula is derived which results in a very efficient algorithm.

1 Introduction

Due to electric current in the human body a magnetic field is induced which can be detected outside the body. From this information the cause of the current and its location have to be identified. In that way the focus of epileptic fits or the reason for cardiac infarction can be observed. The magnetic field of the earth is stronger than those fields by a factor of 10^8. Hence it is extremely difficult to measure with a sufficiently high precision the necessary information, namely the magnetic field. As a consequence the devices are technically demanding and therefore expensive.

The observed magnetic induction, the vector field B, is related to the total current density J by the Biot – Savart law

$$B(x) = \int_\Omega J(y) \times \frac{x-y}{|x-y|^3} dy \quad . \tag{1}$$

The searched – for impressed source current J^i appeares in a nonlinear way in

$$J = J^i + \sigma E \quad ,$$

where the Ohmic current σE depends on J^i. Instead of approaching the fully nonlinear problem we follow Sarvas, [7], and, as in the first commercial scanners, see Gudden et al. [2], we assume that the part of the patient to be examined is a homogeneous ball with a dipole distribution.

In Section 2 we describe the mathematical model, then in the following section we study the nonuniqueness problem where we see that besides the already known problem with magnetic silent current sources only the cross product of position and dipole can be determined. Hence the strength of the dipole is not computable, at most its position. Also there is no reconstruction in the center of the ball possible. This is different than in the situation of x–ray computerized tomography where the nonuniqueness is a consequence of insufficiently many data. Here the mathematical model contains the nonuniqueness even in the case of all possible data.

The last chapter is devoted to the numerical solution where based on ill – posed problems we put the reconstruction using lead fields on a mathematical basis. Finally an approximate inversion formula is derived using the mollifier method of [5].

2 A Simple Mathematical Model

In the following we assume that the part of the body under examination is a spherically symmetric conductor. Then, as done in Sarvas, [7], the magnetic field B is much simpler to compute. We determine B outside the ball Ω at a point x for a dipole Q at the point y inside Ω. Outside Ω the total current J vanishes, hence from Maxwell's equations we get $\nabla \times B = 0$. The magnetic field can thus be expressed outside Ω in terms of the magnetic scalar potential U as

$$B(x) = -\mu_0 \nabla U(x) , \tag{2}$$

where μ_0 denotes the magnetic permeability. With the magnetic field B_0 in the homogeneous space,

$$B_0(x) = \frac{\mu_0}{4\pi} Q(y) \times \frac{x-y}{|x-y|^3} , \tag{3}$$

where $Q(y)$ is a dipole at position y, we consider a line integral of ∇U along the direction $e_x = \frac{x}{|x|}$ of x resulting in

$$\begin{aligned} U(x) &= \frac{1}{\mu_0} \int_0^\infty B_0(x+te_x) e_x dt \\ &= \frac{1}{4\pi} \int_0^\infty Q(y) \times \frac{x+te_x-y}{|x+te_x-y|^3} \cdot e_x dt \\ &= -\frac{1}{4\pi} Q(y) \cdot y \times e_x \int_0^\infty |x+te_x-y|^{-3} dt \end{aligned}$$

where we used $x \times e_x = e_x \times e_x = 0$. The integration gives

$$U(x) = -\frac{1}{4\pi} Q(y) \cdot y \times e_x \frac{1}{(|x-y| + <x-y, e_x>)|x-y|} \tag{4}$$

where $< \cdot, \cdot >$ denotes the scalar product in $\mathbb{R}^3$. Multiplication with $|x|/|x|$ and using $Q \cdot y \times x = Q \times y \cdot x$ we get

$$U(x) = -\frac{1}{4\pi} Q(y) \times y \cdot x \cdot \frac{1}{F(x,y)} \tag{5}$$

where

$$F(x,y) = |x-y|(|x-y||x| + < x-y, x >)$$
$$= |x-y|^2|x|(1+\cos\angle(x-y,x)) \ .$$

With (2) we finally derive

$$B(x) = \frac{\mu_0}{4\pi F^2(x,y)}\Big(F(x,y)Q(y)\times y - < Q(y)\times y, x > \nabla_x F(x,y)\Big) \quad (6)$$

where

$$\nabla_x F(x,y) = \alpha(x,y)x - \beta(x,y)y \ ,$$
$$\alpha(x,y) = \frac{|x-y|^2}{|x|} + \frac{< x-y, x >}{|x-y|} + 2|x-y| + 2|x| \ ,$$
$$\beta(x,y) = |x-y| + 2|x| + \frac{< x-y, x >}{|x-y|} .$$

This is the mathematical model relating in the case of a homogeneous ball the dipole at y to the magnetic field at x, see, as mentioned above, [7].

3 Mathematical Results

In the following we start from the mathematical model given in Formula (6) where we assume that we have a whole distribution of dipoles in the domain Ω, leading to the linear integral equation of the first kind

$$B = T_1 Q \quad (7)$$

where

$$T_1Q(x) = \frac{\mu_0}{4\pi}\int_\Omega \Big(\frac{1}{F(x,y)}Q(y)\times y - \frac{1}{F^2(x,y)} < Q(y)\times y, x > \nabla_x F(x,y)\Big)dy \ . \quad (8)$$

The field B is measured outside Ω, after a rescaling we assume that Ω is contained in the unit ball; i.e., $\Omega \subset V(0, 1-\delta)$, and the measurements are taken on the unit sphere S^2.

Theorem 1. *The operator T_1 is compact as mapping between the spaces*

$$(L_2(\Omega))^3 \to (L_2(S^2))^3$$

and

$$(C(\Omega))^3 \to (C(S^2))^3 \ .$$

Proof. The function F is continuous and because of $y \in \Omega \subset V(0, 1-\delta)$ and $x \in S^2$ it is bounded away from 0. Hence the kernel of the integral operator is continuous and so the integral operator is compact between the mentioned spaces. □

Theorem 2. *The above given integral operator* T_1 *has a nontrivial null – space, namely*

$$\mathcal{N}(T_1) \supseteq \{Q : Q(y) = q(y) \cdot y, q \ scalar\} \tag{9}$$

Proof. The vector field Q appeares only in the vector product $Q(y) \times y$. Hence for multiples of y, $Q(y) = q(y)y$, we see that $Q(y) \times y = 0$. □

Next we factorize the null – space by introducing

$$f(y) = Q(y) \times y \tag{10}$$

and consider

$$Tf(x) = \frac{\mu_0}{4\pi} \int_{\Omega} \Big(\frac{1}{F(x,y)} f(y) - \frac{1}{F^2(x,y)} < f(y), x > \nabla F(x,y) \Big) dy \ . \tag{11}$$

Again T is a compact linear operator between the spaces used in Theorem 1. The solution of our original problem can be achieved in two steps. Solve

$$Tf = B$$

for f and

$$Q(y) \times y = f(y)$$

for Q. The above mentioned nonuniqueness is contained in the second step. This equation is solvable if $f(y)$ is perpendicular to y. Then the solution is determined in the following way.

Let z be the unit – vector perpendicular to y and f such that z, y, f form a right – hand system. Then the solution of

$$Q \times y = f$$

is

$$Q = \alpha y + \frac{||f||}{||y||} z \text{ for all } \alpha \in \mathbb{R} \ . \tag{12}$$

This means that Q is any vector in the plane perpendicular to f with the exemption that Q is a multiple of y if $f \neq 0$.

The length of Q is then

$$||Q||^2 = \alpha^2 + \frac{||f||^2}{||y||^2} \text{ for all } \alpha \in \mathbb{R} \ , \tag{13}$$

what means that it can take on any value notless than $||f||/||y||$. Only if bounds of the modulus are given we can get statements restricting the possible directions.

As a consequence it makes only sense to decide whether there is a dipole at a given point or not. In that case it is sufficient to determine $f(y)$ and decide whether it is 0 or not.

In addition the solution of the system of first kind integral equations $Tf = B$ is ill – posed which leads to a possible amplification of the data error, see e.g. [4].

To summarize the dipole distribution with direction and strength cannot be determined even in the ideal situation of infinitely many noiseless data. Only the spatial distibution of them is computable.

4 Lead Field Reconstruction

In the following we first assume that as data the fields $B(x_k)$ are given at N points $x_k \in S^2$, $k = 1, \ldots, N$. Then, of course, the problem is underdetermined, and instead of introducing artificially any discretization we compute the minimum norm solution of the problem. We consider the mapping

$$T : \left(L_2(\Omega)\right)^3 \to \left(\mathbb{R}^3\right)^N$$

with

$$Tf = B_N$$

where each component B_k of B_N is a threedimensional vector. The minimum norm solution f_M of the problem is determined as

$$f_M = T^* u$$

where $u \in \mathbb{R}^{3N}$ solves

$$TT^* u = B_N \ .$$

We now first determine the adjoint operator $T^* : \mathbb{R}^{3N} \to \left(L_2(\Omega)\right)^3$. With K we denote the 3×3 matrix function defining the kernel of the integral operator T; i.e.,

$$K(x,y) = \frac{\mu_0}{4\pi}\left(\frac{1}{F(x,y)} I_3 - \frac{1}{F^2(x,y)} \nabla F(x,y) x^\top\right) \tag{14}$$

where I_3 is the 3×3 identity matrix and $\nabla F x^\top$ is the dyadic product defined as $(uv^\top)_{k\ell} = u_k v_\ell$. The adjoint operator is then computed to

$$\begin{aligned}
< Tf, u >_{\mathbb{R}^{3N}} &= \sum_{k=1}^{N} < Tf(x_k), u_k >_{\mathbb{R}^3} \\
&= \sum_{k=1}^{N} < \int_\Omega K(x_k, y) f(y) dy, u_k >_{\mathbb{R}^3} \\
&= \int_\Omega < f(y), \sum_{k=1}^{N} K^\top(x_k, y) u_k >_{\mathbb{R}^3} dy \\
&= < f, T^* u >_{\left(L_2(\Omega)\right)^3} \ .
\end{aligned}$$

This means

$$T^* u(y) = \sum_{k=1}^{N} K^\top(x_k, y) \cdot u_k$$

or in components

$$T^* u(y)_m = \sum_{k=1}^{N} \sum_{\ell=1}^{3} K(x_k, y)_{\ell,m} u_{k,\ell}$$

where $u_{k,\ell}$ denotes the ℓ – th component of the vector $u_k \in \mathbb{R}^3$.

The $3N \times 3N$ matrix representing the operator TT^* consists of $N \times N$ blocks of 3×3 matrices

$$(TT^*)_{k\ell} = \int_\Omega K(x_k, y) K^\top(x_\ell, y) dy \tag{15}$$

After solving the system of equations with $3N$ unknowns the minimum norm solution is represented as

$$f_M(y) = \sum_{k=1}^{N} K^\top(x_k, y) u_k \tag{16}$$

Next we consider the case that instead of the vector field B at position x_k only components or linear combination of the components are measured. Then this can be incorporated in the following way. Say the data are

$$g_k = < a_k, B(x_k) > = a_k^\top B(x_k) \tag{17}$$

for given vectors $a_k \in \mathbb{R}^3$. We do not discuss here the consequences concerning a possible loss of information in the reconstruction. The operator that we face now is

$$A : (L_2(\Omega))^3 \to \mathbb{R}^N$$

with

$$(Af)_k = < a_k, Tf_k >_{\mathbb{R}^3} = \int_\Omega a_k^\top K(x_k, y) f(y)\, dy\ .$$

In order to compute the minimum norm solution we have to build up the $N \times N$ matrix

$$(AA^*)_{k\ell} = a_k^\top (TT^*)_{k\ell} a_\ell$$

with $(TT^*)_{k\ell}$ from (15). The vector $\alpha \in \mathbb{R}^N$, $\alpha = (\alpha_1, \ldots, \alpha_N)$, solves

$$AA^* \alpha = G$$

where $G = (g_1, \ldots, g_N)^\top$ is the data vector. The solution is then represented as

$$f_M(y) = \sum_{k=1}^{N} \alpha_k K^\top(x_k, y) a_k \tag{18}$$

The vector fields $K^\top(x_k, y) a_k$ are often called lead fields, see [6], [7].

An approximate inversion formula can be derived using methods of [5]. The aim is to determine the $3 \times N$ matrix V such that

$$VG \in \mathbb{R}^3$$

is an approximation to f in a point $y \in \Omega$. To this end we fix $y \in G$ and choose a regularization parameter γ such that

$$V_{\gamma y} G \simeq E_{\gamma y} f$$

where $E_{\gamma y}f$ is a mollified version of f at the point y. For the sake of simplicity we choose

$$E_{\gamma y}f = e_{\gamma y}I_3 f$$

which means that each component of f is treated the same way. As an example of e_γ we consider the three – dimensional sinc - function

$$e_{\gamma y}(z) = \frac{\gamma^3}{\pi^3}\text{sinc } \gamma(z-y) \ .$$

Another possiblity is to use wavelets and scaling functions for computing a wavelet decomposition of the searched – for distribution. An introduction to wavelets can be found in Lemarié, [3].

Then we determine $V_{\gamma y}$ such that

$$AA^* V_{\gamma y}^{\mathsf{T}} = AE_{\gamma y} \ .$$

This means that a Cholesky decomposition of the $N \times N$ matrix AA^*, or possibly $AA^* + \delta I_N$, has to be computed once. The ℓ - th row of V is the solution of the equation with right – hand side $AE_{\gamma y}^{\ell}$, where $E_{\gamma y}^{\ell}$ is the ℓ – th column of $E_{\gamma y}$. The approximation of f_γ is then achieved by matrix – vector multiplication which can be performed in parallel, which is very efficient if the $V_{\gamma y}$ are precomputed and stored.

Finally we want to mention a parametric model of the problem. If the number of dipoles is known a priori, say one or two as in typical medical applications, then it is possible to treat the position y and $f = Q \times y$ as unknowns. The dependence of y is nonlinear and of f linear. So for one dipole we have three nonlinearly appearing variables, y, and two linearly, namely $f \in y^\perp$ because of $f = Q \times y$. Hence the method regarding this fact and described by Golub – Pereyra, [1], is appropriate.

References

[1] Golub, G.H., Pereyra, V.: The differentiation of pseudo – inverses and nonlinear least squares problems whose variables separate. SIAM J. Numer. Anal. **10** (1973) 413-432

[2] Gudden, F., Hoenig, E., Reichenberger, H., Schittenhelm, R., Schneider, G.: Ein Vielkanalsystem zur Biomagnetischen Diagnostik in Neurologie und Kardiologie : Prinzip, Methode und erste Ergebnisse. electromedica **57** (1989) 2-7

[3] Lemarié, P.G.(ed.): Les Ondelettes en 1989. Springer LNM 1438, Berlin 1990

[4] Louis, A.K.: Inverse und schlecht gestellte Probleme. Teubner, Stuttgart, 1989

[5] Louis, A.K., Maaß,P.: A mollifier method for linear operator equations of the first kind. Inverse Problems **6** (1990) 427-440

[6] Robinson, S.E.: Theory and properties of lead field synthesis analysis. Proc. of the 7th International Conference on Biomagnetism, 14-18 Aug 1989, New York, 35-36

[7] Sarvas, J.: Basic mathematical and electromagnetic concepts of the biomagnetic inverse problem. Phys. Med. Biol. **32** (1987) 11-22

ON VARIABLE BLOCK ALGEBRAIC RECONSTRUCTION TECHNIQUES

Yair Censor*
Department of Mathematics and Computer Science
University of Haifa, Mt. Carmel, Haifa 31905, Israel.

Abstract

The variable block ART algorithmic scheme allows the processing of groups of equations (i.e., blocks) which need not be fixed but may rather vary dynamically throughout iterations. The number of blocks, their sizes and the assignment of equations to blocks may all vary, provided that the weights attached to the equations do not fade out in a certain technical sense. Besides encompassing row-action ART, Block-ART and Cimmino-type SIRT, the variable block ART scheme opens new, and as yet unexplored, vistas in algebraic image reconstruction techniques.

1. Introduction.

This paper reviews the variable block Algebraic Reconstruction Technique (ART) algorithmic scheme for solving systems of linear equations that arise from the fully discretized model of transmission tomography. Mathematically speaking, this scheme is a special instance of the more general Block-Iterative Projections (BIP) method of Aharoni, Butnariu and Censor [1,4] or the even more general scheme of Flam and Zowe [11]. However, the variable block ART scheme deserves to be looked at separately because of its importance to image reconstruction from projections. It includes the classical row-action ART of Gordon et al. [13], the fixed block ART (i.e., block Kaczmarz algorithms) of Eggermont et al. [9], as well as the Cimmino version of SIRT (Simultaneous Iterative Reconstruction Technique) of Gilbert [12] (see also Lakshminarayanan and Lent [20] and van der Sluis and van der Vorst [22]) - as special cases and serves as a unifying framework for the description of all these popular iterative reconstruction techniques.

---

* This work was supported by NIH grant HL-28438 while visiting the Medical Image Processing Group (MIPG) at the Department of Radiology, Hospital of the University of Pennsylvania, Philadelphia, PA., USA.

The novelty added to all those by the variable block ART scheme lies in the fact that it allows the processing of blocks (i.e., groups of equations) which need not be fixed in advance, but may rather change dynamically throughout iterations. The number of blocks, their sizes and the assignment of equations to blocks may all vary, provided that the weights attached to the equations are not allowed to fade out, i.e., they have to fulfill the technical condition (2.2) given below.

The behavior of iterative reconstruction algorithms when the underlying system of equations is inconsistent is an interesting question because noise and other inaccuracies in data would usually make any consistency assumption unrealistic. We briefly survey results related to the behavior of ART, fixed block ART and SIRT when applied to an inconsistent system. This question is still open, in general, for the variable block ART.

Another important issue is the implementation and practical performance of block iterative reconstruction algorithms with fixed or variable blocks. In addition to studying the algorithms in terms of quality of reconstructed images there is a potential of using block-iterative algorithms on a parallel architecture machine. We briefly survey some recent results on these matters.

2. The Variable Block Algebraic Reconstruction Scheme.

Consider a system of linear equations obtained from the fully discretized model for transmission tomography image reconstruction, see, e.g., [5]:

$$\sum_{j=1}^{n} x_j a_j^i = y_i , \qquad i=1,2,\ldots,m. \tag{2.1}$$

Here $y=(y_i)\in\mathbb{R}^m$ (the m-dimensional Euclidean space) is the <u>measurements vector</u>, $x=(x_j)\in\mathbb{R}^n$ is the (unknown) <u>image vector</u>, and, for each i, the vector $a^i=(a_j^i)\in\mathbb{R}^n$ is the i-th column of A^T, the transpose of the m×n <u>projection matrix</u> A. Unless otherwise stated we assume that the system (2.1) is consistent, i.e., that, given A and y, the set $\{x\in\mathbb{R}^n \mid Ax=y\}$ is nonempty. Algorithmic behavior for inconsistent systems is discussed separately below.

A vector $w=(w_i)\in\mathbb{R}^m$ is called a <u>weight vector</u> if $w_i\geq 0$ for all i and

$\sum_{i=1}^{m} w_i=1$. A sequence $\{w^k\}_{k=0}^{\infty}$ of weight vectors is called <u>fair</u> if for every i, there exist infinitely many values of k for which $w_i^k>0$. This guarantees that no equation is zero-weighted indefinitely. To prevent equations from fading away by positive but steadily diminishing weights we require that, for every i, the stronger condition

$$\sum_{k=0}^{\infty} w_i^k = +\infty , \tag{2.2}$$

holds.

The sequence of weight vectors $\{w^k\}$ actually determines which block is used at each iteration by attaching positive weights to equations that belong to the current block and zero weights to the rest.

<u>Algorithm 1.</u> <u>Variable block ART - the general scheme.</u>

<u>Initialization.</u> $x^0 \in \mathbb{R}^n$ is arbitrary.

<u>Iterative Step.</u>

$$x^{k+1} = x^k + \lambda_k \sum_{i=1}^{m} w_i^k \left(\frac{y_i - \langle a^i, x^k \rangle}{\| a^i \|^2} \right) a^i . \tag{2.3}$$

Here $\langle a^i,x^k\rangle = \sum_{j=1}^{n} x_j^k a_j^i$ is the standard inner product in $\mathbb{R}^n$ and $\{\lambda_k\}_{k=0}^{\infty}$ is a sequence of <u>relaxation parameters</u> choosen by the user. As a direct corollary of [1, Theorem 1] we obtain

<u>Theorem 1.</u> If the system (2.1) is consistent and $\{w^k\}$ are weight vectors with property (2.2), and if the relaxation parameters $\{\lambda_k\}$ are such that $\tau_1 \le \lambda_k \le 2-\tau_2$, for all $k \ge 0$, with $\tau_1,\tau_2>0$, then any sequence $\{x^k\}$ generated by Algorithm 1 coverges to a solution of (2.1).

The variable block ART algorithm allows processing of the information contained in groups of equations, called <u>blocks</u>. The number of blocks, their sizes (i.e., the number of equations in each block) and their specific structure (i.e., which equations are assigned to each block), may all vary from one iterative step to the next. The following special cases of Algorithm 1 have been studied separately in the past.

(i) Row-action ART. This classical sequential ART of [13] is obtained by choosing the weight vectors as $w^k=e^{i(k)}$ where $e^t \in \mathbb{R}^n$ is the t-th standard basis vector (having one in its t-th coordinate and zeros elsewhere). Each block contains a single equation and the index sequence $\{i(k)\}$ with $1 \le i(k) \le m$, for all k, is the control sequence of the algorithm which determines the index of the single equation upon which the algorithm operates at the k-th iterative step. If $i(k)=k(\mathrm{mod}\ m)+1$ then the control is cyclic. See e.g., [7,15] for more details and references. The iterative steps take obviously the form

$$x_j^{k+1} = x_j^k + \lambda_k \frac{b_{i(k)} - \langle a^{i(k)}, x^k \rangle}{\|a^{i(k)}\|^2} a_j^{i(k)}, \qquad (2.4)$$

for all $j=1,2,\dots,n$.

(ii) Cimmino-type SIRT. In this fully simultaneous reconstruction algorithm [12,20,22] all equations are lumped, with fixed weights, into a single block and are acted upon simultaneously in every step. The iteration formula is precisely (2.3) with $w^k=w$ for all $k \ge 0$ and $w_i \ne 0$ for all $i=1,2,\dots,m$.

(iii) Fixed block ART. Here the index set $I=\{1,2,\dots,m\}$ is partitioned as $I=I_1 \cup I_2 \cup \dots \cup I_M$ into M blocks. $\{t(k)\}$ is a control sequence over the set $\{1,2,\dots,M\}$ of block indices and the weight vectors are of the form $w^k = \sum_{i \in I_{t(k)}} w_i^k e^i$. This guarantees that equations outside the t(k)-th block are not operated upon in the k-th iterative step. The block-Kaczmarz procedure of [9] is thus obtained.

In addition to these well-known special cases the variable block ART enables the implementation of dynamic ART algorithms in which the block formation strategy might vary during the iterative process itself. Such variations in the block formation strategy may be used to accelerate the initial convergence towards an acceptable reconstructed image. It is possible under the regime of the variable block ART to perform multilevel image reconstruction, as suggested by Herman et al. [16] where the authors state: "We are investigating multilevel approaches, since we hope that they have the potential to speed up iterative reconstruction procedures so that they become competitive with the convolution method. By multilevel approaches we mean methods in which we repeatedly change during the iterative process the system of equations to be solved and/or the way the system is organized into blocks".

Yet another aspect of variable block ART is the possibility to exploit its ultimate flexibility towards parallel computations, see, e.g., [5].

3. Variable Block ART in Image Reconstruction.

In this section we briefly review some of the recent literature which reports on experimental work with special versions of ART which are derivable from the variable block ART algorithmic scheme.

3.1 The fixed block-Kaczmarz algorithm.

Motivated by an application in truly three dimensional image reconstruction, Eggermont et al. developed in [9] their fixed-block-Kaczmarz method, gave an analysis of its convergence in the consistent case and proved its cyclic convergence for inconsistent systems. The performance of this algorithm on a realistic three-dimensional image reconstruction problem is reported in Altschuler et al. [2]. Earlier theoretical work on the fixed-block-Kaczmarz method includes the papers of Elfving [10] and Peters [21].

The effects of different fixed block sizes on the initial performance of the fixed-block-Kaczmarz algorithm was investigated by Herman and Levkowitz in [17]. In spite of the limited scope of their reported experiments Herman and Levkowitz noticed significant dependence on the block size. They found that block sizes which are intermediate to the extremes of "row-action" (one equation per block) and "fully simultaneous" (all equations in one block) implementations - show better initial performance according to several calculated measures of merit.

3.2 Variable block ART.

In an experiment entitled "Multiblock" Herman et al. [16] used variable block sizes in the block-Kaczmarz algorithm without really having at hand a mathematical framework that would justify it. They say there [16, p. 133]: "As can be seen from Figures 9.4 and 9.5, multiblock outperforms all the variants of ART reported here, if it is run long enough". The variable block ART scheme presented here (Algorithm 1) and its convergence analysis lay down the mathematical foundation for such multiblock implementaions.

It is not difficult also to envision an algorithm that will use information about the iterate x^k, the current approximation to the reconstructed image, to affect subsequent choices of equations and their weights in forthcoming block formations. Such "iteration-dependent evolutionary" algorithms can be developed only after we gain a firm knowledge about the possible merits of various variable block schemes in ART.

3.3 Parallel computation.

Possible ways of exploiting the variable block ART algorithmic scheme for parallel computations were discussed in [5]. We are, however, not aware of any computational efforts in this direction. Our recent report [25] does include some preliminary experimental image reconstruction work on a parallel computer, but with a different block-iterative algorithm, namely, the fixed-block-MART (Multiplicative Algebraic Reconstruction Technique) of [8] for entropy optimization. Recent experimental work on parallel soluion of linear systems is reported by Sameh and co-workers, of which we mention just a sample [3, 19]. Those results, however, are not specific for image reconstruction problems.

3.4 The inconsistent case.

Because of their computational appeal (simplicity, row-action nature, etc.) and their efficacious performance in some specific situations, ART methods have been applied to inconsistent systems of equations as well. The surprisingly good results prompted studies of the behavior of the algorithms when applied to such systems. For row-action Kaczmarz's method Tanabe [23,24] proved "cyclic convergence" i.e., the convergence of the subsequences of iterates lying on each of the hyperplanes of the system. This result was extended to the fixed block Kaczmarz method by Eggermont et al. [9] who also incorporated periodic relaxation parameters. Following this latter result, Censor et al. [6] were able to analyze the effect of strong underrelaxation in Kaczmarz's method for inconsistent systems. This was recently studied and further generalized by Hanke and Niethammer [14] who also discuss acceleration of the method.

For the fully simultaneous Cimmino method, Iusem and De Pierro [18] showed the local convergence to a weighted least squares solution if the system is inconsistent. We are not aware of any study that would in any way unify these results by making a statement about the behavior of the variable block ART method for inconsistent systems.

References.

[1] R. Aharoni and Y. Censor, "Block-iterative projection methods for parallel computation of solutions to convex feasibility problems", Linear Algebra and Its Applications, 120:165-175, (1989).

[2] M.D. Altschuler, Y. Censor, P.P.B. Eggermont, G.T.Herman, Y.H. Kuo, R.M. Lewitt, M. McKay, H.K. Tuy, J.K. Udupa and M.M. Yau, "Demonstration of a software package for the reconstruction of the dynamically changing structure of the human heart from cone beam x-ray projections," Journal of Medical Systems, 4:289-304, (1980).

[3] R. Bramley and A. Sameh, "Domain decomposition for parallel row projection algorithms", Technical Report CSRD No. 958, Center for Supercomputing Research and Development, University of Illinois, Urbana, Ill., January 1990.

[4] D. Butnariu and Y. Censor, "On the behavior of a block-iterative projection method for solving convex feasibility problems", International Journal of Computer Mathematics, 34: 79-94, (1990).

[5] Y. Censor, "Parallel application of block-iterative methods in medical imaging and radiation therapy", Mathematical Programming, 42: 307-325, (1988).

[6] Y. Censor, P.P.B. Eggermont and D. Gordon, "Strong underrelaxation in Kaczmarz's method for inconsistent systems", Numerische Mathematik, 41:83-92, (1983).

[7] Y. Censor and G.T. Herman, "On some optimization techniques in image reconstruction from projections", Applied Numerical Mathematics, 3:365-391, (1987).

[8] Y. Censor and J. Segman, "On block-iterative entropy maximization", Journal of Information and Optimization Sciences, 8:275-291, (1987).

[9] P.P.B. Eggermont, G.T. Herman and A. Lent, "Iterative algorithms for large partitioned linear systems, with applications to image reconstruction", Linear Algebra and Its Applications, 40:37-67, (1981).

[10] T. Elfving, "Block-iterative methods for consistent and inconsistent linear equations", Numerische Mathematik, 35: 1-12, (1980).

[11] S.D. Flam and J. Zowe, "Relaxed outer projections, weighted averages and convex feasibility", BIT, 30:289-300, (1990).

[12] P.F.C. Gilbert, "Iterative methods for the three-dimensional reconstruction of an object from projections", Journal of Theoretical Biology, 36:105-117, (1972).

[13] R. Gordon, R. Bender and G.T. Herman, "Algebraic Reconstruction Techniques (ART) for three-dimensional electron microscopy and X-ray photography", Journal of Theoretical Biology, 29:471-481, (1970).

[14] M. Hanke and W. Niethammer, "On the accelaration of Kaczmarz's method for inconsistent linear systems", Linear Algebra and Its Applications, 130:83-98, (1990).

[15] G.T.Herman, Image Reconstruction From Projections: The Fundamentals of Computerized Tomography, Academic Press, New York, 1980.

[16] G.T. Herman, H. Levkowitz, H.K. Tuy and S. McCromick, "Multilevel image reconstruction", in: Multiresolution Image Processing and Analysis, (A. Rosenfeld, Editor), Springer-Verlag, Berlin, 1984, pp. 121-135.

[17] G.T. Herman and H. Levkowitz, "Initial performance of block-iterative reconstruction algorithms", in: Mathematics and Computer Science in Medical Imaging, (M.A. Viergever and A. Todd-Pokropek, Editors), Springer-Verlag, Berlin, 1987, pp. 305-318.

[18] A.N. Iusem and A.R. De Pierro, "Convergence resutls for an accelerated nonlinear Cimmino algorithm", Numerische Mathematik, 49: 367-378, (1986).

[19] C. Kamath and A. Sameh, "A projection method for solving non-symmetric linear systems on multiprocessors", Parallel Computing, 9:291-312, (1988/89).

[20] A.V. Lakshminarayanan and A. Lent, "Methods of least squares and SIRT in reconstruction", Journal of Theoretical Biology, 76:267-295, (1979).

[21] W. Peters, "Lösung linearer Gleichungssysteme durch Projektion auf Schnitträume von Hyperebenen und Berechnung einer verallgemeinerten Inversen", Beiträge zur Numerische Mathematik, 5:129-146, (1976).

[22] A. van der Sluis and H.A. van der Vorst, "SIRT-and CG-type methods for the iterative solution of sparse linear least-squares problems", Linear Algebra and Its Applications, 130:257-302, (1990).

[23] K. Tanabe, "Projection method for solving a singular system of linear equations and its applications", Numerische Mathematik, 17: 203-214, (1971).

[24] K. Tanabe, "Characterization of linear stationary iterative processes for solving a singular system of linear equations", Numerische Mathematik, 22: 349-359, (1974).

[25] S.A. Zenios and Y. Censor, "Parallel computing with block-iterative image reconstruction algorithms", Applied Numerical Mathematics, to appear.

On Volterra–Lotka differential equations and Multiplicative Algorithms for Monotone Complementarity Problems

P.P.B. EGGERMONT

Abstract. We study multiplicative iterative algorithms for the solution of strongly inverse monotone complementarity problems. The guiding principle in our analysis is the connection with differential equations of Volterra–Lotka type and their Lyapunov functions. The results are applied to linear complementarity problems with monotone resp. diagonally dominant coefficient matrices.

1. Introduction. We study multiplicative iterative algorithms for the solution of monotone complementarity problems. The recent interest in multiplicative iterative algorithms stems from the seminal papers by SHEPP and VARDI [12] and VARDI *et al.* [14], in which the Expectation–Maximization (EM) algorithm was proposed for the approximate computation of the intensity field maximizing the likelihood functional. Applied to an arbitrary differentiable function $\ell : I\!R^N_+ \longrightarrow I\!R$ the algorithm takes the form

$$x_j^{n+1} = x_j^n - \omega_n x_j^n [\ell'(x^n)]_j \ , \quad j = 1, 2, \cdots, N \ , \tag{1.1}$$

for $n \geq 1$, where $x^1 > 0$ (component wise) is an initial guess. Here $\omega_n > 0$ is a suitable *relaxation* parameter. The algorithm (1.1) purports to solve the constrained minimization problem

$$\text{minimize} \quad \ell(x) \quad \text{subject to} \quad x \geq 0 \ . \tag{1.2}$$

For the minimum negative log-likelihood problem it can be shown rather elegantly that the algorithm (1.1) converges, see SHEPP and VARDI [12], VARDI *et al.* [14]. For general convex functions $\ell(x)$ it is still an open problem. However, for the slightly modified algorithm

$$x_j^{n+1} = \frac{x_j^n}{1 + \omega_n [\ell'(x^n)]_j} \ , \quad j = 1, 2, \cdots, N \ , \tag{1.3}$$

a complete and elegant convergence theory is possible, see [7].

We raise the question whether algorithms of this type can be used for problems where there is no (apparent) function that is being minimized. The natural extension of the convex minimization problem is the monotone complementarity problem, viz. for $F : I\!R^N_+ \longrightarrow I\!R^N$ a monotone mapping, find x such that

$$x \in I\!R^N_+ \ , \quad F(x) \in I\!R^N_+ \ , \quad \langle F(x), x \rangle = 0 \ . \tag{MCP}$$

We assume troughout that F is continuous on $I\!R^N_+$. Every convex minimization problem over $I\!R^N_+$ can be formulated as a monotone complementarity problem with $F(x)$ the gradient of the objective function. The conditions (MCP) are precisely the Karash-Kuhn-Tucker conditions for a minimum. However, it is obvious that something is lost in the translation of a minimization problem into a complementarity problem, so that we need more than *mere* monotonicity for our multiplicative iterative algorithms to work. We assume that a solution of (MCP) exists, and make the following ***strict inverse monotonicity*** assumption:

$$\langle F(x) - F(y), x - y \rangle > 0 \ , \ \text{whenever } F(x) \neq F(y) \ . \tag{1.4}$$

This is satisfied, e.g., if F is strictly monotone, or $F(x) = A^T\Phi(Ax)$, where Φ is strictly monotone, and $A \in I\!R^{N\times N}$. Later on we shall need to strengthen this to the assumption of ***locally strongly inverse monotonicity***, viz. to the assumption

(1.5) For every compact subset $K \in I\!R_+^N$ there exist a positive constant $\gamma = \gamma(K)$ such that $\langle F(x) - F(y), x - y\rangle \geq \gamma\,|F(x) - F(y)|^2$ for all $x, y \in K$.

In case γ is independent of K, this says formally that the inverse mapping F^{inv} is strongly monotone, whence the appellation of *strongly inverse monotone.*

The multiplicative algorithms for (MCP) we have in mind are

$$x_j^{n+1} + \omega_n x_j^{n+1} F_j(x^{n+1}) = x_j^n \ , \quad j = 1, 2, \cdots, N \ , \quad \text{and} \tag{1.6}$$

$$x_j^{n+1} = \frac{x_j^n}{1 + \omega_n F_j(x^n)} \ , \quad j = 1, 2, \cdots, N \ . \tag{1.7}$$

For both algorithms we assume throughout that the starting point x^1 has strictly positive components. Both the explicit algorithm (1.7) and the implicit algorithm (1.6) are related to the differential equation of Volterra-Lotka type

$$\frac{dx_j}{dt} = -x_j F_j(x) \ , \quad j = 1, 2, \cdots, N \ , \tag{1.8}$$

see, e.g., HOFBAUER and SIGMUND [8]. There is a rich stability theory for Volterra-Lotka equations, and our aim is to study analogues for the algorithms (1.6) and (1.7).

Before proceeding, we note that the complementarity problem (MCP) is amenable to diagonal scaling, as follows. Let Λ be a strictly positive, diagonal matrix with diagonal elements λ_j, $j = 1, 2, \cdots, N$, and let $x_j = \lambda_j y_j$ for all j. Then (MCP) may be formulated in terms of y as

$$y \in I\!R_+^N \ , \quad \Lambda F(\Lambda y) \in I\!R_+^N \ , \qquad \langle \Lambda F(\Lambda y), y\rangle = 0 \ . \tag{MCPy}$$

Now, e.g., algorithm (1.7) applied to (MCPy) reads

$$y_j^{n+1} = \frac{y_j^n}{1 + \omega_n \lambda_j F_j(\Lambda y^n)} \ , \quad j = 1, 2, \cdots, N \ , \tag{1.9}$$

and translating this back in terms of x yields

(1.10) $$x_j^{n+1} = \frac{x_j^n}{1+\omega_n\lambda_j F_j(x^n)}\ , \quad j=1,2,\cdots,N\ .$$

The additional factors λ_j *cannot* change the classification of F, so properties of F such as monotonicity, or diagonal dominance or symmetry of the matrix A when $F(x) = Ax - b$ must be taken modulo diagonal matrices Λ. An interesting case arises if in (1.10) we take $F(x) = Ax - b$ and we set $\omega_n \equiv 1$ and $\lambda_j = 1/b_j$, viz.

(1.11) $$x_j^{n+1} = x_j^n \frac{b_j}{[Ax^n]_j}\ , \quad j=1,2,\cdots,N\ .$$

This is known as CHAHINE's algorithm, [3]. See also TWOMEY [13], DAUBE-WITHERSPOON and MUEHLLEHNER [6].

We now summarize the remainder of the paper. In §2, we discuss the stability properties of the Volterra-Lotka differential equation for the general monotone problem and for linear problems. In §3 we consider the implicit algorithm for monotone complementarity problems with the inverse monotonicity property. In §4 we study the convergence of the explicit algorithm for *locally strongly inverse monotone* problems, and give conditions on the relaxation parameters ω_n. In §5 and §6 we consider the explicit algorithm (1.7) and CHAHINE's algorithm for the linear complementarity problem, both with monotone and with diagonally dominant matrices.

2. Some Lyapunov functions for Volterra-Lotka differential equations. We consider the differential equation of Volterra-Lotka type

(VL) $$\frac{dx_j}{dt} = -x_j F_j(x)\ , \quad j=1,2,\cdots,N\ ,$$

with initial point $x(0) \in \operatorname{int} I\!R^N_+$. Equations of this type occur, e.g., in theoretical biology (with affine linear $F(x)$), see VOLTERRA [15], and HOFBAUER and SIGMUND [8], §21. Here we summarize the theory concerning the convergence of the solution $x(t)$ of (VL) towards a limit x^*, and whether x^* solves the monotone complementarity problem (MCP). We consider various classes of mappings F(x), to wit gradient type mappings, strictly inverse monotone mappings, and (affine) linear maps $F(x) = Ax - b$, with strictly monotone and diagonally dominant matrices $A \in I\!R^{N\times N}$. The Lyapunov function for the classical (VL) already known to VOLTERRA [15] is given by

(2.1) $$I(x|y) = \sum_j x_j \log\frac{x_j}{y_j} + y_j - x_j\ ,$$

where $x,\ y \in I\!R^N_+$. This is well defined, provided we take 0/0 to be 1, $0\log 0$ to be 0, and we allow the value $+\infty$ (observe that each term $x_j \log x_j/y_j + y_j - x_j$ is nonnegative). We quote the following inequalities, CSISZÁR [5],

(2.2) $$2\,I(X_0|Y_0) + X_0\,|X-Y|_1^2 \le 2\,I(x|y) \le 2\sum_j \frac{(x_j-y_j)^2}{y_j}\ ,$$

with $I(X_0|Y_0) = X_0 \log(X_0/Y_0) + Y_0 - X_0$ in conformance with (2.1), and

$$X_0 = \sum_i x_i\,, \quad X_j = \frac{x_j}{X_0}\,, \quad Y_0 = \sum_i y_i\,, \quad Y_j = \frac{y_j}{Y_0}\,. \tag{2.3}$$

This says that $I(x|y)$ measures the distance between x, $y \in \mathbb{R}^N_+$, be it in a peculiar way.

2.1. Gradient type mappings. We briefly mention the case where $F(x)$ is the gradient of a convex, differentiable function $\ell(x)$ on $\mathbb{R}^N_+$, which attains its infimum on $\mathbb{R}^N_+$, i.e. there exists an $x^0 \in \mathbb{R}^N_+$ such that

$$\ell(x^0) = \inf\{\ \ell(x)\ :\ x \in \mathbb{R}^N_+\ \}\,. \tag{2.4}$$

With $x(t)$ the solution of (VL) we have that $\ell(x)$ and $I(x^0|x)$ are Lyapunov functions for (VL), see HOFBAUER and SIGMUND [8],

$$\frac{d}{dt}\ell(x) = -\sum_j x_j\,|\ell'_j(x)|^2 \le 0\,, \tag{2.5}$$

$$\frac{d}{dt}I(x^0|x) = -\langle \ell'(x), x - x^0\rangle \le -[\ell(x) - \ell(x^0)] \le 0\,. \tag{2.6}$$

In the second inequality the convexity of $\ell(x)$ is used. The first inequality says that $\ell(x(t))$ decreases along each trajectory of (VL), and the second one says that for *every* solution x^0 of (2.4), the solution $x(t)$ of (VL) gets closer and closer to x^0. In particular, this implies the boundedness of the trajectory $x(t)$, $t \ge 0$, and also that any ω-limit point of $x(t)$, $t > 0$ is in fact a solution of (2.4). This then implies that $x(t) \longrightarrow x^*$ as $t \longrightarrow \infty$, where x^* is a solution of (2.4), and hence also of (MCP).

2.2. Strictly inverse monotone mappings. We note that in §2.1 the gradient $\ell'(x)$ of a convex function $\ell(x)$ is monotone, i.e.

$$\langle \ell'(x) - \ell'(y), x - y\rangle \ge 0\,, \quad \forall x, y \in \mathbb{R}^N_+\,.$$

In case $F(x)$ is not the gradient of a convex functional, then (2.5) is not available, and (2.6) only partly, with the result that we cannot prove that an ω-limit point of $x(t)$, $t > 0$ solves (MCP). This is the reason why we assume that F is strictly inverse monotone rather than merely monotone. Then (2.6) takes on a slightly different form, viz. with x^0 any solution of (MCP)

$$\frac{d}{dt}I(x^0|x) = -\langle F(x) - F(x^0), x - x^0\rangle - \langle F(x^0), x\rangle \le 0\,. \tag{2.7}$$

This shows that once again $I(x^0|x)$ is a Lyapunov function for (VL). Once more it can be shown that $x(t) \longrightarrow x^*$ as $t \longrightarrow \infty$, where x^* is a solution of (MCP), as follows. From (2.7) we have that $I(x^0|x)$ is a decreasing function of t, and is bounded below (by 0). It follows that $x(t)$, $t > 0$ is bounded. If x^* is an ω-limit point, then from (2.7) we have

$$\langle F(x^*) - F(x^0), x^* - x^0\rangle = 0\,, \quad \langle F(x^0), x^*\rangle = 0\,.$$

The first equality implies that $F(x^*) = F(x^0)$ and hence $F(x^*) \in I\!R^N_+$, and then the second one gives that $\langle F(x^*), x^*\rangle = 0$. Since obviously $x^* \in I\!R^N_+$, this shows that x^* solves (MCP). Then we may replace x^0 with x^* in (2.7), so that $I(x^*|x)$ is a decreasing function of t. It follows that $I(x^*|x) \longrightarrow 0$, and so, by (2.3), that $x(t) \longrightarrow x^*$ as $t \longrightarrow \infty$. The above, well known reasoning will be referred to later on to show the convergence of the algorithms (1.6)–(1.7)–(1.11), and is crucial to this paper.

2.3. Affine linear mappings. For the remainder of §2 we let $F(x) = Ax - b$, with $A \in I\!R^{N\times N}$, $b \in I\!R^N$. If A is symmetric, semi-positive definite then $F(x)$ is strictly inverse monotone, and it is even a gradient mapping. If A is strictly monotone, then F is strictly inverse monotone. So the material of §2.1 and §2.2 applies. We point out here that the assumption (1.5) in this case translates to $\langle Ax, x\rangle > 0$ unless $Ax = 0$, which is equivalent to the existence of a positive constant γ such that

$$\langle Ax, x\rangle \geq \gamma\,|Ax|^2\ ,\ \forall x \in I\!R^N\ . \tag{2.8}$$

2.4. Diagonally dominant matrices – I. We assume that the matrix A is (strongly) diagonally dominant and has a positive diagonal, so that for some positive δ

$$a_{jj} - \sum_{i\neq j} |a_{ji}| \geq \delta\ ,\quad j = 1, 2, \cdots, N\ . \tag{2.9}$$

It can be proved, see BERMAN and PLEMMONS [2], that there exist a strictly positive diagonal matrix D such that DA is strictly monotone. Then

$$\frac{d}{dt} I(Dx^0|Dx) = -\langle DA(x - x^0), x - x^0\rangle - \langle D(Ax - b), x^0\rangle\ ,$$

and, as in §2.2, we get that $x(t) \longrightarrow x^0$ as $t \longrightarrow \infty$. In this case the solution is unique.

2.5. Diagonally dominant matrices – II. A more straight forward Lyapunov function which is more *classically* related to the diagonal dominance of A is $|x - x^0|_\infty$. The proof is as follows. Let the index j be such that $|x_j - x^0_j| = |x - x^0|_\infty$. Without loss of generality we assume that $x \neq x^0$ so that then $s_j = \text{sign}(x_j - x^0_j)$ equals ± 1, and

$$\frac{d}{dt}|x - x^0|_\infty = \frac{d}{dt}|x_j - x^0_j| = \frac{d}{dt} s_j\,(x_j - x^0_j) = -s_j x_j [Ax - b]_j\ .$$

Now we write $Ax - b = A(x - x^0) + Ax^0 - b$. Since $x^0_j [Ax^0 - b]_j = 0$ for all j, we get

$$-s_j x_j [Ax^0 - b]_j = -s_j (x_j - x^0_j)\,[Ax^0 - b]_j = -|x_j - x^0_j|\,[Ax^0 - b]_j \leq 0$$

since $Ax^0 - b \in I\!R^N_+$). Also

$$\begin{aligned} -s_j x_j [A(x - x^0)]_j &= x_j\{\,-a_{jj}|x_j - x^0_j| + s_j \sum_{i\neq j} a_{ji}(x_i - x^0_i)\,\} \\ &\leq x_j |x - x^0|_\infty \{\,-a_{jj} + \sum_{i\neq j} |a_{ji}|\,\} \leq -\delta x_j |x - x^0|_\infty\ . \end{aligned}$$

Since $x(t) \in \text{int}\, I\!R^N_+$ always, we have shown that

$$\frac{d}{dt}|x - x^0|_\infty < 0\ , \text{ as long as } x \neq x^0\ . \tag{2.10}$$

It follows that if x^* is an ω-limit point of $x(t)$, $t > 0$ then

$$|x^* - x^0|_\infty = \liminf_{t \longrightarrow \infty} |x - x^0|_\infty\ , \quad \text{and so} \quad \limsup_{t \longrightarrow \infty} \frac{d}{dt}|x - x^0|_\infty = 0\ .$$

Now (2.10) implies that $x^* = x^0$, and so once more $x(t) \longrightarrow x^* = x^0$.

2.6. Diagonally dominant matrices – III. In this section we consider column wise diagonally dominant matrices with positive diagonal, i.e. matrices A that satisfy

$$a_{ii} - \sum_{j \neq i} |a_{ji}| \geq \delta\ , \quad i = 1, 2, \cdots, N\ . \tag{2.11}$$

We note that if A is (row wise) diagonally dominant in the sense of (2.9), then there exist a positive diagonal matrix Λ such that ΛA is column wise diagonally dominant in the sense of (2.11).

When the solution x^0 of (MCP) is strictly positive, so that $Ax^0 = b$, then it can be shown that $\sum_j |\log(x_j/x_j^0)|$ is also a Lyapunov function. One verifies in a way similar to the derivation of (2.10), that

$$\frac{d}{dt}\sum_j \left| \log \frac{x_j}{x_j^0} \right| < -|x - x^0|_1 \max_i \{\, a_{ii} - \sum_{j \neq i} |a_{ji}|\, \}\ . \tag{2.12}$$

As before, this implies that $x(t) \longrightarrow x^0$ as $t \longrightarrow \infty$.

3. The implicit algorithm – the monotone case. In this section we study the implicit algorithm (1.6) under the *strict inverse monotonicity* assumption (1.4) and assuming (MCP) has a solution. The analysis closely resembles that for differential equations of Volterra–Lotka type, see §2.2. We begin by showing that the implicit algorithm indeed defines the sequence $\{x_n\}_n$.

LEMMA 3.1. *For any $\omega_n > 0$ the implicit algorithm (1.6) determines the sequence $\{x^n\}_n \subset I\!R^N_+$ uniquely.*

PROOF: We define $G : I\!R^N_+ \longrightarrow I\!R^N$ by $G_j(x) = F_j(x) + \omega_n(-x_j^n/x_j + 1)$, $j = 1, 2, \cdots, N$, so that (1.6) amounts to $G(x) = 0$. Since F s monotone, G is *strictly* monotone. It follows that *if* a solution to $G(x) = 0$ exists, then it is unique. To prove the existence of a solution, let x^0 be the solution of (MCP), and let $x^n \in \text{int}\, I\!R^N_+$. We define $I\!K = \{x \in \text{int}\, I\!R^N_+ : I(x^0|x) \leq I(x^0|x^n)\}$, and denote its boundary by $\partial I\!K$. Then $I\!K$ is bounded, closed, and convex, and has nonempty interior. We define a projector P onto $I\!K$ as follows. If $x \notin I\!K$ then $P(x)$ is the point on the line segment $[x^0, x] = \{\theta x^0 + (1-\theta)x : 0 \leq \theta \leq 1\}$ that lies on $\partial I\!K$ and is closest to x. If $x \in I\!K$ then $P(x) = x$, of course. Now define the map $T : I\!R^N_+ \longrightarrow I\!K$ by $T(x) = P(x - G(x))$. Then

T is continuous (even though $G(x)$ is not continuous when x has a zero component), and T maps $\mathbb{K}$ into itself. By Brouwer's theorem, see [9], T has a fixed point. We show that the fixed point does not lie in $\partial\mathbb{K}$. Let $x \in \partial\mathbb{K}$. Then $I(x^0|x) = I(x^0|x^n)$. Now consider

$$\langle x - x^0, G(x)\rangle = \langle x - x^0, F(x)\rangle + \omega \sum_j (x_j - x_j^n)\left(-\frac{x_j^0}{x_j^n} + 1\right) . \tag{3.1}$$

The first term on the right may be written as $\langle x - x^0, F(x) - F(x^0)\rangle + \langle x, F(x^0)\rangle - \langle x^0, F(x^0)\rangle$. By (1.4) the first term of this last expression is nonnegative. Since x^0 solves (MCP) the last term vanishes, and $F(x^0) \in \mathbb{R}_+^N$. Since x is in $\mathbb{R}_+^N$ as well, then the second term is nonnegative also. Thus $\langle x - x^0, F(x)\rangle \geq 0$. By strict convexity, the last sum of (3.1) strictly dominates $\omega\,(I(x^0|x) - I(x^0|x^n))$ which vanishes. We have shown that $\langle x - x^0, G(x)\rangle > 0$, for all $x \in \partial\mathbb{K}$. We now show that $P(x - G(x)) \neq x$. Let L denote the line through x^0 and x, i.e. $L = \{\lambda x^0 + (1-\lambda)x : \lambda \in \mathbb{R}\}$. If $x - G(x)$ does *not* lie on the line L then surely $P(x - G(x)) \neq x$. On the other hand if $x - G(x)$ *does* lie on the line L, then $\langle x^0 - x, x - G(x) - x\rangle = \langle x - x^0, G(x)\rangle > 0$, so that x and $x - G(x)$ lie on opposite sides of x^0 on the line L. Since $x - G(x)$ and $P(x - G(x))$ lie on the same side of x^0 on the line L this shows that $x \neq P(x - G(x))$. So we have shown that if $x \in \partial\mathbb{K}$ then $x \neq T(x)$, so the fixed point(s) of T do not lie on $\partial\mathbb{K}$, so they must lie in the interior of $\mathbb{K}$. It follows that if x^* is the fixed point, then $x^* = x^* - G(x^*)$, and $G(x^*) = 0$. So x^{n+1} exists, and lies in the interior of $\mathbb{R}_+^N$. This proof is very similar to the proof of the existence of solutions of complementarity problems resp. variational inequalities, see Theorem 4.2 and Corollary 4.3 of KINDERLEHRER and STAMPACCHIA [9]. Q.E.D.

We now state the analogue of the material in §2.3.

LEMMA 3.2. *Let x^0 be the solution of the complementarity problem (MCP). Then*

$$I(x^0|x^n) - I(x^0|x^{n+1}) \geq \omega_n \langle F(x^{n+1}) - F(x^0), x^{n+1} - x^0\rangle + \omega_n\langle F(x^0), x^{n+1}\rangle , \tag{3.2}$$

and the right hand side is positive, unless x^n solves the complementarity problem.

PROOF: Since all $x^n > 0$ component wise, the $I(x^0|x^n)$ are finite. Then

$$\begin{aligned} I(x^0|x^n) - I(x^0|x^{n+1}) &= \sum_j x_j^0 \log\frac{1}{1+\omega_n F_j(x^{n+1})} + x_j^{n+1} - x_j^n \\ &\geq \sum_j -\omega_n x_j^0 F_j(x^{n+1}) + \omega_n x_j^{n+1} F_j(x^{n+1}) \\ &= \omega_n\langle F(x^{n+1}) - F(x^0), x^{n+1} - x^0\rangle + \omega_n\langle F(x^0), x^{n+1} - x^0\rangle . \end{aligned} \tag{3.3}$$

The inequality is due to the fact that $-\log t \geq 1 - t$. In the second term the contribution $\langle F(x^0), x^0\rangle$ vanishes, since x^0 solves the complementarity problem. Since $F(x^0) \geq 0$ element wise it is obvious that the last member of (3.3) is nonnegative. Moreover, it vanishes if and only if $F(x^{n+1}) = F(x^0)$ and $\langle F(x^0), x^{n+1}\rangle = 0$, but then $\langle F(x^{n+1}), x^{n+1}\rangle = 0$ as well, and since both x^{n+1} and $F(x^{n+1})$ $(= F(x^0))$ are nonnegative element wise it follows that x^{n+1} is a solution of the complementarity problem. But then also $x^{n+1} = x^n$, so already x^n solves the complementarity problem. Q.E.D.

THEOREM 3.3. *The sequence $\{x^n\}_n$ generated by the implicit algorithm (1.6) converges, provided $\inf_n \omega_n > 0$.*

The proof is similar to the material in §2.2, and is omitted. To prepare for the next section, we note that under the assumption of (locally) strong inverse monotonicity (1.5) we get from Lemma 3.2 that

$$I(x^0|x^n) - I(x^0|x^{n+1}) \geq \gamma_{n+1}\omega_n\,|F(x^{n+1}) - F(x^0)|^2 + \omega_n\langle F(x^0), x^{n+1}\rangle\,, \tag{3.5}$$

where γ_{n+1} is any positive number satisfying

$$\gamma_{n+1}\,|F(x^{n+1}) - F(x^0)|^2 \leq \langle F(x^{n+1}) - F(x^0), x^{n+1} - x^0\rangle\,. \tag{3.6}$$

4. The explicit algorithm – the monotone case. Here we develop results for the explicit algorithm (1.7) under the assumption of locally strongly inverse monotonicity (1.5), analogous to those of the previous section. It is obvious that there will be some restraints on the stepsize parameter ω_n. We begin by stating the analogue of Lemma 3.2. where x^0 is any solution of the complementarity problem. As already remarked, $F(x^0)$ is unique.

LEMMA 4.1. *Let x^0 be the solution of the complementarity problem (MCP). Let ω_n satisfy*

$$0 < \omega_n \leq \min\left\{-\frac{1}{2F_j(x^n)} : F_j(x^n) < 0\right\}\,,$$

and let k_n, c_n and γ_n be given as

$$c_n = 2\,|F(x^n)|_\infty\,, \qquad k_n = 2\,|x^n|_\infty\,, \qquad \gamma_n = \frac{\langle F(x^n) - F(x^0), x^n - x^0\rangle}{|F(x^n) - F(x^0)|^2}\,.$$

Then the sequence $\{x_n\}_n$ generated by the explicit algorithm (1.7) satisfies

$$I(x^0|x^n) - I(x^0|x^{n+1}) \geq \omega_n\,\{[\gamma_n - k_n\omega_n]\,|F(x^n) - F(x^0)|^2 + [1 - c_n\omega_n]\,\langle F(x^0), x^n\rangle\}\,.$$

PROOF: Similar to the proof of Lemma 3.2 we have

$$I(x^0|x^n) - I(x^0|x^{n+1}) \geq \omega_n\langle F(x^n), x^n - x^0\rangle - \omega_n\langle x^n - x^{n+1}, F(x^n)\rangle\,.$$

The first term on the right can be estimated as in (3.5)–(3.6), and dominates

$$\gamma_n\omega_n\,|F(x^n) - F(x^0)|^2 + \omega_n\langle F(x^0), x^n\rangle\,.$$

The second term equals (using (1.7) to get an expression for $x_j^{n+1} - x_j^n$)

$$\omega_n^2\sum_j \frac{x_j^n|F_j(x^n)|^2}{1 + \omega_n F_j(x^n)} \leq 2\omega_n^2\sum_j x_j^n\,\{|F_j(x^n) - F_j(x^0)|^2 + 2F_j(x^n)F_j(x^0) - |F_j(x^0)|^2\}$$

$$\leq \omega_n^2\,\{k_n|F(x^n) - F(x^0)|^2 + c_n\langle F(x^0), x^n\rangle\}\,.$$

Putting everything together proves the theorem. Q.E.D.

We are now ready to prove the convergence of the explicit algorithm. The idea is to choose ω_n such that $\{I(x^0|x^n)\}_n$ is a decreasing sequence. Then, obviously, all x^n belong to the compact set A,

$$A = \{y \in \mathbb{R}_+^N : I(x^0|y) \leq I(x^0|x^1)\}\,, \tag{4.1}$$

and the ω_n, k_n and c_n can be chosen the same for all n.

THEOREM 4.2. *Let $\gamma(A)$ be such that (1.5) holds with $K = A$, and let $\gamma_0 = \min\{1, \gamma(A)\}$. Let k_0 and c_0 be defined as*

$$k_0 = 2 \max_{y \in A} |F(y)|_\infty , \qquad c_0 = 2 \max_{y \in A} |y|_\infty .$$

and choose ω_n such that $\inf_n \omega_n > 0$ and $\omega_n \le \frac{1}{2} \min\{\gamma_0/k_0, 1/c_0\}$. Then

$$(4.2) \qquad I(x^0|x^n) - I(x^0|x^{n+1}) \ge \tfrac{1}{2}\gamma_0 \omega_n \{ |F(x^n) - F(x^0)|^2 + \langle F(x^0), x^n \rangle \} ,$$

and $\{x_n\}_n$ converges to a solution of the complementarity problem.

PROOF: Note that $\gamma_0 \le \gamma_n$, $k_0 \ge k_n$, $c_0 \ge c_n$, see Lemma 4.1, so that with the given choice of ω_n, it follows that $\gamma_n - k_n\omega_n \ge \gamma_0/2$, and likewise for $1 - c_n\omega_n$. The inequality (4.3) then follows from Lemma 4.1. The convergence of $\{x^n\}_n$ to a solution of the complementarity problem follows now just as in §2.2. Q.E.D.

. On Chahine's algorithm. The material above shows that the algorithm

$$(5.1) \qquad x_j^{n+1} = \frac{x_j^n}{1 + \omega_n([Ax^n]_j - b_j)} , \quad j = 1, 2, \cdots, N ,$$

onverges for suitable ω_n to a solution of the linear complementarity problem

$$(5.2) \qquad x \in I\!R_+^N , \qquad Ax - b \in I\!R_+^N , \qquad \langle x, Ax - b \rangle = 0 ,$$

rovided A is strongly inverse monotone. It is not clear to this author whether mere nonotonicity is sufficient for the convergence.

For the remainder of this section we assume that A is diagonally dominant with a positive diagonal, see (2.9). Then we have the following result for the explicit algorithm.

LEMMA 5.1. *Let A be diagonally dominant with a positive diagonal. Let the relaxation parameters ω_n satisfy*

$$1 + \omega_n[Ax^n - b]_j > 0 , \qquad \frac{\omega_n a_{jj}}{1 + \omega_n[Ax^n - b]_j} \le 1 , \quad j = 1, 2, \cdots, N .$$

Then the sequence $\{x_n\}_n$ generated by the explicit algorithm (5.1) satisfies

$$|x^{n+1} - x^0|_\infty < |x^n - x^0|_\infty \quad \text{for all } n \ge 1 , \text{ as long as } x^n \ne x^0 .$$

The proof is similar to that of Lemma 5.2 below, and is omitted.

Recently Chahine's algorithm (1.11) has gained attention, see CHAHINE [3], BARCILON [1], CHU [4], DE PIERRO [10],[11], EGGERMONT [7], and TWOMEY [13]. It is quite natural to assume that A is nonnegative element wise, with a strictly positive diagonal, and that b is strictly positive. DE PIERRO [10],[11] has studied the convergence of this algorithm when A is symmetric. See also [7]. BARCILON [1] has shown the convergence if A is diagonally dominant and the system $Ax = b$ has a strictly positive solution. Here we show that this extra solvability condition is not necessary, by slightly modifying BARCILON's proof [1] in the style of §2.6. This also covers *triangular* matrices with a positive diagonal, [4], since these are diagonally similar to diagonally dominant matrices.

LEMMA 5.2. *Let A be diagonally dominant, with a positive diagonal. Then the sequence generated by Chahine's algorithm (1.11) satisfies*

$$|x^{n+1}-x^0|_\infty < |x^n - x^0|_\infty \qquad \text{for all } n \geq 1 \text{ , as long as } x^n \neq x^0 \text{ .}$$

PROOF: We need to distinguish between those indices j with $x_j^0 > 0$, and those with $x_j^0 = 0$. So first let j be such that $x_j^0 > 0$. Then

$$\begin{aligned} x_j^{n+1} - x_j^0 &= x_j^n - x_j^0 - \frac{x_j^n}{[Ax^n]_j}\{[Ax^n]_j - b_j\} \\ &= x_j^n - x_j^0 - \frac{x_j^n}{[Ax^n]_j}\left[A(x^n - x^0)\right]_j - \frac{x_j^n}{[Ax^n]_j}[Ax^0 - b]_j \text{ .} \end{aligned}$$

Since $x_j^0 > 0$ then $[Ax^0 - b]_j = 0$ by complementarity, so the last term in the above expression vanishes. Now straightforward estimation gives

$$|x_j^{n+1} - x_j^0| \leq |x^n - x^0|_\infty \left\{ \left| 1 - \frac{x_j^n}{[Ax^n]_j} a_{jj} \right| + \sum_{i\neq j} \frac{x_j^n}{[Ax^n]_j} |a_{ji}| \right\} \text{ ,}$$

and since $a_{jj}x_j^n / [Ax^n]_j \leq 1$ we get that

$$|x_j^{n+1} - x_j^0| \leq |x^n - x^0|_\infty \left\{ 1 - \frac{x_j^n}{[Ax^n]_j} \left[a_{jj} - \sum_{i\neq j} |a_{ji}| \right] \right\} < |x^n - x^0|_\infty \text{ ,} \tag{5.3}$$

where we used the diagonal dominance. Now let j be such that $x_j^0 = 0$. Then by complementarity $[Ax^0 - b]_j \geq 0$. Then we have that

$$x_j^{n+1} = x_j^n \frac{b_j}{[Ax^n]_j} = x_j^n - \frac{x_j^n}{[Ax^n]_j}[A(x^n - x^0)]_j - \frac{x_j^n}{[Ax^n]_j}[Ax^0 - b]_j \text{ .}$$

The last term is nonpositive, and since $x_j^0 = 0$, we get that

$$|x_j^{n+1} - x_j^0| = x_j^{n+1} \leq x_j^n - x_j^0 - \frac{x_j^n}{[Ax^n]_j}[A(x^n - x^0)]_j \text{ ,}$$

and estimating as in the first case gives $|x_j^{n+1} - x_j^0| < |x^n - x^0|_\infty$. Q.E.D.

The proof of the convergence of the Chahine algorithm for diagonally dominant matrices A now proceeds as in §2.2.

6. The implicit algorithm – diagonally dominant case. Here we consider the discrete analogue for the material in §2.6. Such an analogue does not seem to be readily available for the original algorithm (5.1) or (1.11), but for the *implicit* analogues of these algorithms it works with some additional constraints on the relaxation parameter. The *implicit version* reads

$$x_j^{n+1} = \frac{x_j^n}{1 + \omega_n[Ax^{n+1} - b]_j} \text{ ,} \qquad j = 1, 2, \cdots, N \text{ .} \tag{6.1}$$

We have the following

LEMMA 6.1. *Let A be column wise diagonally dominant with a positive diagonal, see (2.11), and assume that the system $Ax = b$ has a strictly positive solution x^0. Assume that $\omega_n|Ax^{n+1} - b|_\infty \leq \eta$, where η satisfies $\eta < 1$ as well as*

$$\frac{4\eta}{1-\eta} \leq \frac{\delta}{\max_i \sum_{j\neq i} |a_{ji}|} . \tag{6.2}$$

Then the sequence $\{x_n\}_n$ generated by the implicit algorithm (6.1) satisfies

$$\sum_j \left| \log \frac{x_j^{n+1}}{x_j^0} \right| < \sum_j \left| \log \frac{x_j^n}{x_j^0} \right| , \quad \text{as long as } x^n \neq x^0 .$$

PROOF: Let $e_j = x_j^{n+1} - x_j^0$, and set $s_j = +1$ if $e_j \geq 0$, and $= -1$ otherwise. Then

$$\sum_j \left| \log \frac{x_j^{n+1}}{x_j^0} \right| = \sum_j s_j \log \frac{x_j^{n+1}}{x_j^0} = \sum_j s_j \log \frac{x_j^n}{x_j^0} + \sum_j s_j \log \frac{1}{1+\omega_n r_j} .$$

where $r = Ax^{n+1} - b$. Obviously, $\sum_j |\log(x_j^n/x_j^0)|$ dominates the first sum on the right. One verifies for all possible combinations of signs of $x_j^{n+1} - x_j^0$ and r_j that $s_j \log[1/(1+\omega_n r_j)] \leq -\omega_n s_j r_j/(1+\eta t_j)$, where $t_j = 0$ if $s_j = -1$, and $t_j = \operatorname{sign} r_j$ otherwise. Now $-s_j r_j = -a_{jj}|e_j| - s_j \sum_{i\neq j} a_{ji} e_i \leq -a_{jj}|e_j| + \sum_{i\neq j} |a_{ji}|\,|e_i|$, and so we get after changing the order of summation that

$$\sum_j s_j \log \frac{1}{1+\omega_n r_j} \leq -\omega_n \sum_i \frac{|e_i|}{1+\eta t_i} \left\{ -a_{ii} + \sum_{j\neq i} |a_{ji}| \frac{1+\eta t_i}{1+\eta t_j} \right\} \tag{6.3}$$

Now $(1+\eta t_i)/(1+\eta t_j) \leq (1+\eta)/(1-\eta)$, and one verifies that with the choice (6.2) for η we get from (2.11) that

$$-a_{jj} + \sum_{i\neq j} \frac{1+\eta}{1-\eta} |a_{ij}| \leq -\tfrac{1}{2}\delta .$$

It follows that the right hand side of (6.3) is dominated by $-\frac{1}{2}\delta\,(1-\eta)^{-1}\,\omega_n\,|x^{n+1} - x^0|_1$, and the conclusion follows. Q.E.D.

References

[1] V. Barcilon. *On Chahine's relaxation method for the radiative transfer equation.* J. Atmospheric Sciences 27: 960–967 (1970)

[2] A. Berman, and R.J. Plemmons. *Nonnegative matrices in the mathematical sciences.* New York: Academic Press (1979)

[3] M.T. Chahine. *Inverse problems in radiative transfer: determination of atmospheric parameters.* J. Atmospheric Science 27: 960–967 (1970)

[4] W.P. Chu. *Convergence of Chahine's nonlinear relaxation method used for limb viewing remote sensing.* Applied Optics 24: 445–447 (1985)

[5] I. Csiszár. *I-divergence geometry of probability distributions and minimization problems.* Annals of Probability 3: 146–158 (1975)

[6] M.E. Daube-Witherspoon, and G. Muehllehner. *An iterative space reconstruction algorithm suitable for volume* ECT. IEEE Trans. Medical Imaging MI-5: 61–66 (1986)

[7] P.P.B. Eggermont. *Multiplicative iterative algorithms for convex programming.* Linear Algebra Appl. 130: 25–42 (1990)

[8] J. Hofbauer, and K. Sigmund. *The theory of evolution and dynamical systems.* Cambridge: Cambridge University Press (1988)

[9] D. Kinderlehrer, and G. Stampacchia. *An introduction to variational inequalities and their applications.* New York: Academic Press (1980)

[10] A.R. de Pierro. *On the convergence of the iterative image space reconstruction algorithm for volume* ECT. IEEE Trans. Medical Imaging MI-6: 174–175 (1987)

[11] A.R. de Pierro. *Nonlinear relaxation methods for solving symmetric linear complementarity problems.* J. Optimiz. Theory Appl. 64: 87–99 (1990)

[12] L.A. Shepp, and Y. Vardi. *Maximum likelihood reconstruction in emission tomography.* IEEE Trans. Medical Imaging MI-1: 113–122 (1982)

[13] S. Twomey. *Introduction to the mathematics of inversion in remote sensing and indirect measurements.* Amsterdam: Elsevier (1977)

[14] Y. Vardi, L.A. Shepp, and L. Kaufman. *A statistical model for positron emission tomography.* J. Amer. Statist. Assoc. 80: 8–38 (1985)

[15] V. Volterra. *Leçons sur la théorie mathématique de la lutte pour la vie.* Paris: Gauthier–Villars (1931)

Department of Mathematical Sciences
University of Delaware
Newark, DE 19716 / USA
e-mail: eggermont@brahms.udel.edu

Constrained regularized least squares problems

Tommy Elfving
Department of Mathematics. Linköping University.
S-581 83 Linköping, Sweden.

1 Introduction.

We consider the discrete linear model,

$$A_{k+1}x = a_{k+1} + e$$

where x is the unknown, A_{k+1} a given $q_{k+1} \times n$ matrix, a_{k+1} a vector of observations and e an unknown noise vector. (The meaning of the integer k will be explained in the next section). The model is assumed to arise from the discretization of an ill-posed problem, such as the Radon transform, $Rf = g$, used for modelling the X-ray attenuation in tomography, [5]. Then x_j denotes an approximation to f at the j:th gridpoint.

In ill-posed problems small changes in the observation vector can make large changes in the solution vector. One important technique to deal with this problem is Tichonov regularization, see e.g. [8], which favors solutions which are smooth in a certain sense (usually measured by a Sobolev norm). If the true solution also is known to be nonnegative ,which is the case for the attenuation function in tomography,[5], it is natural to use this information to eliminate undesired solutions.

In section 2 we formulate the Tichonov regularization problem using a discrete Sobolev norm. We also impose constraints of the general type $x \in C$, a closed convex set in R^n. The constraints include , in 1-D, nonnegativity, monotonicity and convexity and in 2-D nonnegativity. The problem is reformulated as a minimum norm problem with linear constraints. By using a dual formulation we show how the solution may be retrieved by solving a convex unconstrained optimization problem. We investigate the structure of the problem and derive expressions for the objective, the gradient and the Hessian potentially useful for computational purposes.

*The author benfitted from discussions with Dr. Lars-Erik Andersson.The research was done with support from the Swedish Natural Science Research Council under contract F-FU 9443-302

In section 3 the details of some important special cases, e.g. box-constraints and general linear inequality constraints, are studied.

In the last section an algorithmic schema is proposed which includes the steepest descent method, the nonlinear Conjugate Gradient method and Newton's method. In particular we consider the steplength calculation and outline how it can be efficiently done. We also discuss the implementation of the Newton iteration for some special cases.

The algorithmic part needs further research both from a theoretical and an experimental point of view. At this stage no numerical experiments have been made.

2 The problem

Before stating the problem some notation will be introduced. Let k be a fixed integer and

$$\{A_j\}, q_j \times n, \quad and \quad \{a_j\}, q_j \times 1, \quad j = 0, 1, ..., k+2$$

be given matrices and vectors. The index set J is a subset of the first $k+2$ nonnegative integers,

$$J \subseteq \{0, 1, ..., k+1\}.$$

We will consider the following constrained regularized least squares problem,

$$\min_x \left\{ \sum_{j=0}^{k} \|A_j x - a_j\|_2^2 + \sigma \|A_{k+1} x - a_{k+1}\|_2^2 \right\}, \tag{2.1}$$

with constraints

$$\bar{l}_j \leq A_j x \leq \bar{u}_j, j \in J, \quad A_{k+2} x = a_{k+2}, \tag{2.2}$$

where

$$\{\bar{l}_j, \bar{u}_j\}, q_j \times 1, \quad \bar{l}_j < \bar{u}_j, \quad j = 0, 1, ..., k+1, \tag{2.3}$$

are given upper and lower bounds and $\sigma \geq 0$ is a regularization parameter (usually $\sigma > 0$). Here we define

$$[\bar{l}_j]_i = -\infty, \quad [\bar{u}_j]_i = \infty, \quad i = 1, 2, .., q_j, \quad j \notin J,$$

using the notation $[l_j]_i$ for the $i:th$ component of a vector l_j.

We assume that the matrix A_{k+2} has full row-rank and that there exists an x^* such that

$$A_{k+2} x^* = a_{k+2}, \quad \bar{l}_j < A_j x^* < \bar{u}_j, j \in J. \tag{2.4}$$

Under this assumption and condition (5) below problem (1) has a unique solution.

The matrices $\{A_j\}_0^k$ correspond to a discrete Sobolev norm of order k. In accordance we assume that the matrix A_0 is the identity, i.e.

$$A_0 = I. \tag{2.5}$$

Note that we allow $A_j = 0 (a_j = 0)$ for $j > 0$.

Here and in the sequel I denotes the identity matrix, the order of which will be apparent from the context. As mentioned in the introduction the matrix A_{k+1} is normally ill-conditioned, e.g. resulting from the discretization of an integral equation of the first kind. There may also be additional constraints on the vector x which are expressed as a linear system of equations, $A_{k+2}x = a_{k+2}$. The index set J is used for imposing certain physically plausible constraints on the solution vector x. If e.g. $J = \{0\}, \bar{l}_0 = 0, \bar{u}_0 = \infty$ then problem (1) ,due to (5), is positively constrained. We will discuss some other applications in the following section.

To introduce a dual formulation of problem (1) we first let

$$y_j = \begin{cases} A_j x - a_j & j = 0, 1, ..., k, \\ (A_{k+1}x - a_{k+1})\sqrt{\sigma} & j = k+1, \end{cases} \tag{2.6}$$

and

$$y \in R^{\bar{q}}, \quad \bar{q} = \sum_0^{k+1} q_i, \qquad y^T = (y_0^T, y_1^T, ..., y_{k+1}^T).$$

Note that from (5)

$$x = y_0 + a_0.$$

The closed convex set C_J is

$$C_J = \begin{cases} \{y \in R^{\bar{q}} | l_j \le y_j \le u_j, j \in J\} & \text{if} J \ne \emptyset, \\ R^{\bar{q}} & \text{else}, \end{cases} \tag{2.7}$$

with

$$l_j = \bar{l}_j - a_j, \quad u_j = \bar{u}_j - a_j, \quad j = 0, 1, ..., k+1,$$

$$l_{k+1} = \sqrt{\sigma} l_{k+1}, \quad u_{k+1} = \sqrt{\sigma} u_{k+1}.$$

Then problem (1) becomes,

$$\min_y \|y\|_2^2, \qquad y \in C_J, \qquad By = b. \tag{2.8}$$

Put $k_0 = k$ if the constraint $A_{k+2}x = a_{k+2}$ is present in (2) and $k_0 = k - 1$ else.

Then

$$B = \begin{pmatrix} B_1 & -I \\ A_{k+2} & 0 \end{pmatrix}, \quad if \quad k = k_0, \qquad B = (B_1 \quad -I), \quad else. \tag{2.9}$$

Here

$$B_1^T = (A_1^T, A_2^T, ..., A_{k+1}^T), b^T = (b_1^T, b_2^T, ..., b_{k_0+2}^T), \quad b_j = a_j - A_j a_0, \tag{2.10}$$

where we have defined,

$$a_{k+1} := \sqrt{\sigma} a_{k+1}, A_{k+1} := \sqrt{\sigma} A_{k+1}.$$

The matrix B has dimension $\hat{q} \times \bar{q}$ with $\hat{q} = \sum_1^{k_0+2} q_i$. Note that $\hat{q} - \bar{q} = q_{k_0+2} - n$ and hence $By = b$ is underdetermined since $A_{k+2}x = a_{k+2}$ is so. It is easily seen that B has full row-rank and hence $By = b$ is a consistent system. Further

$$int(C_J) \cap \{y | By = b\} \neq \emptyset. \tag{2.11}$$

This follows from (4) (pick $(y_o + a_o) = x^*$). Now necessary and sufficient conditions for y to be the solution of (8) are,

$$y^T(z - y) \geq 0, \quad \forall z \in C_J \cap \{v | Bv = b\}.$$

Hence

$$(y^T - \lambda^T B)(z - y) \geq 0,$$

which are the necessary and sufficient conditions for the problem,

$$\min \|y - B^T\lambda\|_2^2, \qquad y \in C_J, By = b. \tag{2.12}$$

We have the following result.

Lemma 1 *Problem (8) has a unique solution y, which is related to the unique solution x of (1) by $x = y_0 + a_0$. Further y satifies the equations,*

$$BP_{C_J}(B^T\lambda) = b, \qquad y = P_{C_J}(B^T\lambda), \tag{2.13}$$

where P_C is the orthogonal projection onto the closed convex set C. Here $\lambda^T = (\lambda_1^T, \lambda_2^T, ..., \lambda_{k_0+2}^T)$, where $\lambda \in R^{\hat{q}}$ ($\lambda_j \in R^{q_j}$) is the dual vector corresponding to the constraints $By = b$. Conversely if for a given λ, $y = P_{C_J}(B^T\lambda)$ satisfies $By = b$ then y is the solution of problem (8) and $x = y_0 + a_0$ is the solution to problem (1).

Lemma 1 is valid for any closed convex set C_J.This Lemma was proved in [9] for the case $C = \{x|x \geq 0\}$. In [7], [1] generalizations to infinite dimensional cases are given.

Put

$$g(z) = \|z\|_2^2 - \|z - P_{C_J}(z)\|_2^2. \tag{2.14}$$

Let

$$f(\lambda) = 0.5g(B^T\lambda) - b^T\lambda \tag{2.15}$$

so that,

$$f(\lambda) = \lambda^T B P_{C_J}(B^T\lambda) - 0.5\|P_{C_J}(B^T\lambda)\|_2^2 - b^T\lambda. \tag{2.16}$$

Consider the *problem*

$$\min f(\lambda). \tag{2.17}$$

Then

Lemma 2 *$f \in C^1$, f is convex and $\nabla f = BP_{C_J}(B^T\lambda) - b$.*

Proof. Put $C = \{t \in R|a \leq t \leq b\}$. Then $P_C(t) = min(max(a,t),b)$. The function

$$r(t) = t^2 - (t - P_C(t))^2 \tag{2.18}$$

is easily shown to be convex and belonging to C^1. Now $g(z)$ decomposes into a sum of functions of type (18). It follows that $g(z)$, and by (15), $f(\lambda)$ are both convex and belong to C^1. By direct differentiation, $r'(t) = 2P_C(t)$. But $f'(\lambda) = 0.5Bg'(B^T\lambda) - b$. The expression for ∇f follows easily.

Remark 1. If $t \neq a, b$ in (18) then $r(t) \in C^\infty$. It follows that $f(\lambda) \in C^\infty$ at $\lambda = \lambda^*$ provided that with, $z^* = B^T\lambda^*$, $[z^*]_i \neq [l]_i, [u]_i$.

Lemma 3 *Problem (17) has at least one solution. For any solution λ of problem (17) $x = [P_{C_J}(B^T\lambda)]_0 + a_0$ is the unique solution of problem (1).*

Proof. If λ is a solution to (17) then $\nabla f(\lambda) = 0$ and the result follows from Lemma 2 and Lemma 1.

To show the existence of a solution it suffices to show that $f(\lambda)$ is coercive, i.e.

$$f(\lambda) \to \infty, \quad \|\lambda\|_2 \to \infty.$$

Take y^* such that $l_j < y_j^* < u_j, j \in J$ and $By^* = b$ (this is possible due to (11)). Then

$$f(\lambda) = < B^T\lambda, P_{C_J}(B^T\lambda) - y^* > -0.5\|P_{C_J}(B^T\lambda)\|_2^2 = \sum r_i(\lambda),$$

where

$$r_i(\lambda) = [B^T\lambda]_i[P_{C_J}(B^T\lambda) - y^*]_i - 0.5[P_{C_J}]_i^2,$$

and $< .,. >$ denotes the Euclidean scalarproduct. In this proof $[v]_i$ denotes the i:th (scalar) component of a vector v. Fix the value of λ and consider a specific i. We can distinguish between three cases.

Case (a). $[B^T\lambda]_i \geq [u]_i$. Then

$$r_i(\lambda) = [B^T\lambda]_i[u - y^*]_i - 0.5[u]_i^2.$$

Case (b). $[B^T\lambda]_i \leq [l]_i$. Then

$$r_i(\lambda) = [B^T\lambda]_i[l - y^*]_i - 0.5[l]_i^2.$$

Case (c). $l_i \leq [B^T\lambda]_i \leq [u]_i$. Then

$$r_i(\lambda) = 0.5[B^T\lambda]_i^2 - [B^T\lambda]_i[y^*]_i.$$

Now $\|B^T\lambda\|_2^2 \geq \sigma_{min}^2(B^T)\|\lambda\|_2^2$, where $\sigma_{min}(B^T) > 0$ is the smallest singular value of B^T. Hence at least one component $[B^T\lambda]_i$ must be unbounded as $\|\lambda\|_2 \to \infty$. It follows that

$$f(\lambda) = \sum r_i(\lambda) \to \infty, \quad \|\lambda\|_2 \to \infty.$$

We remark that proofs of Lemma 2 and 3 are given by Michelli and Utreras (Lemma 3.1 and Theorem 3.2 in [7]) for C_J a closed convex set in a Hilbert space. We believe it is instructive to provide separate proofs for our special set C_J (7). It also makes this paper selfcontained.

We now consider the specific convex set (7) in more detail. Put

$$z = B^T\lambda.$$

Let D_l, D_u be diagonal matrices of order $\bar{q}\times\bar{q}$, and D_l^j, D_u^j diagonal matrices of order $q_j \times q_j$ defined as follows,

$$D_l(z) = diag(D_l^j), \quad D_u(z) = diag(D_u^j), \quad j = 0, 1, ..., k+1. \tag{2.19}$$

$$D_l^j = \begin{cases} diag(\rho_j^i), & j \in J, \\ I, & j \notin J. \end{cases} \tag{2.20}$$

$$D_u^j = \begin{cases} diag(\mu_j^i), & j \in J, \\ I, & j \notin J. \end{cases} \tag{2.21}$$

Here

$$\rho_j^i = \begin{cases} 1, & if \quad [z_j]_i \geq [l_j]_i, \\ 0 & else, \end{cases}$$

$$\mu_j^i = \begin{cases} 1, & if \quad [z_j]_i \leq [u_j]_i, \\ 0 & else. \end{cases}$$

Define

$$[(I - D_l^j)l_j]_i = 0, \quad [(I - D_u^j)u_j]_i = 0, \tag{2.22}$$

when $[l_j]_i = -\infty$ and $[u_j]_i = \infty$ repectively. Then

$$P_{C_J}(z) = D_l D_u z + (I - D_l)l + (I - D_u)u, \tag{2.23}$$

where

$$u = (u_0^T, u_1^T, ..., u_{k+1}^T)^T, l = (l_0^T, l_1^T, ..., l_{k+1}^T)^T.$$

Also as is easily checked,

$$\|P_{C_J}(z)\|_2^2 = z^T D_l D_u z + l^T (I - D_l)l + u^T (I - D_u)u.$$

Hence the following expression holds,

$$f(\lambda) = 0.5\lambda^T B D_l D_u B^T \lambda + (\lambda^T B - 0.5 l^T)(I - D_l)l \tag{2.24}$$
$$+(\lambda^T B - 0.5u^T)(I - D_u)u - b^T \lambda,$$

and

$$\nabla f(\lambda) = B D_l D_u B^T \lambda + B(I - D_l)l + B(I - D_u)u - b. \tag{2.25}$$

If the conditions in *Remark* 1 hold then $f \in C^\infty$ and

$$\nabla^2 f(\lambda) = B D_l D_u B^T. \tag{2.26}$$

Put $d_1 = \bar{q} - \hat{q}$ and let d_2 be the number of zero elements in the diagonal of the matrix $D_l D_u$. If $d_2 > d_1$ then $\nabla^2 f(\lambda)$ is always singular.

By Lemma 3,

$$x = [D_l D_u B^T \lambda + (I - D_l)l + (I - D_u)u]_0 + a_0. \tag{2.27}$$

We now utilize the special structure of the matrix B to decompose the expressions for f, its gradient and Hessian further. Put

$$B_2^T = (A_1^T, A_2^T, ..., A_{k_0+2}^T).$$

Note that $B_1 = B_2$ if $k_0 = k - 1$. Then

$$z^T = (B^T \lambda)^T = ((B_2^T \lambda)^T, -\lambda_1^T, ..., -\lambda_{k+1}^T).$$

It follows from (20) that,

$$[D_l^0(\lambda)]_i = [D_l^0]_i = \begin{cases} 1 & if \quad [B_2^T \lambda]_i \geq [l_0]_i, \\ 0 & else. \end{cases} \tag{2.28}$$

and for $j > 0$,

$$[D_l^j(\lambda)]_i = [D_l^j]_i = \begin{cases} 1 & if \quad [-\lambda_j]_i \geq [l_j]_i, \\ 0 & else. \end{cases} \tag{2.29}$$

Similiar expressions hold for $D_u^j(\lambda)$. Using the above expression the formulas for f and ∇f become,

$$\begin{aligned} f = {} & 0.5\lambda^T B_2 D_l^0 D_u^0 B_2^T \lambda + 0.5\lambda^T \bar{D}_l \bar{D}_u \lambda + \lambda^T B_2 (I - D_l^0) l_0 \\ & -\lambda^T (I - \bar{D}_l)\bar{l} - 0.5 l^T (I - D_l) l + \lambda^T B_2 (I - D_u^0) u_0 \\ & -\lambda^T (I - \bar{D}_u)\bar{u} - 0.5 u^T (I - D_u) u - b^T \lambda, \end{aligned} \tag{2.30}$$

and

$$\begin{aligned} \nabla f = {} & B_2 D_l^0 D_u^0 B_2^T \lambda + \bar{D}_l \bar{D}_u \lambda + B_2 (I - D_l^0) l_0 - (I - \bar{D}_l)\bar{l} \\ & + B_2 (I - D_u^0) u_0 - (I - \bar{D}_u)\bar{u} - b, \end{aligned} \tag{2.31}$$

where

$$\begin{aligned} \bar{D}_l &= diag(D_l^j), j = 1, 2, ..., k_0 + 2, \quad D_l^{k+2} = 0, \\ \bar{l} &= (l_1^T, l_2^T, ..., l_{k_0+2}^T), \quad l_{k+2} = 0. \end{aligned} \tag{2.32}$$

Similiar definitions hold for $\bar{D}_u, \bar{l}_u$. If the conditions in *Remark* 1 hold then $f \in C^\infty$ and

$$\nabla^2 f(\lambda) = B_2 D_l^0 D_u^0 B_2^T + \bar{D}_l \bar{D}_u. \tag{2.33}$$

Note that $\nabla^2 f(\lambda)$ is non singular iff

$$N(B_2 D_l^0 D_u^0) \cap N(\bar{D}_l \bar{D}_u) = \emptyset, \tag{2.34}$$

where $N(B)$ denotes the nullspace of the matrix B. Further,

$$x = D_l^0 D_u^0 B_2^T \lambda + (I - D_l^0) l_0 + (I - D_u^0) u_0 + a_0. \tag{2.35}$$

3 Applications

We now consider in more detail some special instances of problem (2.1). Take $k = 1$ in (2.1). Then the objective function becomes,

$$\min_x \|x - a_0\|_2^2 + \|A_1 x - a_1\|_2^2 + \sigma \|A_2 x - a_2\|_2^2. \tag{3.1}$$

It follows,

$$B_2^T = \begin{cases} (A_1^T, \sqrt{\sigma} A_2^T), & k_0 = k-1, \\ (A_1^T, \sqrt{\sigma} A_2^T, A_3^T), & k_0 = k. \end{cases} \tag{3.2}$$

The second case occurs when equality constraints are present.

We will investigate different constraint sets (2.2) associated with (1) and start with two types of box constraints. First let $J = \{0\}$, $k_0 = k - 1 = 0$ i.e.

$$\bar{l}_0 \le x \le \bar{u}_0. \tag{3.3}$$

Then it follows from (2.31), (2.33),

$$\nabla f(\lambda) = B_2 D_l^0 D_u^0 B_2^T \lambda + \lambda + B_2(I - D_l^0)(\bar{l}_0 - a_0) + B_2(I - D_u^0)(\bar{u}_0 - a_0) - b, \tag{3.4}$$

$$\nabla^2 f(\lambda) = B_2 D_l^0 D_u^0 B_2^T + I, \tag{3.5}$$

where $b^T = (b_1^T, b_2^T)$ and

$$b_1 = a_1 - A_1 a_0, \quad b_2 = (a_2 - A_2 a_0)\sqrt{\sigma}. \tag{3.6}$$

A possible application arises with A_2 equal a discretization of the 2-D Radon transform and A_1 a 2-D discrete Laplacian. The constraints (3) come from physical considerations [5].

Next let $J = \{1\}$, $k_0 = k - 1$, i.e.

$$\bar{l}_1 \le A_1 x \le \bar{u}_1. \tag{3.7}$$

Then again it follows by (2.31), (2.33),

$$\nabla f(\lambda) = B_2 B_2^T \lambda + \bar{D}_l \bar{D}_u \lambda - (I - \bar{D}_l)\bar{l} - (I - \bar{D}_u)\bar{u} - b, \tag{3.8}$$

$$\nabla^2 f(\lambda) = B_2 B_2^T + \bar{D}_l \bar{D}_u. \tag{3.9}$$

Here b is defined from (6) and

$$\bar{D}_l = diag(D_l^1, I), \quad \bar{l}^T(I - \bar{D}_l) = (l_1^T(I - D_l^1), 0^T),$$

with $l_1 = \bar{l}_1 - a_1$. Similiar definitions hold for $\bar{D}_u$. The solution is obtained from (2.35),

$$x = B_2^T \lambda + a_0. \tag{3.10}$$

A possible application would be the computation of discrete monotone or convex 1-D splines. Then $a_0 = a_1 = 0, A_1 =$ bidiag(1,-1) (the monotone case) or $A_1 =$ tri(1,-2,1) (the convex case) and A_2 a subset of the rows of the identity matrix of order n. Note that this choice of norm does not correspond to polynomial splines.

Consider next $J = \{0, 2\}, k_0 = k - 1$ and only lower constraints of the following form,

$$x \geq 0, \quad A_2 x \geq a_2. \tag{3.11}$$

Then

$$D_l = diag(D_l^0, I, D_l^2), \quad \bar{D}_l = diag(I, D_l^2),$$

and one can easily derive expressions for $f, \nabla f, \nabla^2 f$. A possible application is the calculation of the dose plan in radiation therapy. Here $\bar{l}_2 = a_2$ is the wanted dose and $A_2 x$ the injected one. From a medical point of view it is important that $A_2 x \geq a_2$. Since x has the physical meaning of irradiation density nonnegativity is also a natural constraint ,[6].

In our next example $J = \{0, 1\}, \quad k_0 = k = 1$ with only lower constraints i.e.

$$x \geq \bar{l}_0, \quad A_1 x \geq \bar{l}_1, \quad A_3 x = a_3. \tag{3.12}$$

Then by (2.31), (2.33),

$$\nabla f = B_2 D_l^0 B_2^T \lambda + \bar{D}_l \lambda + B_2 (I - D_l^0) l_0 - (I - \bar{D}_l) \bar{l} - b, \tag{3.13}$$

$$\nabla^2 f(\lambda) = B_2 D_l^0 B_2^T \lambda + \bar{D}_l. \tag{3.14}$$

Here

$$\bar{D}_l = diag(D_l^1, I, 0), \quad \bar{l}^T (I - \bar{D}_l) = (l_1^T (I - D_l^1), 0^T, 0^T),$$

with $b^T = (b_1^T, b_2^T, b_3^T)$ as defined in (2.10) and $l_j = \bar{l}_j - a_j$.

We next observe specially the case $k = 0$ in (2.1), under nonnegativity constraints,

$$\min_{x \geq 0} \quad \|x - a_0\|_2^2 + \sigma \|A_1 x - a_1\|_2^2. \tag{3.15}$$

Here $k_0 = k - 1 = -1$ and

$$B_2 = \sqrt{\sigma} A_1, b = \sqrt{\sigma}(a_1 - A_1 a_0), l_0 = -a_0,$$

and by (2.31)

$$\nabla f = \sigma A_1 D_l^0 A_1^T \lambda + \lambda + \sqrt{\sigma} A_1 D_l^0 a_0 - \sqrt{\sigma} a_1. \tag{3.16}$$

Again if the conditions in *Remark* 1 i.e.

$$[A_1^T \lambda]_i \neq [-a_0]_i$$

are satisfied then,

$$\nabla^2 f(\lambda) = I + \sigma A_1 D_l^0 A_1^T.$$

The expression for the solution is by (2.35),

$$x = \sqrt{\sigma} D_l^0 A_1^T \lambda + D_l^0 a_0. \tag{3.17}$$

As the final example we mention the minimum norm problem with non-negativity constraints,

$$\min_{x \geq 0} \|x\|_2^2, \quad A_1 x = a_1. \tag{3.18}$$

Then

$$f(\lambda) = 0.5\|(A_1^T \lambda)_+\|_2^2 - a_1^T \lambda. \tag{3.19}$$

$$\nabla f = A_1 (A_1^T \lambda)_+ - a_1, \quad \nabla^2 f = A_1 D_l^0 A_1^T, \quad x = (A_1^T \lambda)_+. \tag{3.20}$$

Here $(x)_+$ denotes the positive part of x.

4 Algorithms

Consider the following gradient type algorithm for solving problem (2.17).

$$p^0 = -M^0 \nabla f(\lambda^0) \tag{4.1}$$

$$\lambda^{n+1} = \lambda^n + \alpha_n p^n \tag{4.2}$$

$$p^{n+1} = -M^{n+1} \nabla f(\lambda^{n+1}) + \beta_{n+1} p^n. \tag{4.3}$$

Here λ^n is the n :th iterate. The vector p^n is the n :th search direction. We shall assume that $\{p^n\}$ are descent directions, i.e. fulfill

$$p^{n^T} \nabla f(\lambda^n) < 0. \tag{4.4}$$

The matrix $[M^n]^{-1}$ is a positive definite approximation to the second derivative of $f(\lambda^n)$. The choice of the preconditioning matrix M^n affects the rate of convergence of the algorithm. If no second derivative information is available a simple choice is $M^n = I$. We shall consider the following choices of the iteration parameter β.

$$\beta = \begin{cases} 0 \\ \frac{<\nabla f^{n+1}, M^{n+1} \nabla f^{n+1}>}{<\nabla f^n, M^n \nabla f^n>} \\ \frac{<y^n, M^{n+1} \nabla f^{n+1}>}{<\nabla f^n, M^n \nabla f^n>}, \qquad y^n = \nabla f^{n+1} - \nabla f^n. \end{cases}$$

$(\nabla f^n = \nabla f(\lambda^n).)$ The choice $\beta_n = 0, \quad M^n = I$ gives a gradient type method. In [2] such an algorithm was considered for a problem (solution of linear inequalities) resembling the problem treated here. Newton's method arises for the choice $M^n = [\nabla^2 f^n]^{-1}$ and $\beta_n = 0$. The other two choices of β is picked in analogy with the quadratic case where, as is well known , convergence occurs after a finite number of iterations and the two choices give mathematically identical iterates. In the non quadratic case the last choice has the potential advantage of, in case of slow convergence , giving automatic restart along the gradient direction, [3],[4].

Put

$$h(\alpha) = f(\lambda + \alpha p).$$

The steplength α is at each iteration picked as the solution to the problem

$$\min_{\alpha > 0} h(\alpha). \tag{4.5}$$

Now $f(\lambda)$ is convex and it follows easily that $h(\alpha)$ also is convex. Also

$$h(\alpha) \to \infty, \quad \alpha \to \infty. \tag{4.6}$$

This follows from the corresponding result for $f(\lambda)$, Lemma 3,(note also that $p \neq 0$ by assumption (4)). Let

$$h'(\alpha) = p^T \nabla f(\lambda + \alpha p) := \varphi(\alpha). \tag{4.7}$$

Then $\varphi(0) < 0$ by (4), $\varphi(\infty) > 0$ by (6) and $\varphi(\alpha)$ is monotone increasing. Hence $h(\alpha)$ has a global minimum which can be found by solving the equation

$$\varphi(\alpha) = 0. \tag{4.8}$$

We now show that assumption (4) is fulfilled and first observe as in [4] that (8) implies,

$$< p^1, \nabla f^1 >= - < \nabla f^1, M^1 \nabla f^1 >< 0.$$

Hence p^1 and by induction p^n are all descent directions.

We now return to the step length calculation and remark that in our application $\varphi(\alpha)$ is piecewise linear and from Lemma 2,

$$\varphi(\alpha) = p^T B P_{C_J}(B^T(\lambda + \alpha p)) - p^T b.$$

Using expression (2.23) with $z = B^T(\lambda + \alpha p)$ and putting

$$v = B^T \lambda, \quad w = B^T p$$

the following equivalent formulation of (8) appears,

$$\alpha = \psi(\alpha). \tag{4.9}$$

Here

$$\psi(\alpha) = (p^T b + w^T (D_l - I)l + w^T (D_u - I)u - w^T D_l D_u v)/w^T D_l D_u w, \quad (4.10)$$

where $D_l = D_l(v + \alpha w)$, $D_u = D_u(v + \alpha w)$.

We briefly outline how the nonlinear equation (9) can be solved. Compute the sequence $\{\alpha_j\}$, $\alpha_1 < \alpha_2 < .. < \alpha_p$, such that, at each interval $int(j) = (\alpha_j, \alpha_{j+1})$, the matrices D_l, D_u are fixed. Evaluate $\psi(\alpha)$, $\alpha \in int(j)$. This can be done efficiently by updating only the component of $D_l(D_u)$ that has been changed. If $\psi(\alpha) \in int(j)$ the solution has been found else proceed to interval $int(j+1)$. The computation of $\{\alpha_j\}$ involves forming two new vectors ($ll_i = [l - v]_i / w_i, w_i \neq 0$ for D_l and similarly for D_u) and sorting them after size.

We end this section by considering specifically one algoritmic example: Newton's method. Then in each step we must solve for Δ in

$$\nabla^2 f(\lambda^n)\Delta = -\nabla f(\lambda^n), \quad (4.11)$$

and iterate as

$$\lambda^{n+1} = \lambda^n + \Delta.$$

Using (2.25) and (2.26) the Newton iteration becomes,

$$BD_l^{[n]} D_u^{[n]} B^T \lambda^{n+1} = -B[(I - D_l^{[n]})l + (I - D_u^{[n]})u] + b. \quad (4.12)$$

Consider in particular the case with only lower constraints, the lower bound being the zero vector, and with no equality constraints (i.e. $k_0 = k - 1$). Then it is easy to verify that the right hand side vector in the iteration (12) becomes $-BD_l a$. Hence at each iteration a linear least squares problem arises,

$$\min \|X\lambda^{n+1} - d\|_2$$

with

$$X^T = BD_l^{[n]}, \quad d^T = (-a_0^T, -a_1^T, .., -\sqrt{\sigma} a_{k+1}^T).$$

As an example consider problem (3.15) where

$$X^T = (\sqrt{\sigma} A_1 D_l^0, I), \quad d^T = (-a_0^T, -\sqrt{\sigma} a_1^T).$$

References

[1] L-E.Andersson, T.Elfving:*Interpolation and Approximation by Monotone Cubic Splines.* LiTH-MAT-R-1990-03. Linköping University (1990).(To appear in J. of Approx. Theory).

[2] Y.Censor, T.Elfving, G.T.Herman: *Regularized least squares solution of linear inequalities.* Technical Report MIPG97. Dept. of Radiology, University of Pennsylvania (1985).

[3] P.Concus, G.H.Golub, D.P.O'Leary: *Numerical Solution of Nonlinear Elliptic Partial Differential Equations by a Generalized Conjugate Gradient Method.* Computing 19, 321-339 (1978).

[4] P.E.Gill, W.Murray, M.H.Wright:*Practical Optimization.* Academic Press 1981.

[5] G.T.Herman:*Image Reconstruction from Projections: The fundamentals of computerized tomography.* Academic Press 1980.

[6] B.K.Lind: *Properties of an algorithm for solving the inverse problem in radiation theraphy.* Inverse Problems 6, 415-426 (1990).

[7] C.A.Micchelli, F.I.Utreras: *Smoothing and Interpolation in a convex Subset of a Hilbert Space.* SIAM J.Sci.Stat.Comput.9, 728-747 (1988).

[8] F.Natterer: *The Mathematics of Computerized Tomography.* Teubner,Wiley 1986.

[9] P.W.Smith, H.Wolkowicz:*A nonlinear equation for linear Programming.* Math.Programming 34, 235-238 (1986).

MULTIPLICATIVE ITERATIVE METHODS IN COMPUTED TOMOGRAPHY

Alvaro R. De Pierro
Instituto de Matemática, Estatística e Ciência da Computação
Universidade Estadual de Campinas
13081 Campinas, SP, Brazil

- Introduction

The problem of image reconstruction from projections (reconstructing a function from its line integrals) has arisen independently in many scientific fields: astrophysics, geophysics, medicine and others. Particularly in medicine, computerized tomography (CT) has been a revolutionary technique for clinical diagnosis [33].

We are concerned here with methods for solving two important versions of this problem: transmission computerized tomography (TCT) and emission computed tomography (ECT). In TCT we aim to obtain the density distribution within a cross-section of the human body from multiple x-ray projections; i.e., mathematically speaking, there is an unknown compact-supported function f defined in $\mathbb{R}^2$ representing relative tissue density, a finite number of measurements are given approximating integrals of f along lines and we have to reconstruct f from these data. Two approaches have been used to solve this problem. The first one deals with methods aiming to approximate the inverse of the transformation defined by the line integrals (the Radon Transform); this type of methods are called transform methods [47] and one of them, convolution-backprojection, has been universally adopted for medical purposes. The second approach consists of discretizing the model at an early stage of the process, leading to a finite dimensional algebraic system of linear equations (equalities or inequalities depending on noise considerations) from which a solution has to be chosen using some optimization criterion (or not); the huge size of those systems of equations leads to the use of row-action iterative methods [5] for solving such systems.

In spite of the fact that transform methods in TCT are in practice more efficient than iterative methods, they are still recognized as useful tools in several specific situations in medical imagining and in non-medical applications of image reconstruction (see [34], [1] and [29] for example). A complete discussion of the advantages and disavantages of both approaches can be found in [6], [10] and [50].

In ECT, advantages of transform methods are not so clear and convolution-backprojection doesn't work so well. In this case, the objective is to reconstruct the distribution of radioactivity inside the body [59] and, in recent years, important experimental research has been done using iterative methods since the paper by Shepp and Vardi [53] on the EM algorithm.

Beyond the polemics on what is better to be used in each particular situation, it is clear that in inverse problems solving, incorporating "a priori" information is crucial to obtain better results and this is easier for iterative methods that enable us to handle this information in a flexible way through the use of constraints or penalization terms in the objective function. One of these constraints, always essential in image reconstruction, is nonnegativity; so, several iterative methods have been proposed preserving this property in a natural way. This is done up-dating current iterates multiplicatively instead of additively.

In this work we present a brief review of those multiplicative methods in CT, we generalize some of them and analyse and prove some of their convergence properties. Finally we point out similarities and differences with related methods used for solving other inverse problems, especially in image restoration [48], [52] and remote sensing ([14], [15] and [60]). An almost exhaustive list of these type of methods in image restoration can be found in [49].

In the following two sections we describe the optimization or/and feasibility problems, multiplicative methods aim to solve and give general definitions and notation. In section IV we present MART-type algorithms, we generalize Log-MART [9] to blocks and prove its convergence and we give convergence proofs for QMART1 and QMART 2 [27].

In section V we present the EM algorithm and its sequential version [22].

Section VI is devoted to the Image Space Reconstruction Algorithm (ISRA) [19] and in section VII we give a general scheme for adapting the EM algorithm for penalized maximum likelihood [46].

II – Optimization and Feasibility Problems

In TCT we usually deal with the problem of finding a solution of the system

$$Ax = b\,, \tag{1}$$

$$x \geq 0\,, \tag{2}$$

where $A = \{a_{ij}\} \in \mathbb{R}_+^{m\times n}$ is the projection matrix (nonnegative) and $b \in \mathbb{R}_+^m$ is the projection data vector. In the presence of noise, (1) may be replaced by finding nonnegative solutions of the system of inequalities

$$b - \varepsilon \leq Ax \leq b + \varepsilon\,, \tag{3}$$

where ε is an error vector.

Frequently, solutions of (1-2) and (2-3) are not unique. So, one should be chosen using some optimization criterion, and problem (1-2) becomes

$$\begin{aligned} &\text{minimize} \quad f(x)\,, \\ &\text{subject to} \quad Ax = b\,,\ x \geq 0\,. \end{aligned} \tag{4}$$

or (2-3)

$$\begin{aligned} &\text{minimize} \quad f(x)\,, \\ &\text{subject to} \quad b_i \leq Ax \leq b_2\,,\ x \geq 0\,. \end{aligned} \tag{5}$$

Two common choices of F giving rise to multiplicative methods are

$$f(x) = -\text{ent}x = \sum_{j=1}^{n} x_j \log x_j \,, \tag{6}$$

and

$$f(x) = -\log\text{-ent}x = -\sum_{j=1}^{n} \log x_j \,, \tag{7}$$

being the first option the well known Shannon's entropy [45] and the second the Burg's entropy [4]. An extensive literature can be found theoretically and practically justifying the use of (6) or (7) in many areas of application (see [38], [39], [40] and [45]). In image reconstruction, use of these criteria has been proposed on a more experimental basis (see [10], [30] and [44]).

In ECT, low photon statistics and attenuation gave rise to different models, based on the Poisson nature of the underlying problem ([43], [54]) or a least squares fitting [21]. So, the mathematical optimization problem to be solved is

$$\begin{aligned} &\text{minimize} \quad f(x)\,, \\ &\text{subject to} \quad x \geq 0\,, \end{aligned} \tag{8}$$

where

$$-f(x) = \sum_{i=1}^{n} b_i \log\langle a_i, x\rangle - \langle a_i, x\rangle \tag{9}$$

is the log-likelihood function associated with the emission process to be maximized or

$$f(x) = \|b - Ax\|^2 = \sum_{i=1}^{n} (b_i - \langle a_i, x\rangle)^2 \,, \tag{10}$$

the least squares function to be minimized. $\langle\cdot\rangle$ denotes the standard inner product and $\|\cdot\|$ the associated norm; a_i are the column vectors of A and the conditions

$$\sum_{i=1}^{m} a_{ij} = 1 \quad \text{for } j = 1, \ldots, n \tag{11}$$

and

$$\sum_{i=1}^{m} b_i = 1\,, \tag{12}$$

hold. A complete description of the model for positron emission tomography (PET) using (9) can be found in [54].

Sometimes, the use of penalization containing "a priori" information is recommended to cope with noise that produces disturbing effects in the image [46]. In those situations the function f takes the form

$$f(x) = g(x) - \gamma p(x)\,, \tag{13}$$

where f is the function defined by (9) or (10), p is a real valued convex function (concave for least squares) and γ a real positive number. Different functions p have been proposed in the literature ([31], [35]).

III – Multiplicative or Nonlinear Relaxation Methods

Most of the existing methods in optimization and feasibility problems consist in generating a sequence in such a way that the current iterate x^k is up-dated adding a direction vector d^k as follows

$$x^{k+1} = x^k + \alpha_k d^k \ , \tag{14}$$

where α_k is a search parameter, or, coordinate-wise

$$x_j^{k+1} = x_j^k + \alpha_k d_j^k \ , \quad \text{for } j = 1, \ldots, n \ . \tag{15}$$

d^k is a descent (or ascent) direction and α_k is computed in order to satisfy the feasibility conditions.

Multiplicative methods instead, are generated using a multiplicative up-dating in such a way that nonnegative constraints are automatically satisfied and no parameter's choice has to be done; i.e.,

$$x_j^{k+1} = x_j^k c_j^k \ , \quad \text{for } j = 1, \ldots, n \tag{16}$$

where c_j^k is a positive real number or x_j^{k+1} is the result of solving an equation with positive solutions.

Of course, it is always possible to express (16) in the form

$$x_j^{k+1} = x_j^k + (c_j^k - 1) x_j^k \tag{17}$$

which is equivalent to (15) with relaxation parameter always equal to one. Or

$$x^{k+1} = x^k + D^k d^k \ , \tag{18}$$

where D^k is an iteration dependent diagonal matrix. Because of this interpretation some multiplicative methods are known in other areas of application as nonlinear relaxation methods (see [15], [23] and [24]).

In the same way as additive methods are related with norms (gradient-type methods) and euclidean distances or squares norms, multiplicative methods are related to more general measures sometimes called entropic-distances [58]. One important example of these "distances" is the Kullback-Leibler (KL) information divergence [41]

$$D(x, y) = \sum_{j=1}^{n} x_j \log \frac{x_j}{y_j} + y_j - x_j \ . \tag{19}$$

The KL distance is included in the larger family of Bregman-distances defined as follows [11].

Let Λ be a subset of $I\!R^n$, and let $f : \Lambda \to I\!R$ be a real valued function defined on Λ. Let S be a nonempty convex set such that $\overline{S} \subseteq \Lambda$. Assume that $f(x)$ has continuous first partial derivatives at any $x \in S$ and denote by $\nabla f(x)$ its gradient at x. From f, construct the function $D : \overline{S} \times S \subseteq I\!R^{2n} \to I\!R$ by

$$D(x, y) = f(x) - f(y) - \langle \nabla f(y), x - y \rangle \ . \tag{20}$$

Consider the partial level sets

$$L_1(y, \alpha) = \{x \in \overline{S} = D(x, y) \leq \alpha\} \ , \tag{21}$$

$$L_2(y, \alpha) = \{x \in S = D(x, y) \leq \alpha\} \ . \tag{22}$$

Definition 1: f is called a Bregman function if

i) $f(x)$ is continuously differentiable at every $x \in S$

ii) f is strictly convex on $\overline{S}$

iii) f is continuous on $\overline{S}$

iv) for every $\alpha \in \mathbb{R}$, $L_1(y,\alpha)$ and $L_2(x,\alpha)$ are bounded for every $y \in S$ and every $x \in \overline{S}$ respectively;

v) if $y^k \to y^* \in \overline{S}$, then $D(y^*, y^k) \to 0$

vi) if $D(x^k, y^k) \underset{k\to\infty}{\longrightarrow} 0$, $y^k \to y^* \in \overline{S}$ and $\{x^k\}$ is bounded, then $x^k \underset{k\to\infty}{\longrightarrow} y^*$.

We denote the family of Bregman functions by B and refer to the set S as the zone of the function f. With this definitions -ent$x \in B$ with zone $S = \mathbb{R}^n_+$. A slight generalization of B can be obtained substituting in the Definition above $\overline{S}$ by S. In such a case – log-ent x is an extended Bregman function ($\tilde{B}$), and the associated distance

$$D(x,y) = \sum_{j=1}^{n} \log \frac{y_j}{x_j} + \frac{x_j}{y_j} - n . \tag{23}$$

Proposition 1. For every $f \in \tilde{B}$, $D(x,y) \geq 0$ and $D(x,y) = 0$ iff $x = y$.

Proof. See [11], Lemma 2.1.

Let now

$$H = \{x \in \mathbb{R}^n \ / \ \langle a, x\rangle = b\} , \tag{24}$$

for a given vector $a \in \mathbb{R}^n$ and $b \in \mathbb{R}$. Then we define the D-projection of $y \in \mathbb{R}^n$ onto H as

$$P_H y = \arg \min_{x \in \overline{S} \cap H} D(x,y) . \tag{25}$$

If $P_H y \in S$ for every y, we say that f is zone consistent with respect to H [11], if this is valid for every parallel hyperplane between y and H, f is said to be strongly zone consistent [11]. In this case $P_H y$ is defined by the unique solution of

$$\nabla f(x) = \nabla f(y) + \lambda a , \tag{26}$$

$$\langle a, x\rangle = b , \tag{27}$$

where λ is a real parameter uniquely determined when a and b are fixed ([11] Lemma 3.1).

Before the presentation of the methods we previously need to give some definitions related to block partitions and sequences control as in [13].

Let

$$I = \{1, 2, \ldots, m\} , \tag{28}$$

r a positive integer such that $r \leq m$ and $\{m_t\}_{t=0}^{r}$ a sequence of positive integers such that

$$0 = m_0 < m_1 < m_2 \cdots m_{r-1} < m_r = m \; . \tag{29}$$

For $t = 1, 2, \ldots, r$, $T_t \subseteq I$ is defined by

$$I_t = \{m_{t-1} + 1, m_{t-1} + 2, \ldots, m_t\} \; ; \tag{30}$$

i.e.; $\{m_t\}$ defines a block-partition of I and I_t is the index set for the t-th block.

Definition 2. A sequence i_k is called an almost cyclic control for the set $R = \{1, 2, \ldots, n\}$ if there exists a constant C such that for every k, $R \subseteq \{i_k+1, \ldots, i_k+C\}$. C is the constant of almost cyclicallity [5].

IV – MART-type Algorithms

The relaxed Bregman's algorithm [26] for solving (4) is defined by, given $x^k \in S$,

$$x^{k+1} = P_{i_k} x^k \; , \tag{31}$$

where P_{i_k} is the Bregman projection of x^k onto the hyperplane

$$H_{i_k} = \{x \in I\!R^n \; / \; \langle a_{i_k}, x\rangle = \alpha_k b_{i_k} + (1 - \alpha_k)\langle a_{i_k}, x^k\rangle\} \tag{32}$$

being a_{i_k} the rows of A chosen in an almost cyclic manner and α_k a relaxation parameter less than one and bounded alway from zero. If the function f is strongly zone consistent, convergence of (31) to a solution of (4) is proven in [26] if $\nabla f(x^0) \in R(A^t)$. For a general starting point the limit of the sequence will solve the problem

$$\min_{x \in \bar{S}} D(x, x^0) \; , \quad \text{subject to} \quad Ax = b \tag{33}$$

i.e., the limit will be the Bregman projection of the starting point onto the feasible set.

One of the main drawbacks of (31) is that a nonlinear system derived from (26)-(27) should be solved each step for the parameter λ. For the maximum entropy problem (f given by (6)) if the matrix elements are scaled between zero and one; i.e.,

$$0 \leq a_{ij} \leq 1 \quad \text{for every} \;\; i, j \tag{34}$$

and

$$b_i > 0 \;\; , \text{for} \;\; i = 1, \ldots, m \tag{35}$$

a particular choice of α_k in (32) gives rise to MART (multiplicative algebraic reconstruction technique) the first multiplicative method in image reconstruction, proposed by Gordon et al. [30].

MART.

Given a starting $x^0 > 0$

$$x_j^{k+1} = x_j^k \left(\frac{b_{i_k}}{\langle a_{i_k}, x^k \rangle} \right)^{a_{ij}}, \text{ for } j = 1, \ldots, n \tag{36}$$

Convergence of (36) was first proven in [44] but only in [8] was established the close relation between (36) and Bregman's method. Not any rate of convergence result is known so far, although we conjecture that it is linear except for boundary solution points (x_j and $b_i - \langle a_i, x \rangle = 0$ means that $\lim_{k \to \infty} \frac{x_j^{k+1}}{x_j^k} = 1$, so convergence cannot be linear).

MART is essentially a sequential method since only one equation is processed at a given moment. A block version suitable for parallel computing with its convergence proofs was proposed in [13] based in an algorithm derived in [18].

Parallel MART.

Given a starting $x^0 > 0$

$$x_j^{k+1} = x_j^k \Pi_{i \in I_t} \left(\frac{a_i}{\langle a^i, x^k \rangle} \right)^{\omega_i a_{ij}}, \text{ for } j = 1, \ldots, n \,; \tag{37}$$

where the ω_i's are positive real numbers such that

$$\sum_{i \in I_t} \omega_i = 1 \,, \tag{38}$$

I_t defined in section III and t being an almost cyclic control for R. For the case of I_t being a singleton we retrieve MART, but in the general case not any connection has been established so far between (37) and Bregman's method.

If the function to be minimized is (7), the same convergence results can be proven for algorithm (31) [9]. In that case, as before, it is possible to avoid the computation of the parameter λ of equation (26) and the sequence defined is as follows [9].

Log-entropy MART.

Given a positive starting x^0,

$$x_j^{k+1} = \frac{x_j^k}{1 - a_{ij} x_j^k c_k}, \text{ for } j = 1, \ldots, n \,, \tag{39}$$

where

$$c_k = \lambda_k \left(1 - \frac{\langle a_{i_k}, x^k \rangle}{b_{i_k}} \right) t_k \,, \tag{40}$$

$$t_k = \min_j \left\{ \frac{1}{a_{ij} x_j^k} \;/\; a_{ij} \neq 0 \right\}, \tag{41}$$

and $\lambda_k \in [\varepsilon, 1]$ with $\varepsilon > 0$.

For additive up-dating methods like ART [33], parallel versions ([37]) (Cimmino-like methods) are obtained by computing the new iterate as a convex combination (or arithmetic mean) of the projections. In MART, that is a multiplicative method, this is replaced by a geometric mean. This would suggest to generalize (39) as

$$x_j^{k+1} = x_j^k \Pi_{i\in I_t}\Big(\frac{1}{1-a_{ij}x_jc_k}\Big)^{\omega_i a_{ij}} \quad \text{fot } j=1,\dots,n\,. \tag{42}$$

It can be proven that (42) converges to a solution of the system (1-2) because the log-distance (23) is decreasing, but the limit point not necessarily solves the optimization problem (4). So we introduce the following new algorithm.

Parallel Log-entropy MART.

Given x^0 positive starting point

$$x_j^{k+1} = \frac{x_j^k}{1 - x_j^k \sum\limits_{i\in I_t} \omega_i c_i a_{ij}}\,, \tag{43}$$

c_i as in (40).

We now prove that $\{x^k\}$ defined by (43) converges to a solution of (4).

It is clear because of the conditions on A and b (A nonnegative, $b > 0$, A with no zero rows and columns) that (1) has one strictly positive solution.

Proposition 2. If x^* is a strictly positive solution of (1) then $D(x^*, x^{k+1}) \le D(x^*, x^k)$.

Proof.

$$D(x^*, x^{k+1}) - D(x^*, x^k) = \sum_{j=1}^n -\log\frac{x_j^k}{x_j^{k+1}} + x_j^*\Big(\frac{1}{x_j^{k+1}} - \frac{1}{x_j^k}\Big)$$

$$= \sum_{j=1}^n -\log\Big(1 - x_j^k\sum_{i\in I_t}\omega_i c_i a_{ij}\Big) - x_j^*\sum_{i\in I_t}\omega_i c_i a_{ij}$$

$$\le \sum_{i\in I_t}\omega_i\Big[\sum_{j=1}^n -\log\Big(1 - \lambda_k t_i a_{ij} x_j^k + \lambda_k t_i a_{ij} x_j^k \frac{\langle a_i, x^k\rangle}{b_i}\Big) - b_i c_i\Big]\,,$$

using convexity of $-\log(1-s)$ and the fact that $\langle a_i, x^*\rangle = b_i$. Now, by convexity of $-\log s$

$$\le \sum_{i\in I_t}\omega_i \sum_{j=1}^n -\Big(\lambda_k t_i a_{ij} x_j^k \log\frac{\langle a_i, x^k\rangle}{b_i}\Big) - b_i c_i$$

$$\le \sum_{i\in I_t}\omega_i\Big(-\lambda_k t_i\langle a_i, x^k\rangle\log\frac{\langle a_i, x^k\rangle}{b_i}\Big) - b_i\lambda_k t_i\Big(1 - \frac{\langle a_i, x^k\rangle}{b_i}\Big)$$

$$= \lambda_k\sum_{i\in I_t}\omega_i b_i t_i\Big(-\frac{\langle a_i, x^k\rangle}{b_i}\log\frac{\langle a_i, x^k\rangle}{b_i} + \frac{\langle a_i, x^k\rangle}{b_i} - 1\Big)\,. \tag{44}$$

Calling $z_i^k = \dfrac{\langle a_i, x^k\rangle}{b_i}$, from (44) we get

$$D(x^*, x^{k+1}) \leq D(x^*, x^k) + \lambda_k \sum_{i\in I_t} \omega_i b_i t_i F(z_i^k)\,, \tag{45}$$

where

$$F(z) = -z\log z + z - 1\,. \tag{46}$$

It is easy to verify that F defined by (46) is a concave nonpositive function and the result follows. □

Proposition 3. The sequence generated by (43) converges to a solution of (1-2).

Proof. By Proposition 2

$$D(x^*, x^k) \leq D(x^*, x^0)\,, \tag{47}$$

therefore using Definition 1 (iv), $\{x^k\}$ is bounded. Let $\tilde{x}$ be a limit point of a subsequence $\{x^{k_j}\}$. x cannot belong to the boundary ($\tilde{x}_j = 0$ for some j) because in that case $\lim_{k\to\infty} D(x^*, x^k) = +\infty$, so $\tilde{x}_j > 0$ for $j = 1, \ldots, n$. From (45)

$$D(x^*, x^k) - D(x^*, x^{k+1}) \geq \varepsilon \sum_{i\in I_t} \omega_i b_i (-F(z_i^k)) \geq 0\,, \tag{48}$$

so, $D(x^*, x^k)$ is monotone decreasing bounded below (convergent) and $\sum_{i\in I_t} \omega_i b_i (-F(z_i^k)) \underset{k\to\infty}{\longrightarrow} 0$. Taking into account that for a given i, by almost cyclicallity, i is chosen infinitely many times, $-F(z_i^k) \underset{k\to\infty}{\longrightarrow} 0$, $\dfrac{\langle a_i, x^{k_j}\rangle}{b_i} \to 1$, because $z = 1$ is the maximum of F and $F(1) = 0$. Then $\tilde{x}$ is a strictly positive solution of (1). Taking $x^* = \tilde{x}$, $D(x^*, x^k) \underset{k\to 0}{\longrightarrow} 0$ and the result is a consequence of Definition 1 (vi) applied to (23).

Theorem 1. The sequence generated by (43) converges to a solution of (4) for an appropriate starting point.

Proof. It suffices to prove that if $x^* = \lim_{k\to\infty} x^k$, it satisfies the Kuhn-Tucker conditions (see [2]) for problem (4). By a simple manipulation of (43) we get

$$-\frac{1}{x_j^{k+1}} = -\frac{1}{x_j^k} + \sum_{i\in I_t} \omega_i c_i a_{ij}\,,\ \text{for } j = 1, \ldots, n\,, \tag{49}$$

or

$$\nabla f(x^{k+1}) = \nabla f(x^k) + A^t \tilde{w}^k\,, \tag{50}$$

for some $\tilde{w}^k$. By induction there exists w^k such that

$$\nabla f(x^k) = \nabla f(x^0) + A^t w^k\,. \tag{51}$$

Taking limits in (51)

$$\nabla f(x^*) = \nabla f(x^0) + A^t w^*\,, \tag{52}$$

but this and the fact that $Ax^* = b$, $x^* > 0$ are the Kuhn-Tucker conditions for the problem (33). If $\nabla f(x^0) = A^t w^0$ for some w^0, then x^* solves (4). □

One of the main drawbacks of MART is that exponentials and logarithms should be computed each step, being this very expensive. Recently [27], a modification called QMART was suggested in order to simplify the complexity of the original algorithm. The resulting method was to have reasonable behavior for image reconstruction. The idea consists of, instead of using the Bregman distance $D(x, y)$, expanding by Taylor to second degree in x for the point y to obtain

$$\widetilde{D}(x,y) = \frac{1}{2}(x-y)^t \nabla^2 f(y)(x-y) , \tag{53}$$

and use $\widetilde{D}$-projections in (31). For the KL divergence this gives

QMART$_1$.

Given a starting $x^0 > 0$

$$x_j^{k+1} = x_j^k \left(1 + \beta_{i_k} \frac{b_{i_k} - \langle a_{i_k}, x^k \rangle}{\sum_{j=1}^{n} a_{ij}^2 x_j^k} a_{ij} \right) , \quad \text{for } j = 1, \ldots, n . \tag{54}$$

Unfortunately in this case nonnegativity is not guaranteed by (54) and β_k is a positive number that has to be chosen in such a way that this property is preserved ($x_j^{k+1} > 0$ for $j = 1, \ldots, n$). In [27] a geometric interpretation of (54) and some experiments are shown, but no convergence results are given. Assuming conditions on the β_i^k's some results are presented next.

Proposition 4. If in each step

$$\beta_{i_k} \leq \frac{\sum_{j=1}^{n} a_{ij}^2 x_j^k}{\langle a_i, x^k \rangle} , \tag{55}$$

(54) is well defined and $D(x^*, x^{k+1}) \leq D(x^*, x^k)$ for every x^* solution of (1), where D is the KL divergence.

Proof. Observe first that if $b_{i_k} - \langle a_{i_k}, x^k \rangle < 0$ then

$$\beta_{i_k} \frac{\langle a_{i_k}, x^k \rangle - b_{i_k}}{\sum_{j=1}^{n} a_{ij}^2 x_j^k} a_{ij} \leq \left(1 - \frac{b_{i_k}}{\langle a_{i_k}, x^k \rangle}\right) a_{ij} \leq 1 ,$$

so

$$1 + \beta_{i_k} \frac{b_{i_k} - \langle a_{i_k}, x^k \rangle}{\sum_{j=1}^{n} a_{ij}^2 x_j^k} a_{ij} > 0$$

and (54) is well defined.

Let x^* be a solution of (1), then

$$D(x^*, x^{k+1}) - D(x^*, x^k) = \sum_{j=1}^{n} x_j^* \log \frac{x^k}{x_j^{k+1}} + x_j^{k+1} - x_j^k$$

$$= \sum_{j=1}^{n} -x_j^* \log\left(1 + \beta_{i_k} \frac{b_{i_k} - \langle a_{i_k}, x^k\rangle}{\sum_{j=1}^{n} a_{ij}^2 x_j^k} a_{ij}\right) + \beta_{i_k} \frac{b_{i_k} - \langle a_{i_k}, x^k\rangle}{\sum_{j=1}^{n} a_{ij}^2 x_j^k} a_{ij} x_j^k$$

$$= \sum_{j=1}^{n} -x_j^* \log\left[(1 - a_{ij}) + a_{ij}\left(1 + \beta_{i_k} \frac{b_{i_k} - \langle a_{i_k}, x^k\rangle}{\sum_{j=1}^{n} a_{ij}^2 x_j^k}\right)\right] + \beta_{i_k} \frac{b_{i_k} - \langle a_{i_k}, x^k\rangle}{\sum_{j=1}^{n} a_{ij}^2 x_j^k} a_{ij} x_j^k$$

$$\leq \sum_{j=1}^{n} -x_j^* a_{ij} \log\left(1 + \beta_{i_k} \frac{b_{i_k} - \langle a_{i_k}, x^k\rangle}{\sum_{j=1}^{n} a_{ij}^2 x_j^k}\right) + \beta_{i_k} \frac{b_{i_k} - \langle a_{i_k}, x^k\rangle}{\sum_{j=1}^{n} a_{ij}^2 x_j^k} a_{ij} x_j^k \tag{56}$$

$$= -b_{i_k} \log\left(1 + \beta_{i_k} \frac{b_{i_k} - \langle a_{i_k}, x^k\rangle}{\sum_{j=1}^{n} a_{ij}^2 x_j^k}\right) + \beta_{i_k} \frac{\langle a_{i_k}, x^k\rangle}{\sum_{j=1}^{n} a_{ij}^2 x_j^k} (b_{i_k} - \langle a_{i_k} x^k\rangle) \tag{57}$$

$$\leq b_{i_k}\left[-\log\left(1 + \overline{\beta}\left(\frac{b_{i_k}}{\langle a_{i_k}, x^k\rangle} - 1\right)\right) + \overline{\beta}\left(1 - \frac{\langle a_{i_k}, x^k\rangle}{b_{i_k}}\right)\right], \tag{58}$$

where $\overline{\beta} = \beta_{i_k} \frac{\langle a_{i_k}, x^k\rangle}{\sum_{j=1}^{n} a_{ij}^2 x_j^k}$, inequality (56) is by convexity and (57) is obtained summing on i taking into account that x^* solves (1).

Let $z_{i_k} = \frac{b_{i_k}}{\langle a_{i_k}, x^k\rangle}$ and $F(z) = -\log z + 1 - z^{-1}$, then by convexity (58) is less equal than

$$b_{i_k} \overline{\beta} F(z) . \tag{59}$$

Once again $F(z)$ is a nonpositive function with a unique maximum for $z = 1$ and the result follows.

□

Theorem 2. If (55) holds the sequence defined by (54) converges to a solution of (1).

Proof. The same arguments of Proposition 3 are valid here.

It is very easy to see using a single hyperplane (say $x_1 + x_2 = 1$) that QMART$_1$ no longer maximizes the entropy function. If equality is taken for β_{i_k} in (55), the resulting algorithm will be the following.

Nonlinear Relaxed ART.

Given a starting $x^0 > 0$

$$x_j^{k+1} = x_j^k\left(1 - a_{ij} + \frac{b_{i_k}}{\langle a_{i_k}, x^k\rangle}\right), \quad \text{for } j = 1,\dots,n\,. \tag{60}$$

This algorithm, called QMART$_2$ in [27], was first suggested in [60] by Twomey for solving the Fredholm equation of the first kind modelling the radiative transfer problem. A convergence proof for a generalized version is given in [23].

To complete this section we observe that all the algorithms presented here can be slightly modified to deal with inequalities as in (5). For MART and log-entropy MART this is done in [8] and [9] respectively. For the parallel log-entropy MART, QMART$_1$ and nonlinear relaxed ART these variants will appear in [25], as well as their relations with Bregman's method.

V – The EM Algorithm (Expectation Maximization)

The EM algorithm is a general method for computing maximum likelihood estimates from incomplete data. In image reconstruction, this algorithm was first introduced by Shepp and Verdi [53] for computing emission densities in PET. We briefly describe the fundamentals of the method.

Let Y be the observed data, a random vector with density function $g(Y,x)$, where x represents the parameters to be estimated. Suppose Y is embedded in a richer or larger sample space with associated density function $f(X,x)$. The problem is to estimate x by maximizing the log-likelihood function, i.e., find x solving

$$\max_{x\in\Omega} \ell(x) = \log g(Y,x)\,, \tag{61}$$

being $\Omega \subseteq I\!R^n$ the parameter space. Let

$$k(X/Y,x) = \frac{f(X,x)}{g(Y,x)}\,, \tag{62}$$

$$h(\tilde{x}/x) = E(\log k(X/Y,\tilde{x})/Y,x) \tag{63}$$

the conditional expectation of $\log k$ given (Y,x), and

$$q(\tilde{x}/x) = \ell(x) + h(\tilde{x}/x) = E(\log f(X,x)/Y,x)\,, \tag{64}$$

the expectation of $\log f$ given (Y,x), then, it is very easy to see that

$$\ell(\tilde{x}) - \ell(x) = [q(\tilde{x}/x) - q(x/x)] + [h(x/x) - h(\tilde{x}/x)]\,. \tag{65}$$

The second term between brackets in (65) is always nonnegative (see [20]), so, if we want to increase the likelihood value, it suffices to increase the value of $q(\overline{x}/x)$ as a function of $\overline{x}$. This property suggested Dempster, Laird and Rubin [20] to define the EM algorithm by maximizing $q(\overline{x}/x^k)$ for each k, the first step being the computation of the conditional expectation q.

EM Algorithm

Given $x^0 \in \Omega$

$$x^{k+1} = \arg\max_{x\in\Omega} q(x/x^k) \,. \tag{66}$$

The first full convergence proof for (66) was given in [17].

For the PET problem (see [43] and [54]), the space Y corresponds to the emission data vectors $b = \{b_i\}$ and the richer space X to the vectors $\widetilde{b} = \{b_{ij}\}$, where b_{ij} are the number of emissions by pixel j detected by pair of detectors i [54]. Then the log-likelihood function for the emission Poisson process is given by (9) (with (11) and (12)) and

$$q(x/x^k) = \sum_{i=1}^{m}\Big(\sum_{j=1}^{n} E(b_{ij}/b_i, x^k)\log a_{ij}x_j\Big) - \langle a_i, x\rangle \,, \tag{67}$$

where

$$E(b_{ij}/b_i, x^k) = \frac{b_i a_{ij} x^k}{\langle a_i, x^k\rangle} \,. \tag{68}$$

To find the maximum of (67), we compute the unique zero of the first partial derivatives

$$\frac{\partial q(x/x^k)}{\partial x_j} = \sum_{i=1}^{m} \frac{b_i a_{ij} x_j^k}{\langle a^i, x^k\rangle x_j} - 1 = 0 \;, \text{ for } j = 1,\ldots,n \,, \tag{69}$$

giving rise to the iteration

$$x_j^{k+1} = x_j^k \sum_{j=1}^{m} \frac{b_i a_{ij}}{\langle a_i, x^k\rangle} \,, \text{ for } j = 1,\ldots,n \,. \tag{70}$$

VI – The Iterative Image Space Reconstruction Algorithm (ISRA)

The EM algorithm (68) can be seen as generating the sequence by multiplying the current iterate by a generalized error computed applying the backprojection operator to the multiplicative error vector defined by $\left\{\frac{b_i}{\langle a_i, x^k\rangle}\right\}$. This is the way it was first deduced for solving radiative transfer equations [16] and it was called generalized nonlinear relaxation. One possible modification to (68) to adapt it for some special PET scanners [19] is to up-date each variable multiplying by the ratio between the backprojected data and the backprojection of the approximate projection data. This approach gives rise to

ISRA.

Given $x^0 > 0$,

$$x_j^{k+1} = x_j^k \frac{\sum_{i=1}^{m} b_i a_{ij}}{\sum_{i=1}^{m} a_{ij}\langle a_i, x^k\rangle} \,, \text{ for } j = 1,\ldots,n \,. \tag{71}$$

This algorithm is proven to converge to a solution of (8) for the least squares function (1) [21]. A general convergence proof including the nonunique solution case can be found in [28] and a generalization to other kind of problems in [24].

An additional interesting remark concerning algorithm (68) and (69) is some kind of acceleration or enhancement of each iteration proposed for the EM algorithm [57]. Instead of defining the updating as in (16) we can consider

$$x_j^{k+1} = x_j^k (c_j^k)^\alpha \text{ , for } j = 1, \ldots, n\,, \tag{72}$$

where α is a real parameter. Some convergence results for (68) using this scheme for $\alpha \in (0,2)$ are given in [36]. For (69) this remains open.

VII – Penalized Maximum Likelihood Using Variants of the EM Algorithm.

While the EM algorithm is mathematically correct decreasing the likelihood value each iteration, in its practical application to PET, after some iterations, it begins to show some deteriorating effect. To cope with this problem, the use of priori information through penalization terms has been proposed (see [46], [31] and [32]). In this case (9) is substituted by

$$\max_{x \in \Omega} t(x) = \{\ell(x) - \gamma p(x)\}\,, \tag{73}$$

where $p(x)$ is a convex function such that (71) has a unique solution, and γ is a positive real number. Now, the maximization step (66) is equivalent to solve the system of equations

$$\frac{\partial q(x/x^k)}{\partial x_j} = \sum_{i=1}^m \frac{b_i a_{ij} x_j}{\langle a_i, x^k \rangle} - 1 - \gamma \frac{\partial p(x)}{\partial x_j} = 0 \quad \text{for} \quad j = 1, \ldots, n\,. \tag{74}$$

If p is quadratic with zero off-diagonal terms, (72) is only a second degree equation to be solved for each variable [35], but if p is a quadratic function incorporating more complex information, (72) is a huge nonlinear system of equations to be solved at each step and the EM algorithm becomes absolutely impractical. Several alternatives have been proposed to avoid this inconvenient. The first one, by De Pierro [22], was to up-date variables by blocks instead of simultaneously. This gives rise to the algorithm

Expectation Partial Maximization (EPM).

Given $x^0 > 0$, x^{k+1} is the unique positive solution of

$$\sum_{i=1}^m \frac{b_i a_{ij} x_j^k}{\langle a_i, x^k \rangle} - 1 - \gamma \frac{\partial p(x)}{\partial x_j} = 0\,, \quad \text{for } j \in J_k\,, \tag{75}$$

$$x_j^{k+1} = x_j^k\,, \qquad \text{for } j \notin J_{i_k} \tag{76}$$

where J_{i_k} is a block of variables chosen in such a way that the system (75) is easy to solve (see [35]) and i_k an almost cyclic control. Convergence of the EPM algorithm is proven in [22].

Unfortunately, (73) has an expensive variables updating and other possibilities were considered ([32], [35]). These alternatives are included in the following general scheme (we assume p at least twice differentiable in Ω).

Modified Expectation Maximization (MEM).

Consider a decomposition of p such that

$$p(x) = p_1(x) + p_2(x) , \tag{77}$$

where $p_1(x)$ is a convex function. Then, instead of (66) we define

$$x^{k+1} = \arg\max_{x \in \Omega} F(x) = q(x/x^k) - \gamma p_1(x) - \gamma \nabla p_2(x^k)(x - x^k) , \tag{78}$$

i.e., if p_2 is a component of p introducing heavy calculations in (72), we linearize this component to obtain (76). In our case (76) reduces to find x^{k+1} solving

$$\nabla q(x/x^k) - \gamma \nabla p_1(x) - \gamma \nabla p_2(x^k) = 0 , \tag{79}$$

or

$$\sum_{i=1}^{m} \frac{b_i a_{ij} x_j^k}{\langle a_i, x^k \rangle x_j} - 1 - \gamma \frac{\partial p_1(x)}{\partial x_j} - \gamma \frac{\partial p_2(x^k)}{\partial x_j} = 0 \text{ for } j = 1, \ldots, n . \tag{80}$$

Observe that a unique positive solution if $p_1 \neq 0$ exists for (78) because of the convexity of p_1 and strict concavity of $q(x/x^k)$. If p is a convex quadratic function, p_1 stands for the diagonal terms and p_2 for the off-diagonal terms, (78) is the algorithm proposed by Herman et al. [35]. If $p_1 = 0$, (78) is the One-step-late (OSL) algorithm proposed by P. Green [32]. In the latter case, if p is quadratic, it should be associated with nonnegative matrices in order to the iteration (78) be well defined. The prior suggested by P. Green [32] is $\sum \log \cos h(x_j - x_i)$, where the sum is over neighbouring pairs of pixels. In the following we'll assume that p_1 and p_2 are such that the algorithm is well defined.

Proposition 5. The direction defined by MEM is an ascent direction for (71).

Proof. Using (77)

$$\nabla q(x^{k+1}/x^k) - \gamma \nabla p_1(x^{k+1}) = \gamma \nabla p_2(x^k) . \tag{81}$$

so

$$\nabla F(x^k)^t (x^{k+1} - x^k) = (\nabla q(x^k/x^k) - \gamma \nabla p_1(x^k) - \gamma \nabla p_2(x^k))^t (x^{k+1} - x^k) \tag{82}$$

$$= [(\nabla q(x^k/x^k) - \nabla q(x^{k+1}/k^k) + \gamma(\nabla p_1(x^{k+1}) - \gamma \nabla p_1(x^k))^t](x^{k+1} - x^k) \tag{83}$$

$$= -(x^{k+1} - x^k)^t \nabla^2 q(\tilde{x}^k)(x^{k+1} - x^k) + \gamma (x^{k+1} - x^k)^t \nabla^2 p_1(\tilde{x}^k)(x^{k+1} - x^k) \geq 0 \tag{84}$$

using (79) in equality (81), Taylor in (82) and taking into account convexity of p_1 and concavity of q for the inequality in (82). □

In spite of Proposition 5, it is known [35] that there are values of γ for wich the method is not convergent and only local convergence results can be proven for interior points.

We define now iteration (76) in an explicit form as

$$x^{k+1} = G_\gamma(x^k) , \tag{85}$$

and if

$$x = G_\gamma(\tilde{x}) \tag{86}$$

is the mapping defining the method we need to compute its Jacobian for fixed points in order to analyze local behavior of (83). If D^{ij} denotes the derivatives with respect to the first and second vectors i and j times respectively, differentiating with respect to $\tilde{x}$ in (76)

$$D^{11}q(x/\tilde{x}) + D^{20}q(x/\tilde{x})DG(\tilde{x}) - \gamma D^2 p_1(x)DG(\tilde{x}) - \gamma D^2 p_2(\tilde{x}) = 0 \tag{87}$$

and from (85)

$$DG_\gamma(\tilde{x}) = [-D^{20}q(x/\tilde{x}) + \gamma D^2 p_1)(x)]^{-1}[D^{11}q(x/\tilde{x}) - \gamma D^2 p_2(\tilde{x})] \,. \tag{88}$$

If x is a fixed point of (83)

$$-D^{20}q(x/x) = D^2\ell(x) - D^{20}h(x/x) = B + C \,, \tag{89}$$

and using familiar results about derivatives of log-likelihoods

$$D^{11}q(x/x) = D^{11}h(x/x) = -D^{20}h(x/x) = C \,. \tag{90}$$

Calling $D^2 p_1(x) = K_1$ and $D^2 p_2(x) = K_2$, (86) gives

$$DG_\gamma(x) = (B + C + \gamma K_1)^{-1}(C - \gamma K_2) \,. \tag{91}$$

For $\gamma = 0$, $\rho(DG_0(x)) < 1$ because G_0 defines the EM algorithm. So for γ small enough $\rho(DG_\gamma(x)) < 1$ and the resulting algorithm will be locally convergent.

VIII – Concluding Remarks

We have presented most of the multiplicative methods used or that have been proposed to be used in computerized tomography. Many gaps in the theory and practice of these methods have still to be filled. We have made some contributions in this direction presenting a parallelized version of Log-MART, proving convergence of QMART_1 under suitable conditions and presenting a general scheme for the EM algorithm applied to penalized maximum likelihood.

We point out here that the block Log-MART method presented in section IV is quite interesting from the computational point of view because it is less expensive than MART (approximately same cost of ART) and it maximizes an entropy function.

Some important topics listed below have not been treated in this paper (or nowhere) but will be subject of future research:

(i) MART or Log-MART type methods for inequalities,

(ii) Extensions of ISRA to a regularized least squares approach,

(iii) Convergence rate of the algorithms,

(iv) How to accelerate the algorithms.

References

[1] D.L. Anderson and A.M. Dziewonski, Seismic tomography, Scientific American 251 (1984), pp. 58-66.

[2] M. Avriel, *Nonlinear Programming, Analysis and Methods*, Prentice-Hall, New Jersey, 1976.

[3] L.M. Bregman, The relaxation method of finding the common point of convex sets and its applications to the solution of problems in convex programming, U.S.S.R Computational Mathematics and Mathematical Physics, vol. 7 (1967), pp. 200-217.

[4] J.P. Burg, Maximum entropy spectral analysis, in: *Proceedings of the 37th Annual Meeting of the Society of Exploration Geophysicists*, Oklahoma City, Oklahoma, 1967.

[5] Y. Censor, Row-action methods for huge and sparse systems and their applications, SIAM Review 23 (1981), pp. 444-466.

[6] Y. Censor, On the selective use of iterative algorithms for inversion problems in image reconstruction and radiotherapy, in: Proceedings of the 12th World Congress on Scientific Computation - IMACS 1988 (R. Vichnevetsky, P. Borne and J. Vignes, Editors), Gerfdin, Paris, France, vol. 4 (1988), pp. 563-565.

[7] Y. Censor, M.D. Altschuler and W.D. Powlis, A computational solution of the inverse problem in radiation therapy treatment planning, Applied Mathematics and Computation, 25 (1988), pp. 57-87.

[8] Y. Censor, A.R. De Pierro, T. Elfving, G.T. Herman and A.N. Iusen, On iterative methods for linearly constrained entropy maximization, in: A. Wakulicz, ed., *Numerical Analysis and Mathematical Modelling*, Banach Center Publications, Vol. XXIV, Stefan Banach International Mathematical Center (1989), pp. 147-165.

[9] Y. Censor, A.R. de Pierro and A.N. Iusem, Optimization of Burg's entropy over linear constraints, Applied Numerical Mathematics, to appear.

[10] Y. Censor and G.T. Herman, On some optimization techniques in image reconstruction from projections, Applied Numerical Mathematics 3 (1987), pp. 365-391.

[11] Y. Censor and A. Lent, An iterative row-action method for interval convex programming, J. Optim. Theory Appl. 34 (1981), pp. 321-353.

[12] Y. Censor and A. Lent, Optimization of "$\log x$"-entropy over linear equality constraints, SIAM J. Control Optim. 25 (1987), pp. 921-933.

[13] Y. Censor and J. Segman, On the block-iterative entropy maximization, Journal of Information & Optimization Sciences, vol. 8 (1987), 3, pp. 275-291.

[14] M.T. Chahine, Determination of the temperature profile in an atmosphere from its outgoing radiance, J. Opt. Soc. Amer. 58 (1968) 1634-1637.

[15] M.T. Chahine, Remote sounding of cloud parameters, J. Atmos. Sci., 38, 1, (1982) pp. 159-170.

[16] M.T. Chahine, Generalization of the relaxation method for the inverse solution of nonlinear and linear transfer equations, in *Inversion Methods in Atmospheric Remote Sounding*. A Deepak ed., Academic Press, New York, 1977.

[17] I. Csiszár and G. Tusnády, Information geometry and alternating minimization procedures, in: Statistics & Decisions, Suppl. No. 1 (1984), pp. 205-237.

[18] J.N. Darroch and D. Ratcliff, Generalized iterative scaling for log-linear models. The Annals of Mathematical Statistics, Vol. 43 (1972), pp. 1470-1480.

[19] M.E. Daube-Witherspoon and G. Muehllehner, An iterative image space reconstruction algorithm suitable for volume ECT, IEEE Trans. Med. Imaging, vol. MI-5 (1986), pp. 61-66.

[20] A.P. Dempster, N.M. Laird and D.B. Rubin, Maximum likelihood for incomplete data via the EM algorithm, J.R. Stat. Soc. Series B, 39 (1977), pp. 1-38.

[21] A.R. De Pierro, On the convergence of the iterative image space reconstruction algorithm for volume ECT, IEEE Trans. Med. Imaging, vol. MI-6 (1987), pp. 174-175.

[22] A.R. De Pierro, A generalization of the EM algorithm for maximum likelihood estimates from incomplete data, Tech. Rept. MIPG 119, Medical Image Processing Group, Department of Radiology, Hospital of the University of Pennsylvania, PA, 1987.

[23] A.R. De Pierro, On some nonlinear iterative relaxation methods in remote sensing, Matemática Aplicada e Computacional, vol. 8 (1989), pp. 153-166.

[24] A.R. De Pierro, Nonlinear relaxation methods for solving symmetric linar complementarity problems, J. Optim. Theory Appl. 64 (1990), pp. 87-99.

[25] A.R. De Pierro, Parallel Bregman methods for convex programming and entropy maximization, forthcoming paper.

[26] A.R. De Pierro and A.N. Iusem, A relaxed version of Bregman's method for convex programming, J. Optim. Theory Appl., 51 (1986), pp. 421-440.

[27] N.J. Dusaussoy and I.E. Abdou, Some new multiplicative algorithms for image reconstruction from projections, Linear Algebra Appl., 130 (1990), pp. 111-132.

[28] P.P.B. Eggermont, Multiplicative iterative algorithms for convex programming, Linear Algebra Appl., 130 (1990), pp. 25-42.

[29] H.E. Fleming, Satellite remote sensing by the technique of computed tomography, J. Appl., Metereology 21 (1982), pp. 1538-1549.

[30] R. Gordon, R. Bender and G.T. Herman, Algebraic reconstruction techniques (ART) for three-dimensional electron microscopy and X-ray photography, J. Theoret. Biol. 29 (1970), pp. 471-481.

[31] P.J. Green, Penalized likelihood reconstructions from emission tomography data using a modified EM algorithm, to appear.

[32] P.J. Green, On the use of the EM algorithm for penalized likelihood estimation, to appear.

[33] G.T. Herman, *Image Reconstruction from Projections: The Fundamentals of Computerized Tomography,* Academic Press, New York, 1980.

[34] G.T. Herman, Application of maximum entropy and Bayesian optimization methods to image reconstruction from projections, in: C.R. Smith and W.T. Grandy, Jr., Eds., Maximum-Entropy and Bayesian Methods in Inverse Problems, Reidel, Dordrecht (1985), pp. 319-338.

[35] G.T. Herman, D. Odhner, K.D. Toennies and S.A. Zenios, A parallelized algorithm for image reconstruction from noisy projections, Tech. Rept. MIPG 155, Medical Image Processing Group, Department of Radiology, Hospital of the University of Pennsylvania, PA, 1989.

[36] A.N. Iusem, Convergence analysis for a multiplicatively relaxed EM algorithm, with applications in Position Emission Tomography, to be published.

[37] A.N. Iusem and A.R. De Pierro, Convergence results for an accelerated nonlinear Cimmino algorithm, Numer. Math. 49 (1986), pp. 367-378.

[38] E.T. Jaynes, On the rationale of maximum-entropy methods, Proc. IEEE 70 (1982), pp. 939-952.

[39] R. Johnson and J.E. Shore, Which is the better entropy expression for speech processing: $-S \log S$ or $\log S$?, IEEE Trans. Acoust. Speech Signal Process, 32 (1984), pp. 129-136.

[40] J.N. Kapur, Twenty-five years of maximum-entropy principle, J. Math. Phys. Sci. 17 (1983), pp. 102-156.

[41] S. Kullback, *Information Theory and Statistics*, Wiley, New York, 1959.

[42] K. Lange, M. Bahn and R. Little, A theoretical study of some maximum likelihood algorithms for emission and transmission tomography, IEEE Trans. Med. Imaging., vol. MI-6 (1987), pp. 106-114.

[43] K. Lange and R. Carson, EM reconstruction algorithms for emission and transmission tomography, J. Comput. Assist. Tomog., vol. 8 (1984), pp. 306-316.

[44] A. Lent, A convergent algorithm for maximum entropy image restoration with a medical X-ray application, in: R. Shaw, Ed., *Image Analysis and Evaluation*, Society of Photographic Scientists and Engineers, Washington, DC (1977), pp. 249-247.

[45] R.D. Levine and M. Tribus, Eds., The Maximum Entropy Formalism, MIT Press, Cambridge, MA, 1978.

[46] E. Levitan and G.T. Herman, A maximum a posteriori probability expectation maximization algorithm for image reconstruction in emission tomography, IEEE Trans. Med. Imaging, MI-6 (1987), pp. 185-192.

[47] R.M. Lewitt, Reconstruction algorithms: transform methods, Proc. IEEE, 71 (1983), pp. 390-408.

[48] L.B. Lucy, An iterative technique for the rectification of observed distributions, Astron. J. 79 (1974), pp. 745-754.

[49] E.S. Meinel, Origins of linear and nonlinear recursive restoration algorithms, J. Opt. Soc. Amer. A, vol. 36 (1986), pp. 787-799.

[50] F. Natterer, *The Mathematics of Computerized Tomography,* J. Wiley & Sons, New York, 1986.

[51] D.N. Nychka, Some properties of an EM algorithm that includes a smoothing step, to be published.

[52] W.H. Richardson, Bayesian-based iterative method of image restoration, J. Opt. Soc. Am. 62 (1972), pp. 55-59.

[53] L.A. Shepp and Y. Vardi, Maximum likelihood reconstruction in position emission tomography, IEEE Trans. Med. Imaging, MT-1 (1982), pp. 113-122.

[54] L.A. Shepp, Y. Vardi and L. Kaufman, A statistical model for positron emission tomography, J. of the Am. Stat. Assoc., vol. 80, No. 389 (1985), pp. 8-37.

[55] B.W. Silverman, M.C. Jones, J.D. Wilson and D.W. Nychka, A smoothed EM approach to a class of problems in image analysis and integral equations, to be published.

[56] C.R. Smith and W.T. Grandy, Jr., Eds., *Maximum-Entropy and Bayesian Methods in Inverse Problems,* Reidel, Dordrecht, 1985.

[57] E. Tanaka, A fast reconstruction algorithm for stationary positron emission tomography based on a modified EM algorithm, IEEE Trans. Med. Imaging, MI-6,2 (1987), pp. 98-105.

[58] M. Teboulle, On ϕ-divergence and its applications, Proceedings of the Conference in Honor of A. Charnes 70th. Birthday, Austin, Texas, to appear.

[59] M.M. Ter-Pogossian, M. Raichle and B.E. Sobel, Positron Emission Tomography, Scientific American, 243 (4) (1980), pp. 170-181.

[60] S. Twomey, Comparison of constrained linear inversion and an iterative nonlinear algorithm applied to the indirect estimation of particle size distributions, J. Comput Phys., 18 (1975), pp. 188-200.

[61] S.A. Zenios and Y. Censor, Parallel computing with block iterative image reconstruction algorithms, Tech. Rept. MIPG 134, Medical Image Processing Group, Department of Radiology, University of Pennsylvania, PA, 1990.

REMARK ON THE INFORMATIVE CONTENT OF FEW MEASUREMENTS

P.C. SABATIER
Département de Physique Mathématique
Université Montpellier II, Sciences et Techniques du Languedoc
34095 MONTPELLIER Cedex 5 - FRANCE -

For an ill-posed (essentially underdetermined) problem, with given bounds for their misfit and their "ugliness", the set of solutions is usually characterized by points which minimize a trade-off functional. It is shown that if chains of measurements interpolating each other are used, the minima evolution does not show essentially new creations after a certain order of interpolation is obtained, provided the measurement functionals are smooth enough. Hence there are chains with relatively few measurements, which correspond to a "weak information" on the set of solution, that cannot be dramatically modified by interpolating other measurements. Their appraisal can be done essentially by using the first and second variation of the measurement functionals. This remark suggests for instance practical ways of appraising the ill-posedness of certain problems, by the number of measurements which are necessary to obtain a "weak information".

I - INTRODUCTION AND ASSUMPTIONS

Measurements give numbers. They should be related to points of a normed space $\mathcal{C}$, called parameters. If measurements of the same phenomenon are made at several points of the physical space, they are also related in some way. This way, and the relations to $\mathcal{C}$, determine the informative content of measurements. In this paper, we show that there are cases where the main features of this informative content are obtained after few measurements.

More precisely, let us be given a (nonlinear) functional $\mathcal{M}$ on a Hilbert space $\mathcal{H}$. Let $\mathcal{C} \subset \mathcal{H}$ be the set of "parameters" x, to be inferred

$$\mathcal{M} : \mathcal{C} \subset \mathcal{H} \longrightarrow \mathbb{R} , \tag{1.1}$$

we assume that $\mathcal{M}$ also depends on $y \in \Omega \subset \mathbb{R}^p$, $p = 1,2,3$. y is called the "position" of the measurement.

<u>Assumption 1.</u> We assume that $\mathcal{M}$ is twice differentiable on $\mathcal{C} \times \Omega$

$$x,y \longrightarrow \mathcal{M}(x,y) \in C^2 \quad . \tag{1.2}$$

In this short paper, we only study the case $\Omega = [a,b] \subset \mathbb{R}$. We assume that we successively collect sequences of numbers so defined : the sequence of order n is made of "measurements results" (also called data) collected at the points

$$\begin{cases} y_p^{(n)} = a + (p-1)\, h^{(n)} & \left[p = 1,2,\ldots(2^n+1)\right] \\ h^{(n)} = 2^{-n}\,(b-a) & \end{cases} \tag{1.3}$$

Thus the sequence of order n contains the sequence of order (n-1) and is contained in that of order (n+1) : the measurements are more and more tight, more and more refined. Now we assume that the shifts of these data to the closest related results, ie the measurement errors (or the noise) are bounded. It follows that data should show some regularity that can be appraised by the values of

$$\kappa^{(n)} = h^{(n)} \sum_{p=1}^{2^n+1} \left|m_{p+1}^{(n)} - m_p^{(n)}\right|^2 \tag{1.4}$$

$$\lambda^{(n)} = \operatorname*{Sup}_{q>0} \left| h^{(n)} \sum_{p=1}^{2^n+1} \left[m_p^{(n)}\right]^2 - h^{(n+q)} \sum_{p=1}^{2^{n+q}+1} \left[m_p^{(n+q)}\right]^2 \right| \tag{1.5}$$

where $m_p^{(n)}$ is the measurement result collected at $y_p^{(n)}$. Indeed, if $m_p^{(n)}$ was replaced in the right-hand sides by the value of $\mathcal{M}\left(x,\, y_p^{(n)}\right)$, computed for a given parameter x, taking into account the C^2 assumption on $y \longrightarrow \mathcal{M}(x,y)$ shows that the right-hand side of (1.4) would by asymptotically bounded by $\kappa[h^{(n)}]^2$, κ being an appropriate number depending on x. If $\mathcal{C}$ is compact, it follows in addition that κ would itself be bounded up on $\mathcal{C}$. Similar remarks hold for $\lambda^{(n)}$. Hence we are led to state the following regularity assumptions :

<u>Assumption II.</u> $\mathcal{C}$ is compact.

<u>Assumption III.</u> For $n \geqslant n_0$, there exist positive numbers κ, λ, ϵ_1, ϵ_2 such that

$$\kappa^{(n)} \leqslant \kappa[h^{(n)}]^2 + \epsilon_1 \tag{1.6}$$

$$\lambda^{(n)} \leqslant \lambda[h^{(n)}]^2 + \epsilon_2 \tag{1.7}$$

One should keep in mind that

(a) for "calculated" results $f\left(x,\, y_p^{(n)}\right)$ at a given x, the bound (1.6) holds without ϵ in the right hand side and most often with smaller constant κ. It needs only that $y \longrightarrow f(x,y)$ is continuously differentiable !

(b) for "real data", the values of κ, λ and ϵ may be estimated from the evolution and noise of the first sets of results obtained as measurements become more tight.

Now, our aim is to appraise the evolution of a conveniently described set of solutions as n increases.

II - DEFINITION OF SOLUTIONS

We used the word "solutions" without defining it. Clearly, a "solution" is any element of $\mathcal{C}$ that satisfies "a priori" requirements of reliability and yields a sufficiently good fit. Since it is felt that our main problem does not very much depend on different precise definitions of these statements, we assume for simplicity that being given a reference parameter x_0 in $\mathcal{X}$

(a) the reliability of x is acceptable if the "ugliness" $\|x-x_0\|$ is small :

$$\|x-x_0\| \leqslant \eta \quad . \tag{2.1}$$

Clearly $\mathcal{C}$ can be redefined as being the ball $B(x_0,\eta)$.

(b) for each sequence $y^{(n)}$ of measurements, an acceptable misfit is

$$E(x,\ y^{(n)}) = \left[h^{(n)} \sum_{p=1}^{2^n+1} \left[M\left(x,y_p^{(n)}\right) - m_p^{(n)}\right]^2 w_p\right]^{1/2} \leqslant \theta \tag{2.2}$$

where $m_p^{(n)}$ are data collected at points $y_p^{(n)}$, and the weights w_p are :

$$w_p \begin{cases} 0 & \text{for} \quad p \leqslant 0 \\ \dfrac{1}{2} & \text{for} \quad p = 1 \\ 1 & \text{for} \quad 2 \leqslant p \leqslant 2^n \\ \dfrac{1}{2} & \text{for} \quad p = 2^n+1 \\ 0 & \text{for} \quad p > 2^n+1 \end{cases} \tag{2.3}$$

In the following, we always choose θ definitely larger than the data noise. By allowing such a relatively generous misfit, we hope to be able reducing the number of measurements that are sufficient for a rough information on the set of solutions. The set $X^{(n)} \subset \mathcal{C}$ of "solutions" which satisfy conditions (a) and (b) contains a subset $X_1^{(n)}$:

$$X_1^{(n)} = \left\{x \mid F(x,y^{(n)}) = \theta^{-2}\ E^2(x,y^{(n)}) + \eta^{-2}\|x-x_0\|^2 \leqslant 1\right\} \tag{2.4}$$

and is itself contained in the set $X_2^{(n)}$ defined by the same inequality with 2 in the right-hand side. $X_1^{(n)}$ (resp. $X_2^{(n)}$) may be a void set. If it is not, it certainly contains a point x_M which minimizes $F(x,\ y^{(n)})$ over $\mathcal{C}$, and all the other local minima of F such that $F \leqslant 1$. If $\mathcal{M}$ is linear, x_M is the only minimum and $X_1^{(n)}$ (resp. $X_2^{(n)}$) is an ellipsoid whose x_M is the center. If $\mathcal{M}$ is not linear, the position of other local minima such that $F \leqslant 1$ (resp. $F \leqslant 2$) gives us a qualitative appraisal of the deformation of $X^{(n)}$ We shall say that the evolution of the solutions sets as n varies is <u>smooth</u> if these points evolve slowly and are neither created or delected. As soon as the evolution becomes smooth, we consider that the information we got on the set of solutions and on the resolving power of measurements is qualitatively sufficient.

Using the triangular inequality for norms and bound (1.7) with and without ϵ_1 shows that for large n, $E(x,y^{(n)})$ lies in the neighborhood (radius $2\epsilon_1$) of a limit value. If $2\epsilon_1 \ll \theta$, this means that after $n = n_1$ (say), new increase of n does not increase reliable information, but modifies parameter estimates along with noise. We say that for $n \geqslant n_1$, measurements are saturated.

III - EVOLUTION OF $X_1^{(n)}$ (resp. $X_2^{(n)}$) WITH n

We study $F(x, y^{(n)})$, which is defined by (2.3), for $x \in \mathcal{C}$ and $n = 1,2,\ldots$. Unless $X_1^{(n)}$, (resp. $X_2^{(n)}$) is void for all n, there will be a value of the sequence order, say (n-1), where a minimum value of F, reached at a point $x^{(n-1)}$ (there may be others), is smaller than 1 (resp. 2). The differential of F vanishes for any increase δx from $x^{(n-1)}$

$$\theta^{-2}\, h^{(n-1)} \sum_{p=1}^{2^{n-1}+1} w_p \left[M\left(x^{(n-1)},y_p\right) - m\left(y_p^{(n-1)}\right)\right] \delta\, \mathcal{M}\left(x^{(n-1)},y_p,\, \delta x\right)$$

$$+\ \eta^{-2} \left\langle x^{(n-1)} - x_0,\ \delta x\right\rangle = 0 \tag{3.1}$$

where $\langle\, ,\, \rangle$ is the scalar product, $\delta\mathcal{M}$ is the first variation of $\mathcal{M}$. Assuming $\mathcal{H}$ is a real and separable Hilbert space, it is convenient to write down the definition formula for the first and second variations of $\mathcal{M}$ as

$$\mathcal{M}(x+\delta x,\ y) - \mathcal{M}(x,y) = \tilde{\rho}(x,y)\ \delta x + \frac{1}{2}\ \delta\tilde{x}\ \sigma(x,y)\ \delta x + o(\|\delta x\|^2) \tag{3.2}$$

where $\tilde{\rho}(x,y)$ is an infinite line matrix, $\sigma(x,y)$ an infinite square symmetric real matrix, and the tilda indicates transposition. Hence (3.1) can be rewritten as

$$\theta^{-2}\, h^{(n-1)} \sum_{p=1}^{2^{n-1}+1} w_p\ \Phi\left(x^{(n-1)},\ y_p^{(n-1)}\right) + \eta^{-2}(\tilde{x}^{(n-1)} - \tilde{x}^{(0)}) = 0 \tag{3.3}$$

where

$$\Phi(x,y) = [M(x,y) - m(y)]\ \tilde{\rho}(x,y) \tag{3.4}$$

Proceeding to the measurements of order n, we notice the equalities

$$y^{(n)}_{2p-1} = y^{(n-1)}_{p} \qquad (3.5)$$

$$y^{(n)}_{2p} = \frac{1}{2}\, y^{(n-1)}_{p+1} + \frac{1}{2}\, y^{(n-1)}_{p} \quad . \qquad (3.6)$$

At order n, the equation for a minimum is

$$\theta^{-2}\, h^{(n)} \sum_{p=1}^{2^n+1} w_p\, \Phi\left(x^{(n)},\, y^{(n)}_p\right) + \eta^{-2}\, (\tilde{x}^{(n)} - \tilde{x}^{(0)}) = 0 \quad . \qquad (3.7)$$

Writing down successively the sum on even and on odd order terms and taking into account (3.5) and (2.3), whose values have been chosen for this purpose, we obtain

$$\theta^{-2}\, h^{(n-1)} \sum_{p=1}^{2^{n-1}+1} w_p\, \Phi\left(x^{(n)}, y^{(n-1)}_p\right) + \eta^{-2} (\tilde{x}^{(n)} - \tilde{x}^{(0)})$$

$$\theta^{-2}\, R(x^{(n)},\, y^{(n)}) = 0 \qquad (3.8)$$

where

$$R(x^{(n)},\, y^{(n)}) = h^{(n)} \sum_{p=1}^{2^{n-1}} \left[2\, \Phi\left(x^{(n)},\, y^{(n)}_{2p}\right) - \Phi\left(x^{(n)},\, y^{(n)}_{2p-1}\right) - \Phi\left(x^{(n)},\, y^{(n)}_{2p+1}\right)\right] \qquad (3.9)$$

Setting

$$\delta\tilde{x} = \tilde{x}^{(n)} - \tilde{x}^{(n-1)} \qquad (3.10)$$

it follows from (3.2) that the variation of $\Phi(x,y)$ as x goes from $x^{(n-1)}$ to $x^{(n)}$ is

$$\Phi(x^{(n)},y) - \Phi(x^{(n-1)},y) = \delta\tilde{x}\, \rho(x^{(n-1)},y)\, \tilde{\rho}(x^{(n-1)},y) + Q[\delta\tilde{x}] + o(\|\delta x\|^2) \qquad (3.11)$$

It is easy to calculate the quadratic term $Q[\delta\tilde{x}]$ but we do not need its exact form. Inserting (3.11) into (3.8) and taking into account (3.3), we see that the equation for $\delta\tilde{x}$ reads :

$$\delta\tilde{x}[\eta^{-2} I + \theta^{-2} S] + Q(\delta\tilde{x}) + \theta^{-2} R(x^{(n)},y^{(n)}) = 0 \qquad (3.12)$$

where I is the identity, and

$$S = h^{(n-1)} \sum_{p=1}^{2^{n-1}+1} w_p \, \rho\left(x^{(n-1)}, y_p^{(n-1)}\right) \tilde{\rho}\left(x^{(n-1)}, y_p^{(n-1)}\right) \tag{3.13}$$

Setting

$$M = \eta^{-2} I + \theta^{-2} S \quad . \tag{3.14}$$

We see that M^{-1} is a bounded operator in L^2 so that if the norm of R is small enough, $Q(\delta\tilde{x})$ can be neglected and the leading term for $\delta\tilde{x}$ reads

$$\delta\tilde{x} = \theta^{-2} R \, M^{-1} \quad . \tag{3.15}$$

Now R can be appraised in the following way : we denote $\tilde{\rho}_k(y)$ the kth component of $\tilde{\rho}(x^{(n)}, y)$ and notice that the C^2 assumption (3.2) guarantees that

$$\begin{cases} \tilde{\rho}_k(y^{(n)}) =: \left[h^{(n)} \sum_{p=1}^{2^{n-1}} \tilde{\rho}_k^2\left(y_{2p}^{(n)}\right) \right]^{1/2} \\ \tilde{\sigma}_k(y^{(n)}) =: [h^{(n)}]^{-1} \sum_{p=1}^{2^n+1} \left[\tilde{\rho}_k\left(y_p^{(n)}\right) - \tilde{\rho}_k\left(y_{p-1}^{(n)}\right) \right]^2 \end{cases} \tag{3.16}$$

are finite norms L^2 vector, whereas (1.4) to (1.7) guarantee that if $\mu(y) = M(x^{(n-1)}, y) - m(y)$,

$$h^{(n)} \sum_{q=1}^{2^n} \mu^2 \left(y_q^{(n)}\right) \leqslant \|\mu\|^2 < \infty \tag{3.17}$$

$$h^{(n)} \sum_{q=1}^{2^n} \left[\mu\left(y_{q+1}^{(n)}\right) - \mu\left(y_q^{(n)}\right) \right]^2 \leqslant 2\,\kappa_n [h^{(n)}]^2 + \epsilon_1$$

when these bounds are used in the right hand-<side of (3.9), they yield

$$R(x^{(n)}, y^{(n)}) \leqslant 2\left[2\kappa_n \, [h^{(n)}]^2 + \epsilon_1 \right]^{1/2} \tilde{\rho}_k\,(y^{(n)}) + \|\mu\| \, [h^{(n)}]^2 \, \tilde{\sigma}_k\,(y^{(n)}) \; . \tag{3.18}$$

Hence, for each minimum such that $\|M^{-1}\|$ is not too large (in any case, $\|M^{-1}\| < \eta^2$) and since $\epsilon_1 \ll \theta$, there exists a range of values of n where the position of the minimum is modified only a little bit as the number of measurements increases in the way we describe it. No clearcut minimum disappears or appears and so the range of solutions remains qualitatively the same. This range should not be extended beyond the value n_1 of saturation. It begins around a value n_0 where the set of solutions has already reached its final qualitative aspect. If n_0 is small the informative content of data is qualitatively obtained after a few measurements only.

__Applications__

One may think to several applications.

(a) analyzing the ill-posedness of a problem with finitely many (hopefully few) measurements.

(b) minimizing the number of measurements necessary to take rapidly a decision.

(c) for a given set of possible measurements and a given a priori knowledge on the solutions, making descending algorithms able either to get rapidly the desired result or to decide rapidly the best strategy of measurements.

__Remarks__

(a) In the Oberwolfach lecture, a few slides extracted from Mrs Dolveck-Guilpart work showed that tomographies with 3 or 4 narrow few beams only, could give already a convenient qualitative appraisal of a given object (it was a hollow cube of Alumine and real γ-rays data had been processed),

(b) Professor Natterer called our attention to the fact that if $\mathfrak{M}$ is a linear operator mapping $H_p(X_d)$ into $H_q(Y_d)$, $q = p+a$, $a>0$, the image of $f \in H_p$ being $g \in H_q$, and if the domains of f and g are bounded, a short calculation shows that on the average, n (exact) measurements of g can give f up to an absolute error of the order of

$$\|\Delta f\|_{H_0} \simeq n^{-p/d} \|g\|^{p}_{H_q} \|f\|^{a/q}_{H_p} \quad . \tag{3.19}$$

This result is independent of further details on the operator. For the special case of a linear operator, this remark may apply to our problem in the reconstruction steps where the measurement errors are negligible compared to the discretization ones,ie $\theta >> \epsilon$ and $n << n_1$. Then, for $p = 0$, (3.19) would mean that the relative error on the parameter is of the order of what it would be if the parameters itself was discretized, and if its belonging to H_0 is the only a priori information, bounds on this error are not a priori improved by a strategy of very tight measurements. However, since many parts of the object usually are smooth, they may be retrieved after a few measurements and the __qualitative aspect__ of the solution is obtained (remember that the regularizing way we construct the set of solutions washes out sharp details). Hence Natterer's remark does not contradict ours.

REFERENCES AND ACKNOWLEDGEMENTS

B. Dolveck-Guilpart Tomographic Image Reconstruction from a Limited Set of Projections Using a Natural Pixel Decomposition. p. 54-61 in "Inverse Methods in Action" P.C. Sabatier Ed. Springer 1990.

We wish to thank Mrs Dolveck-Guilpart for communicating us her data and processing results, including (as yet) unpublished ones.

Theorems for the Number of Zeros of the Projection Radial Modulators of the 2D Exponential Radon Transform

W.G. Hawkins, N-C Yang and P.K. Leichner
Johns Hopkins Medical Institutions
402 N. Bond St., Baltimore, MD 21231

ABSTRACT

Theorems and a transformation formula are developed for the 2D exponential Radon transform (ERT) whereby theorems for the number of nodes of radial modulators of the X-ray transform (no attenuation of internal sources) can be extended to the ERT. The results were applied to SPECT simulations with angular under-sampling, and a spectral filter was shown to improve image quality in the region affected by angular aliasing, without altering interior regions that were not affected by angular aliasing.

I INTRODUCTION

The radial modulators of a real-valued function f where $f:\mathbb{R}^2 \rightarrow \mathbb{R}^1$ or $f:\mathbb{R}^1 \times S^1 \rightarrow \mathbb{R}^1$ are defined as follows:

$$f_k(r) = \int_{-\pi}^{\pi} d\phi \; f(r,\theta)\exp(-ik\phi)$$

where (r,θ) are 2D polar coordinates. The function f_k is also called the circular harmonic transform of f. We define the 2D set of projections g of the object f, such that $g:\mathbb{R}^1 \times S^1 \rightarrow \mathbb{R}^1$. We want to determine the minimum number of zeros of the radial modulator g_k. If g is the 2D X-ray transform (XT) of f and f is of bounded support on the unit circle, then it was shown in [1] that the minimum number of nodes or zeros in the interval $0 < p < 1$ was k for $g_{2k}(p)$ and $g_{2k+1}(p)$. Our focus is single-photon computed tomography (SPECT) for the case of uniform attenuation within a convex body (the exponential Radon transform, or ERT), and we will find the equivalent formulation for the ERT.

The motivation for this type of analysis was first given in [2]. If projection radial modulators not possessing the minimum number of zeros were removed from the data, might not this removal improve the quality of the reconstruction, that is, the recovery of f from g? This algorithm or filter is easily implemented and promises to reduce, or at least not increase, the computational burden. For what types of measurement error would a nodal filter be effective? In [3] it was conjectured that a nodal filter would not be effective against random noise, and that it might be effective against systematic errors. We will show that the nodal filter is effective in reducing one type of systematic error, angular undersampling.

II THEORY and METHOD

In $\mathbb{R}^2$, the ERT is defined by

$$g(r,\phi,) = \exp(-\mu\beta(r,\phi)) \int_{S^1}\int_{R^1} f(p,\theta)\, \delta(r-p\cos(\theta-\phi))\exp(-\mu p\sin(\theta-\phi))\; p\,dp\,d\theta \;.$$

It was shown in [1] that the radial modulators of the projections satisfy

$$\int_0^{r_{max}} dr\; g_k(r)\, r^s = 0$$

$$\text{for} \begin{cases} 0 \le s < |k|,\ |k| - s = \textit{even integer}, \\ \textit{or} \\ k - s = \textit{odd integer} \end{cases} \qquad (1)$$

where r_{max} is the radius of the field of view. This statement is often called the consistency condition, because projection data must satisfy this constraint. In [1], condition (1) was used to find the minimum number of nodes. For the ERT, we consider the premultiplied projections

$$p(r,\phi;\mu) = \exp(\mu\beta(r,\phi))g(r,\phi)$$

parameterized by the attenuation coefficient μ, and the 2D Fourier transform of the projections

$$P_k(R;\mu) = \int_{-\infty}^{\infty} p_k(r;\mu)\exp(-irR)\,dr \tag{2}$$

In [4], it was shown that for the continuous limit, the solution for the ERT was

$$f_k(p) = (1/2)i^k\left(\int_{\mu}^{\infty} + \int_{-\infty}^{-\mu}\right) dR\,|R| \left(\frac{R-\mu}{R+\mu}\right)^{k/2} J_k(\,pR(1-(\mu/R)^2\,)^{1/2}\,)P_k(R;\mu) \quad , \tag{3}$$

where J_k is the k-th order Bessel function of the 1st kind.

From eq.(25) in [4], we can prove the following lemma:

$$\left(\frac{R-\mu}{R+\mu}\right)^{k/2} P_k(R;\mu) = (-)^k \left(\frac{R+\mu}{R-\mu}\right)^{k/2} P_k(-R;\mu) \quad . \tag{4}$$

Pf.

From eq(25), we obtain for $|R| \geq \mu$, $k \in Z^+$,

$$P_k(R;\mu) = 2\pi(-i\, sign(R))^k \left(\frac{R+\mu}{R-\mu}\right)^{k/2} \int_0^\infty dp\, p\, f_k(p)\, J_k\left(pR(1-(\mu/R)^2)^{1/2} \right) \quad . \tag{5}$$

Substituting -R for R in (5) and taking into account that J_k is even or odd according as k is even or odd, we obtain (4).

The link to the projection data $p(r,\phi;0)$ that would be obtained from f if
$\mu = 0$ is established by the following theorem:

For the continuous spectrum,

$$P_k(R\,;0) = \exp(-k\,\sinh^{-1}(\mu/R))P_k\!\left(\,sign(R)\sqrt{r^2+\mu^2}\,;\mu\,\right)\;. \tag{6}$$

Pf.

Using eq.(4) in eq.(3) with the change of variable

$$R' = sign(R)\sqrt{R^2-\mu^2}\;\;,$$

and dropping the prime, we obtain

$$\begin{aligned} f_k(p) = i^k\int_0^\infty dR\; R\,\exp(-k\,\sinh^{-1}(\mu/R)) \\ J_k(pR)P_k\!\left(sign(R)\sqrt{R^2+\mu^2};\mu\right)\;, \end{aligned} \tag{7}$$

where

$$\exp(-k\,\sinh^{-1}(\mu/R'\,)) = \left(\frac{R-\mu}{R+\mu}\right)^{k/2}\;.$$

Eq. (7) is still true for $\mu = 0$. Therefore, the property of uniqueness for the Hankel transform implies the theorem, eq. (10). The symmetry conditions follow from

$$p(r,\ \phi;\ 0) = p(-r,\ \phi + \pi;\ 0),$$

which is true if the line integrals exist. From this condition, the Fourier components of $p_k(r;0)$ are

$$a_k(R_m)\cos(R_m r)\ , \qquad a_k(R_m)\sin(R_m r)\ , \tag{8}$$

for k even or odd, respectively. If the object is real-valued (hence the projections are real - valued), then

$$a_k(R) = a^*_{-k}(-R)\ .$$

In order to determine the number of nodes of $p_k(r;\mu)$ given facts about the minimum number of nodes of $p_k(r;0)$, we can trace the transformation

$$p_k(r;0)\ \mid\!\!-\!\!-\!\!>\ p_k(r;\mu)$$

using the theorem, eq.(6). For example, consider k even, then from (2) and (8) we obtain

$$P_k(R;0) = \frac{a_k(R_m)}{2}\ (\ \delta(R-R_m) + \delta(R-R_m)\ )\ . \tag{9}$$

Using transformation (6) in eq. (9), we see that

$$P_k(R;\mu) - \frac{a_k(R_m)}{2}\, \exp\!\left(k\,\sinh^{-1}\!\left(\frac{\mu}{sign(R)\sqrt{R^2-\mu^2}}\right)\right) \tag{10}$$

$$\left\{\, \delta\!\left(sign(R)\sqrt{R^2-\mu^2}-R_m\right) + \delta\!\left(sign(R)\sqrt{R^2-\mu^2}+R_m\right) \right\} \;.$$

Recalling that in the continuous limit,

$$P_k(R;\mu) = 0$$

for

$$|\, R \,| < \mu,$$

We obtain the Fourier inversion integral

$$p_k(r\,;\mu) - \int_{|R|>\mu} dR\; P_k(R\,;\mu)\, \exp(iRr) \;. \tag{11}$$

Using eq.(10) in eq.(11), we obtain

$$p_k(r;\mu) = \frac{a_k(R_m)R_m}{\sqrt{R_m^2+\mu^2}} \left\{ \cosh\left(k \sinh^{-1}\left(\frac{\mu}{R_m}\right)\right) \cos\left(r\sqrt{R_m^2+\mu^2}\right) + \right. \tag{12}$$
$$\left. i \sinh\left(k \sinh^{-1}\left(\frac{\mu}{R_m}\right)\right) \sin\left(r\sqrt{R_m^2+\mu^2}\right) \right\} .$$

A similar result is obtained for k odd.

There are several observations to be drawn from this transformation formula, eq. (12). First, we obtain eq. (8) for $\mu = 0$. Taken individually, neither $Re(p_k(r;\mu))$ nor $Im(p_k(r;\mu))$ have even or odd symmetry. So we will have to determine the number of nodes in the open interval $-r_{max} < r < r_{max}$. Thus $p_k(r;0)$ will possess at least k nodes in the interval $(-r_{max}, r_{max})$.

Most importantly, the effect of uniform attenuation is to shift the frequency R_m of a Fourier component of $p_k(r;\mu)$ to $\sqrt{R_m^2 + \mu^2}$. Since the number of nodes of $p_k(r;0)$ is proportional to the lowest frequency R_l of the Fourier components of $p_k(r;0)$, and the consistency conditions imply

$$R_l \geq \frac{k}{r_{max}} ,$$

for the XT, and

$$R_l \geq \sqrt{\left(\frac{k}{r_{max}}\right)^2 + \mu^2} \tag{13}$$

for the ERT [4], then we have the following

Theorem: In the continuous limit, the minimum number of nodes of Re($p_k(r;\mu)$) or Im($p_k(r;\mu)$) is given by

$$\left[\sqrt{k^2 + (\mu r_{max})^2}\,\right] , \tag{14}$$

where [x] denotes nearest integer $\leq$ x. For R_l expressed on cycles/cm (or cycles/unit length) this formula is modified slightly:

$$\left[\sqrt{k^2 + \left(\frac{\mu r_{max}}{2\pi}\right)}\right] . \tag{14a}$$

Pf.

The fundamental frequency of the radial modulator is shifted upward according to (13). The ratio of this shift is

$$\frac{\sqrt{R_l^2 + \mu^2}}{R_l} . \qquad (15)$$

using eq. (13) and assuming equality to hold for R_l, we obtain from (15) the result (15).

The above theorems are asymptotic results that hold only in the continuous limit, i.e., as Δr, $\Delta\phi$ and ΔR --> 0. But for k and R commensurate with medical applications of SPECT, they are accurate even for small values of R and k.

Another question needing to answered in the implementation of a nodal filter is the effect of bounded support upon the number of nodes. If $f(p,\phi)$ is nonzero only in the disk of radius r_0, and $r_0 < r_{max}$, what is the effect upon the number of nodes of $p_k(r;0)$? Following the proof in [1] we see that

$$\int_0^{r_0} p_k(r\,;\,0)\, r^s\, dr - 2\int_0^{r_0} f_k(\,p\,)\, p^{s-1}\, dp \int_0^1 \frac{t^s\, T_k(\,t\,)}{\sqrt{1-t^2}}\, dt \ ,$$

where T_k is the Tschebyshev polynomial of the 1st kind. The integral on the right determines the number of nodes of $p_k(r;0)$ and it does not depend on r_0.

III APPLICATION TO DATA WITH ANGULAR UNDERSAMPLING

The data set we used was generated from the liver-spleen phantom developed by [5], using a projector code written by B. C. Penney and based on [6]. Planar images of size 64 x 64. were generated for 128 angles in 360°. Pixel size was 0.58 cm. and the diameter D of the region of nonzero support was about 33 cm. The number of projections N required to reconstruct without aliasing is given by [7,8,9,3]

$$N \geq \frac{\pi D}{\Delta X} ,$$

where Δx is the spatial resolution. The data was generated for an attenuation coefficient of $\mu = 0.15\text{cm}^{-1}$. The contour of the attenuating medium was specified, so there would be no misregistration errors in the reconstructed images. Line integrals were convolved in three dimensions with a gaussian point response function with a FWHM of one-half pixel, so $\Delta x = 0.58$ cm. Using these parameters, we see that

$$N \geq 179,$$

so we should encounter angular undersampling outside circle of about 25 cm. The projections were calculate in floating point precision, scaled to realisti values, and Poisson noise was added. There were abou 50,000 counts/sinogram in these data sets, low even fo SPECT.

The data were reconstructed using the CHT algorith based on the energy-distance principle [10,4,11]. Th data were reconstructed with and without the noda filter and are compared in figure 1.

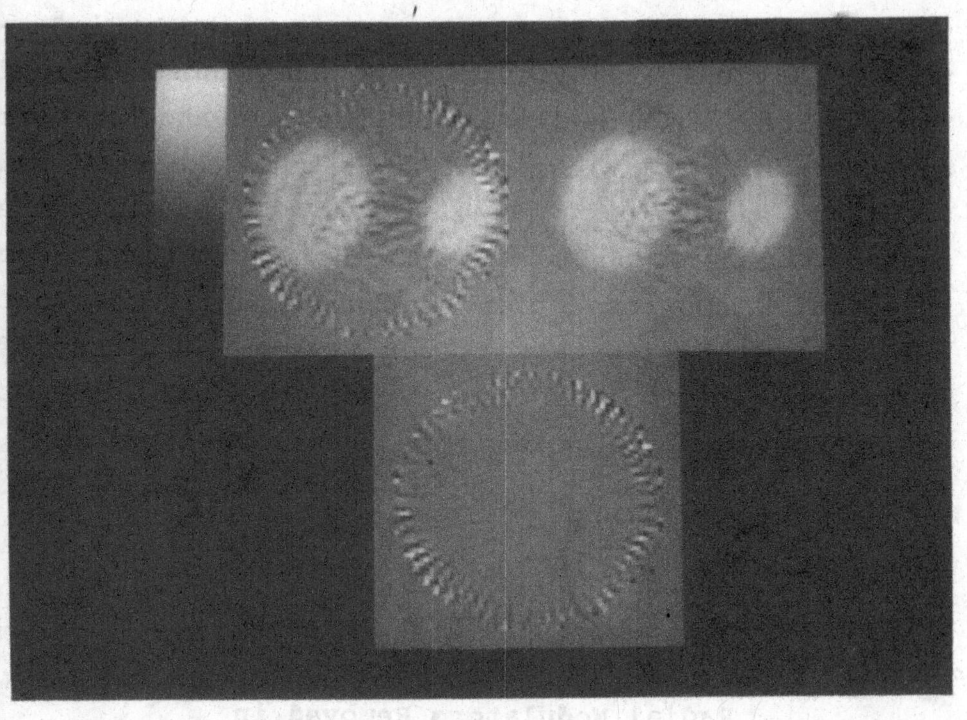

Figure 1

Reconstructions of a typical slice of the liver-spleen phantom. (Upper left) the reconstruction without the nodal filter. (Upper right) reconstruction with the nodal filter. (Center) the difference image, stretched to emphasize differences.

There are probably many ways to implement the information that eq. (14) provides. We have chosen one of the simplest, in order to assess the relevance of this application to clinical SPECT. If both the real and imaginary parts of $p_k(r;\mu)$ failed to possess the minimum number of nodes, then the radial modulator was rejected. Thus the action of the filter is somewhat like that of a low-pass filter with a sharp cutoff frequency. From Table 1, we see that it is not completely accurate to describe the filter this way.

TABLE 1

Radial Modulators Removed in Figure 1

30 - 33, 35 -64

In addition to removing angular streaks, we see in Table 2 that the nodal-filtered image is closer to the reference image than the unfiltered image. We used two different figures of merit to compare the images. In Table 3, an analysis of the signal-to-noise ratio (SNR) for a region of uniform concentration near the center of rotation reveals that there is no difference between the filtered and unfiltered images. In this respect, the nodal filter has a non-stationary character.

TABLE 2

Figures of Merit

Normalized Mean Squared Error	Normalized Cross-Correlation Coefficient
Filtered	
8.42×10^{-2}	0.9604
Unfiltered	
0.5645	0.7995

The statistics for Table 3 were obtained as follows. Three contiguous slices in the center of the phantom were selected. Using computer software for the computer-aided analysis of experiments and clinical data (CAECD?), a region-of-interest (ROI) was drawn by hand near the interior of the large ellipse (the liver) of the nodal filtered images (figure 2). The ROI was saved in memory and transferred to the two other slices, and then to the slices of the unfiltered images. Since all of the image voxels in the ROIs represented the same concentration of isotope in the object, the sample average and standard deviation were calculated. By use of the Student's t-test, we estimated that the observed difference between the two means was statistically insignificant, at the 98% confidence level.

TABLE 3

Statistical Data for an Interior Region of Uniform Concentration

Mean	Per Cent RMS Uncertainty
Filtered	
37.33	30
Unfiltered	
37.31	30

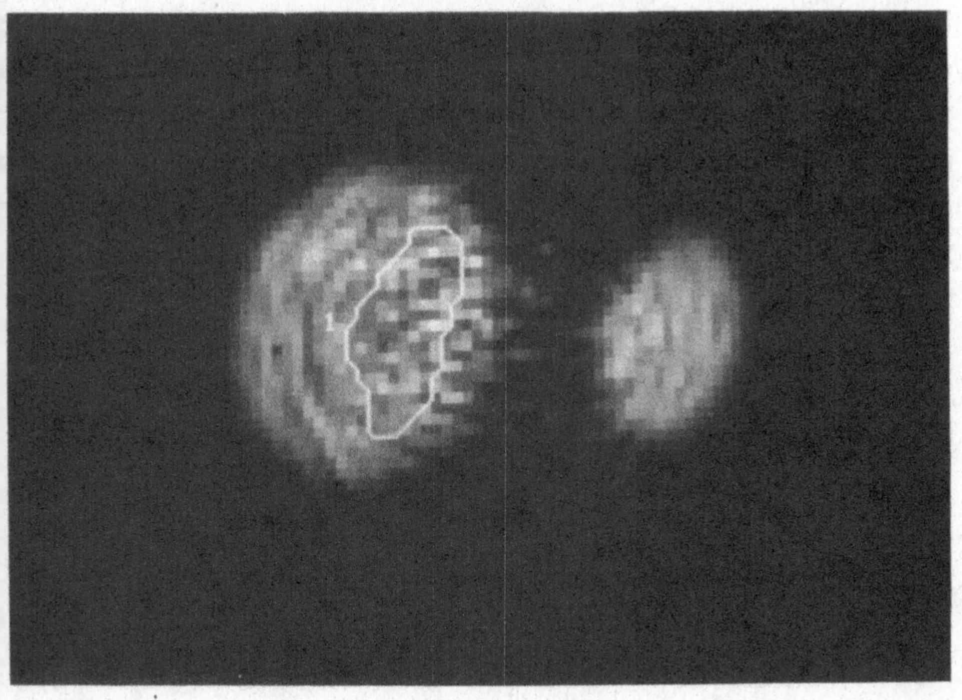

Figure 2

The ROI used in the determination of the means and variances in Table 3.

IV CONCLUSION

We have developed a transformation formula for determining the approximate number of nodes of projection data based on the ERT, and a straightforward application of this information to realistic simulations of SPECT data. We have shown that the implementation offers improvement for the case of angular undersampling, and that the filter has a nonstationary character, by not altering the interior region for which there is sufficient angular sampling.

ACKNOWLEDGMENTS

This work was supported in part by grants from the National Institutes of Health CA43791, CA21661, the National Cancer Institute, and Department of Energy DE-FG02-89ER60867.

REFERENCES

1. Cormack, A.M., "Representations of a Function by its Line Integrals, with some Applications," J. Appl. Phys. 344(9), Sep. 1963. pp. 2722-2727.

2. Cormack, A.M., "Representations of a Function by its Line Integrals, with Some Applications,", J. Appl Phys. 35(10), Oct. 1964, pp 2908-2913.

3. Hawkins, W.G., Dissertation, Dept. of Appl. Math., Univ. of Arizona, Tucson, Az., 1982.

4. Hawkins, W.G., PK Leichner & N-C Yang, "The Circular Harmonic Transform for SPECT and Boundary Conditions on the Fourier Transform of the Sinogram," IEEE Trans. MI 7(2), Jun 1988, pp 135-148.

5. Knesaurek, K, King, MA, Glick, SJ & Penney, BC, "A 3-D non-stationary simulation of SPECT imaging," J. Nucl. Med., 30, pp 1666-1675, May, 1989.

6. Penney, BC, King, MA & Knesaurek, K, "A projector, backprojector pair which accounts for the two dimensional depth and distance dependent blurring in SPECT," IEEE Trans NS, in press.

7. Jaszczak RJ, Coleman RE, Lim CB, "SPECT: Single Photon Emission Computed Tomography," IEEE NS, 27(3), June 1980, pp 1137-1153.

8. Snyder DL, Cox RJ, "An Overview of Reconstructive Tomography and Limitations Imposed by a Finite Number

of Projections," in: <u>Reconstruction Tomography in Diagnostic Radiology and Nuclear Medicine</u>, MM Ter-Pogosian et. al. eds., University Park Press, Baltimore, MD, 1977, pp 3-32.

9. Huesman RH, "The effects of a Finite Number of Projection Angles and Finite Lateral Sampling on the Propagation of Statistical Errors in Transverse Section Reconstruction," Phys. Med. Biol., <u>22</u>(4), 1985, pp 409-415.

10. Edholm PR, Lewitt RW, Lindholm B, "Novel Properties of the Fourier Transform of the Sinogram," SPIE Proc. <u>671</u>, Apr 1986, pp 8-18.

11. Hawkins WG, Leichner PK, Yang N-C, "Validation of the Circular Harmonic Transform for Quantitative SPECT," to appear in J. Nucl. Med.

EVALUATION OF RECONSTRUCTION ALGORITHMS

Gabor T. Herman and Dewey Odhner
Department of Radiology, Hospital of the University of Pennsylvania
3400 Spruce Street, Philadelphia, PA 19104, USA

Abstract. We present a methodology which allows us to experimentally optimize an image reconstruction method for a specific medical task and to evaluate the relative efficacy of two reconstruction methods for a particular task in a manner which meets the high standards set by the methodology of statistical hypothesis testing. We illustrate this by comparing, in the area of Positron Emission Tomography (PET), a Maximum *A posteriori* Probability (MAP) algorithm with a method which maximizes likelihood and with two variants of the filtered backprojection method. We find that the relative performance of techniques is extremely task dependent, with the MAP method superior to the others from the point of view of pointwise accuracy, but not from the points of view of two other PET-related figures of merit. In particular, we find that, in spite of the very noisy appearance of the reconstructed images, the maximum likelihood method outperforms the others from the point of view of estimating average activity in individual neurological structures of interest.

I. ITERATIVE IMAGE RECONSTRUCTION FOR PET

In this article we concentrate on methods motivated by emission computerized tomography, which has as its major emphasis the quantitative determination of the moment-to-moment changes in the chemistry and flow physiology of injected or inhaled compounds labeled with radioactive atoms. In this case the function to be reconstructed is the distribution of radioactivity in a body cross-section and the measurements are used to estimate the total activity along lines of known location. One of the things that distinguishes this problem from that arising from x-ray computerized tomography is that the measurements tend to be much more noisy. For this reason, it appears desirable for an image reconstruction method which is to be used in emission tomography to incorporate an estimation procedure which depends on the statistical nature of the noise in the measurements.

Specifically, we concentrate on *Positron Emission Tomography* (PET). In PET the isotope used emits positrons, which within a few millimeters of their origins annihilate with nearby electrons, resulting in two photons travelling away from each other in (nearly) opposing directions. Near-simultaneous detection of these two photons approximately determines the line along which the emission has taken place. We count such coincidences for a number of lines over a period of time; the number of coincidences for a line is clearly related to the integral of the concentration of the radionuclide along the line. From such measurements we wish to estimate the distribution of the radionuclide at individual points in the cross-section. (In this discussion we have repeatedly idealized the physical situation; e.g., we have talked about cross-sections as if they were infinitesimally thin. The effect of such idealizations on the efficacy of the resulting algorithms is carefully treated in the literature [3, 4, 10–12]; in what follows we work with a mathematically idealized problem without any further justification.)

The emission of positrons is a Poisson process [11], the mean of which is determined by the concentration of the isotope. It is the latter that we wish to determine. More exactly, we are aiming at recovering a function whose value is the expected number of coincidences (generated photon-pairs) along a line per unit length during the data-collection period. (We are assuming, as is physically justified, that the activity is isotropic. Note also that the dimensionality of what we are reconstructing is "inverse length".) The cross-section where the activity takes place can be enclosed by a square-shaped region. We discretize our problem by subdividing this square-shaped region into J small abutting square-shaped picture elements (*pixels*, for short) and assuming that the activity in each pixel is constant. (This is a common approach to image reconstruction from projections [3, 4, 10–12]; for a discussion of what it might mean for the approach taken in this paper see [23], including the printed comments following it.) This approach is represented in Fig. 1, where x_j denotes the expected number of coincidences per unit length in the jth pixel ($1 \leq j \leq J$). We use x to represent the J-dimensional vector whose jth component is x_j and call x the *image vector* [11].

Suppose that we count coincidences along I lines. We use y to represent the I-dimensional vector whose ith element (y_i) is the number of coincidences which are counted for the ith line during the data collection period and call y the *measurement vector* [11]. If l_{ij} denotes the length of intersection of the ith line with the jth pixel, then y_i is a sample from a Poisson distribution whose expected value is

$$\sum_{j=1}^{J} l_{ij} x_j \tag{1}$$

(see Fig. 1).

Based on this, we see that the probability of obtaining the measurement vector y if the image vector is x (the so-called *likelihood* function) is

$$P_L(y/x) = \prod_{i=1}^{I} \left[\frac{1}{y_i!} \left(\sum_{j=1}^{J} l_{ij}\, x_j \right)^{y_i} exp\left(- \sum_{j=1}^{J} l_{ij}\, x_j \right) \right] \tag{2}$$

Our problem, of course, is to estimate x, given y.

One possible approach is the *maximum likelihood* (ML) method, which selects the x that maximizes $P_L(y/x)$ or, equivalently, maximizes

$$\sum_{i=1}^{I} \left[y_i\, ln \left(\sum_{j=1}^{J} l_{ij} x_j \right) - \sum_{j=1}^{J} l_{ij}\, x_j \right] \tag{3}$$

subject to $x \in R_+^J = \{x \mid x_j \geq 0, \ \text{for} \ \ 1 \leq j \leq J\}$. Such an approach was proposed in [21] together with an iterative algorithm for estimating the maximizer of (3). While the algorithm was mathematically correct (the value of (3) was monotonically increasing with the iterations), in its practical application to PET the iterations had to be stopped before a deteriorating "checkerboard effect" (irregular high amplitude patterns) showed up [23]. Thus maximizing likelihood does not, at first sight, appear to be the appropriate optimization formulation for PET.

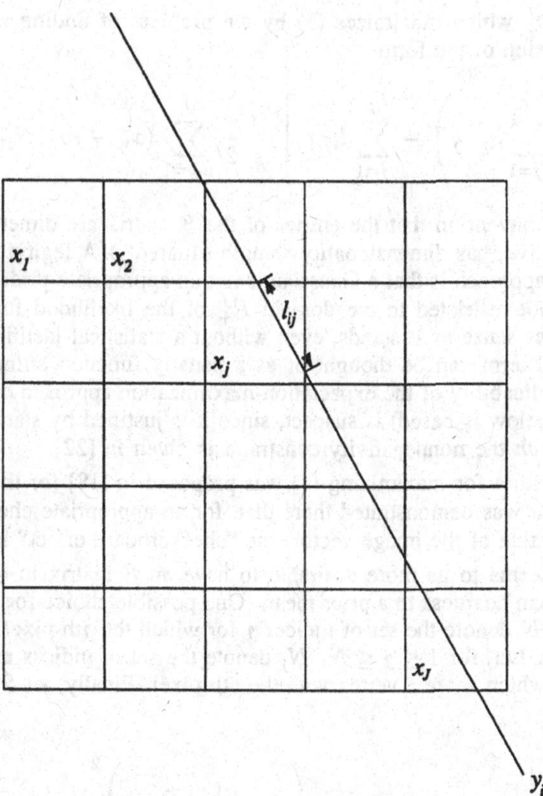

Figure 1. The geometry of data collection for a single line. The expected number of coincidences per unit length in the jth pixel is x_j. The actual number of coincidences counted for the ith line is y_i. The length of intersection of the ith line with the jth pixel is l_{ij}.

To overcome this difficulty, we previously proposed a Maximum *A posteriori* Probability (MAP) maximization approach [18]. We assumed a Gaussian prior probability distribution for the image vector x. (The Gaussian prior had been previously used by us for CT [13] and has also been investigated by others in the PET context; see, e.g., [19]. It is only one of a number of approaches that can be used to overcome the difficulty; among others that have been proposed we mention by the way of examples: MAP with a Gibbs prior [6], the use of sieves [22], and early stopping of a likelihood maximizing iterative process according to some statistical criterion [9]. We did not carry out a careful examination of the relative efficacy of these proposed methods for any particular medical task and so we make no claims whatsoever as to the relative merits of the methods proposed in this paper to the above-mentioned alternatives. It is however the case that the methodology that we propose below for the evaluation of the comparative efficacy of reconstruction algorithms can be used by anyone wishing to demonstrate the statistically significant superiority for a particular task of any one of these methods over any other.) Combining the probability density function of a Gaussian prior with (2) in Bayes' formula for *a posteriori* probability, we replaced the problem of finding an x in R_+^J which maximizes (3) by the problem of finding an x in R_+^J which maximizes an expression of the form

$$\sum_{i=1}^{I}\left[y_i\, ln\left(\sum_{j=1}^{J} l_{ij}\, x_j\right) - \sum_{j=1}^{J} l_{ij}\, x_j\right] - \frac{\gamma}{2}\sum_{u,v=1}^{J}(x_u - m_u)\, S_{uv}\,(x_v - m_v) \qquad (4)$$

(Here we adopt the convention that the entries of the S matrix are dimensionless and so γ, which is always positive, has dimensionality "length squared".) A legitimate objection which can be raised to this approach is that a Gaussian is not an appropriate prior since its probability density function is not restricted to the domain R_+^J of the likelihood function. However, maximizing (4) makes sense as it stands, even without a statistical justification, since (as we shall see) the second term can be thought of as a penalty function enforcing smoothness. Nevertheless, the applicability of the expectation-maximization approach of [18] (on which the algorithm proposed below is based) is suspect, since it is justified by statistical arguments. A method of dealing with the nonnegativity constraint is given in [22].

An iterative algorithm for maximizing (4) was proposed in [18] for the special case when $S_{uv} = 0$ for $u \neq v$. It was demonstrated there that, for an appropriate choice of the m vector (the prior expected value of the image vector) the "checkerboard effect" is prevented.

Nevertheless, it seems to us more desirable to have an S matrix in (4) which enforces smoothness, rather than nearness to a prior mean. One possible choice for such an S is defined as follows [11]. Let N denote the set of indices j for which the jth pixel is not on the border of the picture region. Let, for $1 \leq j \leq N$, N_j denote the set of indices associated with those at most eight pixels which share a vertex with the jth pixel. Finally, let S in (4) be the matrix such that

$$x^T S x = \sum_{j\in N}\left(x_j - \frac{1}{8}\sum_{k\in N_j} x_k\right)^2 \qquad (5)$$

and let m in (4) be the zero vector. (Note that this is less restrictive than it appears at first sight. The functional in (5) would have the same value for any m with constant components. Thus our approach does not bias the reconstruction towards the zero vector, it simply biases it towards a smooth vector.) Choosing S and m in this way, we end up with a MAP approach to PET in which a likelihood maximization term is penalized by a term enforcing smoothness.

For details of derivation, implementation and validation of an efficient iterative algorithm for solving this problem we refer the reader to [16]. Here we just reproduce its iterative step as follows. For $1 \leq j \leq J$, let

$$W_{jj} = \sum_{i=1}^{I} l_{ij} \qquad (6)$$

$$p_j = \frac{W_{jj}}{\gamma S_{jj}} - x_j^{(k)} + \frac{1}{S_{jj}}\sum_{u=1}^{J} S_{ju}\, x_u^{(k)} \qquad (7)$$

$$q_j = \frac{x_j^{(k)}}{\gamma S_{jj}} \sum_{i=1}^{I} \frac{l_{ij}\, y_i}{\sum_{n=1}^{J} l_{in}\, x_n^{(k)}} \tag{8}$$

$$x_j^{(k+1)} = \frac{1}{2}\left(-p_j + \sqrt{p_j^2 + 4q_j}\right) \tag{9}$$

We take the + sign in front of the square root to insure the positivity of $x_j^{(k+1)}$.

II. PERFORMANCE EVALUATION

Iterative image reconstruction methods have been with us for two decades now [7]. Their flexibility, which allows one to adapt them to particular tasks, is usually cited as the justification for choosing them. Nevertheless, they are not nearly as often used as the (non-iterative) transform methods. The main reason for this is that the iterative methods tend to be computationally much more expensive [11]. Cost considerations also influence their efficacy for practical tasks: the experimental adjustment of free parameters in them (such as the number of iterations) so that they become optimal for the task at hand has been considered prohibitively expensive in the past.

The enormous decrease in the cost of computation in recent years substantially changes this situation. It is now feasible to experimentally optimize an iterative image reconstruction method for a specific medical task and to evaluate the relative efficacy of two reconstruction methods for a particular task in a manner which meets the high standards set by the methodology of statistical hypothesis testing [20]. The pioneering work in this direction is due to Hanson; see [8] and its references.

We illustrate our PET-oriented development of this approach by comparing the method of Section I with an expectation maximization (EM) method which maximizes likelihood (ML) [21]. We compare the efficacy of these two methods, for three different numbers of iterations, from the points of view of three tasks: detection of relatively higher uptake on the left vs. the right side of the brain; estimation of the total uptake in various neurological structures; and estimation of uptake at individual points within neurological structures of interest. We also compare the performance of the six iterative techniques (two methods times three iteration numbers) with that of two variants of a transform method (the so-called convolution or filtered-backprojection method).

In order to make our experiments realistic from the point of view of a clinical imaging task, we used a computerized overlay atlas based on average anatomy [1]. This atlas consists of 26 overlays each corresponding to a transaxial slice of the brain. Neuroanatomical structures are represented by ellipses and rectangles at appropriate locations; they are symmetrical with respect to the midline. We made use of this symmetry to set up our experiment as follows.

We created mathematical phantoms in which (in arbitrary units) the activity in the brain background is 1.00 and in the neuroanatomical structures it is 1.95 or 2.00. For each pair of symmetric structures a random number generator chooses exactly one of the pair to have an activity of 2.00. The top left image in Fig. 2 shows the 95×95 digitization of one such phantom. The same digitization (see Fig. 1) was used for all the reconstructions. Since we used 26 different overlays with several structures in each (there are 26 structures, in addition to the background shape, in the overlay shown in Fig. 2), it does not seem reasonable to provide here detailed descriptions of them. These data are available from the authors.

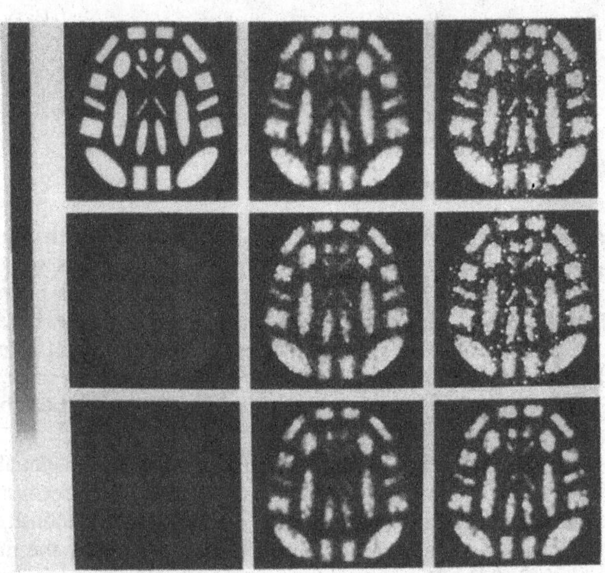

Figure 2. One of our phantoms and eight reconstructions (see text). The grey scale is selected so that we see better the differences inside the brain than outside. (Even so, the small differences between the densities in the neurological structures on the left and the right sides are not visible.) Since all our figures of merit are based solely on the values inside the brain, any artifacts outside the brain have no influence on them.

We generated images and projection data of these phantoms using SNARK89 [14]. In generating the projection data we assumed a ring of 300 detectors with each detector in coincidence with 101 detectors opposite it. (In SNARK89 terminology, we have a divergent ray geometry with 300 views and 101 rays per view. The distance between the detectors was selected so that the fan of rays in a view cover the region of the brain in all phantoms and that the length of the side of a pixel is about the same as the distance between two rays at the center of the reconstruction region.) Poisson noise was introduced into the measurements on the basis of a total of 3,000,000 coincidences collected per slice. Although this averages approximately 100 coincidences per SNARK89 ray (and so it may appear that the normal approximation to the Poisson distribution is justified), we note that for many rays the expected number of coincidences will be much less. All the resulting ray sums were further deteriorated by 10% multiplicative Gaussian noise, to take care of other sources of error besides photon statistics. (Since the ray sums are by far the largest for the center of each projection, adding 10%

multiplicative noise introduces a larger error near the center than elsewhere in the projections. Nevertheless, one can reasonably argue that even such additional noise does not adequately describe noise in real PET data after attenuation correction and scatter deconvolution. However, since our main purpose here is to illustrate our evaluation methodology, rather than to make a final decision regarding the superiority of any particular algorithm for any particular PET instrument and for any particular medical task, we feel that including such additional noise to take care of the errors whose nature we cannot model statistically makes our illustration sufficiently realistic to demonstrate the usefulness of our evaluation approach. We also note that this additional noise is not modeled in the likelihood function. This reasonably reflects the real situation; there will always be some discrepancy between an actual PET instrument and a mathematical/statistical model of its behavior.)

For our evaluation experiments 1,000 phantoms and their projection data were generated: the overlay on which the phantom was based, the sides of elevated activity, and the noise in the data were independently randomly generated each time.

Preliminary experiments were done on an independently generated smaller set of phantoms and projection data (referred to as the *training set*) to find values of the free parameters for the reconstruction methods which are optimal for certain tasks performed on the training set [15]. Some of the details of how the choices were made are given below with the description of the tasks.

The methods that we compared were the convolution method (see, e.g., [11]) and two EM-type algorithms, one for maximizing likelihood (3), and the other is the method of (6)-(9) for MAP estimation (4). We used the computer implementation described in [16]; in the case of ML this results in a pure EM algorithm without any "acceleration" or other tricks. Because of this, there were no free parameters to optimize in the ML case, except the iteration number. Based on the experiments in [15], we picked iteration numbers 2, 28, and 80 as worthy of further study. (A very reasonable question that can be raised is the following: since the different methodologies have been introduced with the justification that they optimize certain functionals, what is the point of even looking at the results of iterative procedures which have been terminated far short of convergence? Our answer to this is two-fold. First, pre-convergence termination is a commonly made recommendation in our field; see [9], which is the most recent, at the time of writing, of a long series of publications discussing the practical appropriateness of early stopping. It seems to us worthwhile to evaluate what is after all common practice. Second, it can be shown for a large family of iterative reconstruction algorithms, see [5] and its references, that truncating the iterative process provides an optimum according to a regularized version of the original functional. Under such circumstances, studying early iterates is similar to studying the optimization problem with varying weights of a smoothness constraint.)

For the convolution method we had to select a filter. Using the training set, we found that a very smoothing filter is the most appropriate for the detection task; it is one which sets all frequencies to be zero beyond eight-tenths of the Nyquist rate (in SNARK89 terms: cutoff=0.8) and otherwise has the shape of the generalized Hamming filter with $\alpha = 0.5$ [11]. This is quite different from what has been found most useful for x-ray CT, which would typically be a generalized Hamming filter with $\alpha = 0.8$ and cutoff = 1.0 [11, 14]. Reconstructions using these two filters are shown in the middle and on the right, respectively, in the top row of Fig. 2.

For the MAP estimation we had to select the weight γ to be given to the smoothing prior in (4). Using the training set we found $\gamma = 10$ to be the most appropriate for the detection task and so we decided to do all our evaluations for only this specific value. (This implies that there may be much more appropriate values for the other tasks; this will have to be looked at prior to making any final recommendations regarding the relative merits of the methods.) The middle and the bottom rows of Fig. 2 show reconstructions by the EM algorithms, for ML and MAP, respectively, after 2, 28, and 80 iterations.

To evaluate the various reconstruction methods we made use of three medically reasonable Figures of Merit (FOMs).

Detection of Relatively Higher Uptake. Here we make use of the fact that structures in our phantoms form symmetric pairs. For each structure we define the *abnormality index* in the reconstruction to be the average of reconstructed pixel values for those pixels whose centers are within that structure in the phantom. A pair of symmetric structures provides us with a *hit*, if the abnormality index in the reconstruction is higher for that structure in the pair for which the activity is higher in the phantom. The FOM is the ratio of hits to the total number of pairs in the data set, and we refer to it as the *hit-ratio*. (One can reasonably hope that this mathematically defined hit-ratio would correlate with human performance in deciding the side of the relatively higher uptake. However, the actual value of the numerical hit-ratio is likely to be considerably higher than that of the corresponding measure for humans, since a human reader would not have knowledge of the exact location of the structures to be compared and would have greater difficulty in perceiving the relative sizes of the average uptake over structures.)

If we find that one method is more accurate than another one according to this FOM, then we are still faced with the problem of deciding whether or not our finding is statistically significant. We adopt the sign test [20] to provide us with a level of significance for rejecting the null-hypothesis that two reconstruction methods are equally good in favor of the hypothesis that the one with the greater hit-ratio is better.

In this approach to statistical significance, we look only at those pairs of structures which have been classified differently by the two reconstruction methods. Let C be the total number of such pairs. Let c be the number of pairs that have been correctly classified by the reconstruction method with the higher hit-ratio. The null-hypothesis that the methods perform equally well implies that c is a random sample from a binomial distribution with total number of items C and equal probabilities assigned to the two classes. We can now use this binomial distribution to see what is the probability of randomly selecting an element from it with value c or higher. This probability provides us with our level of significance for rejecting the null-hypothesis.

The choices for the free parameters in the convolution method and for γ in (4) were made in [15] so as to optimize the algorithms from the point of view of the hit-ratio. In Fig. 3 we plot the average values (over 78 phantoms from the training set) of the hit-ratio. It is based on this plot that we selected iteration 2 as worthy of further study.

Estimation of Total Uptake in Neurological Structures. For each neurological structure, we define the *inaccuracy* to be the absolute value of the difference between the abnormality indices of that structure in the reconstruction and in the phantom. We define the *structural accuracy* to be the FOM which is the negative of the average of the inaccuracy over all structures in all phantoms.

The level of statistical significance for rejecting the null-hypothesis that two reconstruction methods are equally good in favor of the hypothesis that the one with higher structural accuracy is better is calculated as follows. Let β_b and δ_b be the inaccuracies of the bth of altogether B structures as reconstructed by the two methods, respectively. Then, according to the null-hypothesis, $\beta_b - \delta_b$ is a sample of a zero-mean random variable. It follows, for large

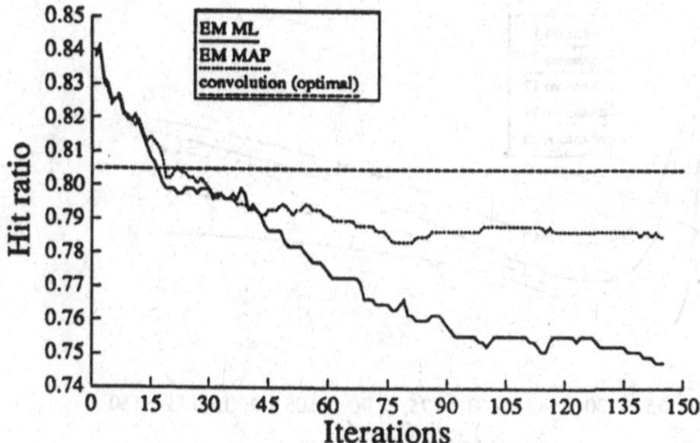

Figure 3. The averages over 78 phantoms of the training set of the hit-ratios.

nough B, that

$$\sum_{b=1}^{B} (\beta_b - \delta_b) \tag{10}$$

s a sample of a normally distributed zero-mean random variable [20]. The variance of this andom variable is B times that of the zero-mean random variable of which the $\beta_b - \delta_b$ are amples for $1 \leq b \leq B$. Hence, for large enough B, it is reasonable to assume that the ull-hypothesis implies that (10) is a sample from normally distributed random variable with nean zero and variance

$$\sum_{b=1}^{B} (\beta_b - \delta_b)^2 \tag{11}$$

We can thus use the normal distribution to calculate significance [20].

Estimation of Pointwise Uptake in Neurological Structures. For this we used the o-called clipped normalized distance provided by SNARK89 [14]. Briefly, both the phantom nd the reconstruction are clipped by setting pixel values which are less than (in our case) .65 to 1.65 and pixel values which are more than (in our case) 2.05 to 2.05. After this a ormalized root mean square distance between the clipped reconstruction and clipped phantom s calculated. The clipping insures that only the accuracy in and around neuroanatomical tructures contributes to the distance measure. The FOM is the average of the negative of the lipped normalized distance over all the phantoms. We call this FOM the *pointwise accuracy*, ince squaring of differences at individual pixels insures that large errors at just a few points vill degrade the FOM.

Statistical significance is calculated in the same way as for structural accuracy, except that ow we compare clipped normalized distances for whole phantoms (rather than inaccuracies or individual structures).

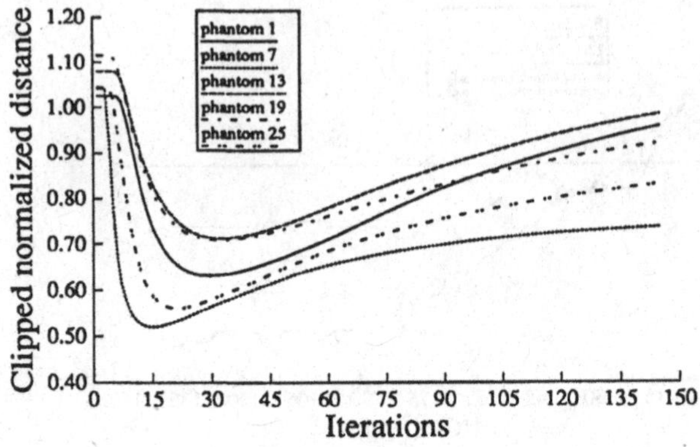

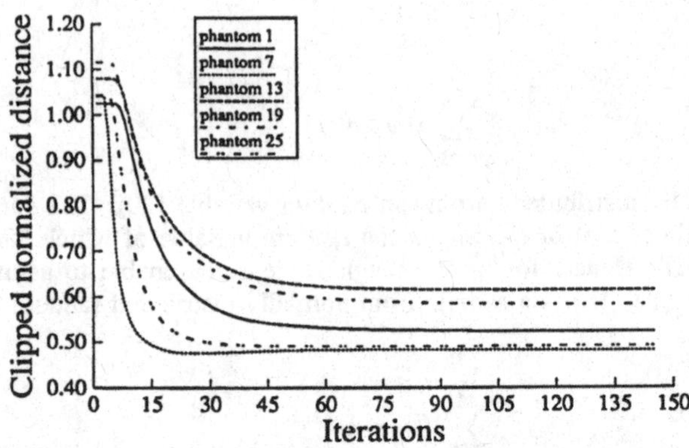

Figure 4. Clipped normalized distances for five phantoms in the training set reconstructed by ML-EM (top) and MAP-EM (bottom).

In Fig. 4 we plot the clipped normalized distances for five different phantoms in the training set both for ML-EM and for MAP-EM with $\gamma = 10$. It is the stability of the MAP approach from the point of view of such distance measures that motivated its study in the first place. In Fig. 5 we plot the average values (over 72 phantoms of the training set) of the clipped normalized distance. For ML-EM this average is minimum at iteration 28, which is why we selected iteration 28 as worthy of further study. The average monotonically decreases for MAP-EM. Based on Figs. 3 and 5, we considered that the performance of MAP-EM does not change significantly after cycle 80.

Table 1 reports on the rank-orderings of the eight reconstruction methods according to the three FOMs. All differences between two successive methods in the ordering are statistically significant at the 0.001 level [20], unless otherwise indicated. If significance is not at the 0.001 level but is at the 0.01 level, that is indicated by a single minus sign after the rank of the

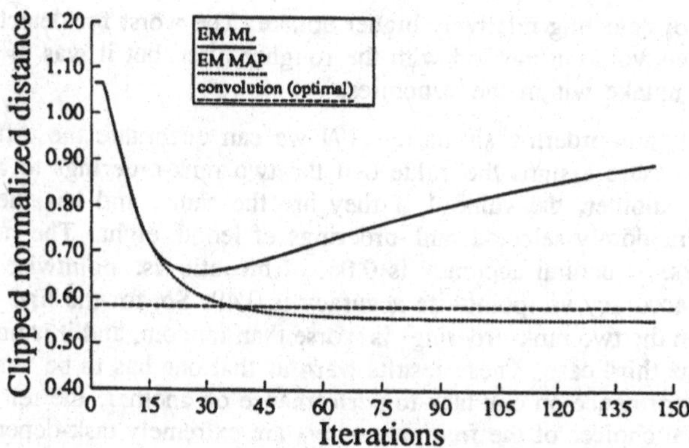

igure 5. The average over 78 phantoms of the training set of the clipped normalized distances.

econstruction with the higher FOM. Similarly, double minus sign indicates significance only t the 0.05 level, and triple minus sign indicates that difference is not significant at the 0.05 evel. We note that in all cases the difference between a method and another which is ranked wo below it was significant at least at the 0.05 level.

The main conclusion to be drawn from this table is the extreme dependence of the relative nerit of two reconstruction methods on the task to be performed. The second iterate of ML-EM was the best for detecting relatively higher uptake, but it had the worst pointwise ccuracy and the second worst structural accuracy. The eightieth iterate of ML-EM was the est for estimating average uptake within structures, but it was the second worst for detecting elatively higher uptake and the third worst for pointwise accuracy. The eightieth iterate of MAP-EM was the best for pointwise accuracy within the neurological structures, nevertheless

		Rank-Order by FOM		
method	parameter	hit-ratio	structural accuracy	pointwise accuracy
ML-EM	2	1 -	7	7.5
	28	4 - - -	4	4
	80	7 -	1	6
MAP-EM	2	2	8	7.5
	28	3 - - -	6	3
	80	6	3	1
convo-lution	smooth	5 - - -	5	2
	rough	8	2	5

Table 1. Rank-ordering of the eight methods by the three different Figures of Merit. Minus signs indicate lesser statistical significance (see text).

it was the third worst for detecting relatively higher uptake. The worst for detecting relatively higher uptake was the convolution method with the rougher filter, but it was the second best for estimating average uptake within the structures.

Using the notion of rank-ordering similarity [17] we can quantitate the differences in rank-orderings. This measure assigns the value 0 if the two rank-orderings to be compared are the reverse of one another, the value 1 if they are the same, and has the expected value of 0.34 for two randomly selected rank-orderings of length eight. The rank-ordering similarity of hit-ratio vs. structural accuracy is 0.06, of hit-ratio vs. pointwise accuracy is 0.25, and of structural accuracy vs. pointwise accuracy is 0.49. So, for the first two cases the correspondence between the two rank-orderings is worse than random, and it is not much better than random even in the third case. These results warn us that one has to be very careful and not generalize from performance on one task to performance on another: the relative merits of methods and the optimal choices of the free parameters are extremely task-dependent. For an interesting theoretical discussion of the relations between FOMs provided by estimation tasks and classification tasks, see [2].

III. DISCUSSION

We have presented an iterative algorithm appropriate for image reconstruction from noisy data. It is designed to find an image which maximizes *a posteriori* probability. The actual function to be maximized consists of a maximum likelihood term (based on the Poisson statistics of the data collection) penalized by a term which is designed to enforce local smoothness. An efficient parallel implementation is reported elsewhere [16]. The efficiency of our implementation means that experiments that we need to carry out (for example for finding the optimal γ for a particular medical problem involving positron emission tomography) can be done in an acceptable period of time even though they involve reconstructing a large number of images. This allows us to adjust our reconstruction algorithm to particular medical needs. It also allowed us to compare our algorithm with ML-EM and the convolution method, to obtain some rather interesting results and to show that these results have a high level of statistical significance. We summarize these results as follows.

First, (the eightieth iterate of) the MAP method outperformed all others that we tried from the point of view of pointwise accuracy. We must note however that the free parameters in the MAP and convolution methods were not selected to optimize this particular FOM, and so the results may well turn out to be different for the optimal choices of the free parameters.

Second, in spite of its relatively large pointwise accuracy, the MAP method is outperformed by both ML-EM and the "rough" convolution method from the point of view of structural accuracy. Although the comment regarding the choice of free parameters applies here as well, this result is nevertheless of great interest as it stands. The reason is that we [16, 18], as well as many others (e.g., [6, 9, 19, 22]), invested a great deal of effort to overcome the perceived deterioration of images produced by the ML-EM algorithm, as demonstrated in Figs. 2, 4 and 5. However, from the point of view of the clinically-used FOM of structural accuracy [1], this deterioration is illusory; the "noise" in the reconstructions averages over the neurological structures of interest, providing us with good structural accuracy in spite of bad pointwise accuracy.

Third, our results on the hit-ratio are also very interesting. What these results imply is that for the detection of relatively higher uptake neither the ML nor the MAP optimization criterion is relevant, since the second iterate of the algorithms (which is optimal according to the hit-ratio) produces pictures with low likelihood (3) and low *a posteriori* probability (4). It is fortuitous that early iterates of the EM algorithms outperform the task-optimized convolution method from this point of view (see Fig. 3), but that has nothing to do with the reasoning behind the EM algorithms.

In conclusion, the method proposed in Section I seems to have great promise if pointwise accuracy in positron emission tomographs is desired. On the other hand, it does not offer an improvement over previously proposed methods for PET reconstruction from the points of view of structural accuracy or the detection of relatively higher uptake. However, more important than any of these specific conclusions is that we have demonstrated a statistically rigorous way of validating claims regarding the superiority of one image reconstruction algorithm over another for a specific task and have illustrated that the relative merit of two reconstruction algorithms can be extremely dependent on the intended medical task.

ACKNOWLEDGMENTS

The research of the authors is supported by NIH grant HL28438. They are grateful to Drs. K.D. Toennies and S.A. Zenios for collaboration in the parallel implementation of the algorithm, to Dr. J. Ollinger for discussions regarding the generation of clinically realistic PET data, to Dr. L. Shepp for discussions regarding statistics and to Dr. C.J. Thompson for comments on an earlier version of the manuscript.

REFERENCES

[1] A. Alavi, R. Dann, J. Chawluk, J. Alavi, M. Kushner, and M. Reivich, *Positron emission tomography imaging of regional cerebral glucose metabolism*, Sem. Nucl. Med., 16 (1986), pp. 2–34.

[2] H. Barrett, *Objective assessment of image quality: effects of quantum noise and object variability*, J. Opt. Soc. Am. A, 7 (1990), pp. 1266–1278.

[3] T. Budinger, G. Gullberg, and R. Huesman, *Emission computed tomography*, in Image Reconstruction from Projections: Implementation and Applications, G. Herman, ed., Springer Verlag, Berlin, 1979, pp. 147–246.

[4] Y. Censor and G. Herman, *On some optimization techniques in image reconstruction from projections*, Appl. Num. Math., 3 (1987), pp. 365–391.

[5] H. Fleming, *Equivalence of regularization and truncated iteration in the solution of ill-posed image reconstruction problems*, Lin. Algeb. Appl., 130 (1990), pp. 133–150.

[6] S. Geman and D. McClure, *Statistical methods for tomographic image reconstruction*, Bull. Int. Stat. Inst., LII-4 (1987), pp. 5–21.

[7] R. Gordon, R. Bender, and G. Herman, *Algebraic reconstruction techniques (ART) for three-dimensional electron microscopy and x-ray photography*, J. Theoret. Biol., 29 (1970), pp. 471–482.

[8] K. Hanson, *Method of evaluating image-recovery algorithms based on task performance*, J. Opt. Soc. Am. A, 7 (1990), pp. 1294–1304.

[9] T. Hebert, *Statistical stopping criteria for iterative maximum likelihood reconstruction of emission images*, Phys. Med. Biol., 35 (1990), pp. 1221–1232.

[10] G. Herman, ed., *Image Reconstruction from Projections: Implementation and Applications*, Springer Verlag, Berlin, 1979.

[11] ——, *Image Reconstruction from Projections: The Fundamentals of Computerized Tomography*, Academic Press, New York, 1980.

[12] ——, *Special issue on computerized tomography*, Proc. IEEE, 71 (1983), pp. 291–435. Guest Ed.

[13] G. Herman and A. Lent, *A computer implementation of a Bayesian analysis of image reconstruction*, Inf. and Control, 31 (1976), pp. 364–384.

[14] G. Herman, R. Lewitt, D. Odhner, and S. Rowland, *SNARK89 – a programming system for image reconstruction from projections*, Tech. Rep. MIPG160, Dept. of Radiol., Univ of Pennsylvania, Philadelphia, 1989.

[15] G. Herman and D. Odhner, *A numerical two-alternative-forced-choice (2AFC) evaluation of imaging methods*, in Computer Applications to Assist Radiology, R. Arenson and R. Friedenberg, eds., Symposia Foundation, Carlsbad, CA, 1990, pp. 549–555.

[16] G. Herman, D. Odhner, K. Toennies, and S. Zenios, *A parallelized algorithm for image reconstruction from noisy projections*, in Large-Scale Numerical Optimization, J. Coleman and Y. Li, eds., SIAM, Philadelphia, to appear.

[17] G. Herman and K. Yeung, *Evaluators of image reconstruction algorithms*, Int. J. Imag. Syst. Techn., 1 (1989), pp. 187–195.

[18] E. Levitan and G. Herman, *A maximum a posteriori probability expectation maximization algorithm for image reconstruction in emission tomography*, IEEE Trans. Med. Imag., 6 (1987), pp. 185–192.

[19] Z. Liang, *Statistical models of a priori information for image processing: Neighboring correlation constraints*, J. Opt. Soc. Amer. A, 5 (1988), pp. 2026–2031.

[20] R. Mould, *Introduction to Medical Statistics*, Adam Hilger, Bristol, England, 2nd ed., 1989.

[21] L. Shepp and Y. Vardi, *Maximum likelihood reconstruction in positron emission tomography*, IEEE Trans. Med. Imag., 1 (1982), pp. 113–122.

[22] D. Snyder and M. Miller, *The use of sieves to stabilize images produced with the EM algorithm for emission tomography*, IEEE Trans. Nucl. Sci., 32 (1985), pp. 3864–3872.

[23] Y. Vardi, L. Shepp, and L. Kaufman, *A statistical model for positron emission tomography*, J. Amer. Statist. Assoc., 80 (1985), pp. 8–35.

Radon Transform and Analog Coding

Hidemitsu Ogawa and Itsuo Kumazawa
Department of Computer Science
Tokyo Institute of Technology
Ookayama 2-12-1, Meguro-ku, Tokyo 152, Japan

1 Introduction

The redundancy in the Radon transform has been pointed out in various forms [4,5,9]. It was applied to several problems, for example, image reconstruction from projections in restricted ranges [6] and image reconstruction from noisy projections [1].

The purpose of this paper is to develop an image reconstruction method, which can detect and correct "errors" and is robust against "noises". The terminologies "error" and "noise" are used for the so-called "impulsive noise" and the "random noise", respectively. Such an error occurs when some X-ray detectors do not work during aquisition of projection data. It also occurs when a computer failes in recalling some of projection data from its storage.

Another example of the "error" appears related to the problem of image reconstruction from incomplete projections such as the limited-angle projections or the restricted-region projections. In such a problem, sample points for the Radon transform are ristricted in a small region on the Radon transformed domain. Such a situation can be considered as that we missed some sample values outside the region.

On the other hand, "noise" is the so-called random noise which is distributed over all sample points. For example, numerical round-off error belongs to that kind of noise.

First we show that the redundancy in the Radon transform leads us to the DFT code [2,7,10,17,18] in a natural way. The DFT code is an analog code which corresponds to the BCH code in digital codes. Following the theory of DFT code, we develop an error detection and correction method for erroneous projections. We also propose to use the series expansion methods developped in [1,5,9] for reconstructing original images after correcting errors, because of its robustness against noises. Those series expansion methods directly provide original images using the Chebyshev moments of the projections. Finally some numerical experiments are demonstrated.

2 General principle of error correction in CT problem

Let $f(x, y)$ be an original image to be reconstructed. It is expressed in the Cartesian coordinates (x, y). We suppose that the support of f is restricted into the unit disk C.

Let (X, Y) be the coordinate system rotated anti-clockwise by an angle α with respect to (x, y). The line integral

$$g(X, \alpha) = \int_{-1}^{1} f(x, y) dY \tag{1}$$

is called the Radon transform which maps $f(x, y)$ to $g(X, \alpha)$ as a function of two variables, X and α. The function $g(X, \alpha)$ is also called the Radon transform of f.

The main purpose of this paper is to develop a reconstruction method which provides a complete original image f from a finite number of sample values of its Radon transform g even when g contains some errors.

The following well-known lemma is our starting point.

[Lemma 1] [1,4,9] If $g(X, \alpha)$ is the Radon transform of an image, then it follows that

$$\int_{0}^{2\pi} \left(\int_{-1}^{1} g(X, \alpha) X^k dX \right) e^{in\alpha} d\alpha = 0 : k < |n|. \tag{2}$$

Eq.(2) means that the k-th moment of the Radon transform g with respect to X is orthogonal to the trigonometric functions of degree n if the absolute value of n is larger than k. In other words, Eq.(2) provides a kind of redundancy in the Radon transform.

Such a redundancy leads to the idea of analog coding [2,3,7,10,17,18]. For reader's convenience, we briefly review the analog coding theory. Let $\mathbf{x}$ be an original signal vector, $\mathbf{y}$ the corresponding code word, and $\mathbf{G}$ the so-called "generating matrix" which transforms the vector $\mathbf{x}$ into the vector $\mathbf{y}$ which belongs to a higher dimensional vector space:

$$\mathbf{y} = \mathbf{G}\mathbf{x}. \tag{3}$$

If $\mathbf{x}$ and $\mathbf{y}$ are restricted to binary vectors, then the analog coding theory reduces to the usual digital coding theory. Almost all results on the digital linear coding theory hold for the analog coding theory.

For example, a matrix $\mathbf{H}$ is called a "parity check matrix" if the null space of $\mathbf{H}$ is equal to the range of $\mathbf{G}$. And the following parity check equation holds:

$$\mathbf{H}\mathbf{y} = \mathbf{0}. \tag{4}$$

Let $\hat{\mathbf{y}}$ be the received vector which is the superposition of the code word $\mathbf{y}$ and an error vector $\mathbf{e}$. Let $\mathbf{s}$ be a vector defined as

$$\mathbf{s} = \mathbf{H}\hat{\mathbf{y}}. \tag{5}$$

The vector $\mathbf{s}$ is called the "syndrome". The syndrome is related to the error vector $\mathbf{e}$ by

$$\mathbf{s} = \mathbf{H}\mathbf{e}, \tag{6}$$

because of Eqs.(4) and (5). Eq.(6) yields the error vector $\mathbf{e}$. Then we can obtain the original code word $\mathbf{y}$ by $\mathbf{y} = \hat{\mathbf{y}} - \mathbf{e}$. Finally, we can obtain the original signal $\mathbf{x}$ from Eq.(3). Comparing the analog coding theory with the Radon transform, we can say

1. Eq.(1) corresponds to Eq.(3). In other words, the Radon transform corresponds to the generating matrix $\mathbf{G}$.

2. Eq.(2) corresponds to the parity check equation (4).

3. We can detect errors in the Radon transform g by checking Eq.(2).

4. We can calculate the syndrome by using Eq.(2).

5. Finally, we can correct errors in g.

That is a general principle of error correction in CT problem. More detail will be discussed in the next section.

3 The Radon transform and the DFT code

This section will show that the redundancy (2) in the Radon transform leads to the DFT code in a natural way.

The DFT code [2,7,10,17,18] is an analog version of the BCH code which is one of the well-established digital codes. The name comes from the Discrete Fourier Transform which is used in the parity check equation for the code. Let $(c_0, c_1, \ldots, c_{2L-1})$ be a DFT code word. The parity check equation for the DFT code is

$$\sum_{l=0}^{2L-1} c_l exp(in_m \frac{\pi l}{L}) = 0 : m = 0, 1, \ldots, M-1, \tag{7}$$

where $n_0, n_1, \ldots, n_{M-1}$ are integers which are successively chosen from the set of integers $\{0, 1, \ldots, 2L-1\}$. Let $[*]$ be the largest integer which does not exceed the bracketted value $*$. We can correct at most $[M/2]$ number of errors by using the DFT code.

For any polynomial $u_k(X)$ of degree k, Eq.(2) yields

$$\int_0^{2\pi} (\int_{-1}^{1} g(X, \alpha) u_k(X) dX) e^{in\alpha} d\alpha = 0 : k < |n|. \tag{8}$$

Almost all results we will mention hereafter are valid for any polynomial $u_k(X)$. However, for some computational reasons, we will use as $u_k(X)$ the k-th Chebyshev polynomial of the second kind defined as

$$u_k(cos\theta) = sin(k+1)\theta / sin\theta. \tag{9}$$

Let $g_k(\alpha)$ be the k-th Chebyshev moment of $g(X, \alpha)$ defined as

$$g_k(\alpha) = \int_{-1}^{1} g(X, \alpha) u_k(X) dX. \tag{10}$$

Then, Eq.(8) yields

$$\int_0^{2\pi} g_k(\alpha) e^{in\alpha} d\alpha = 0 : k < |n|. \tag{11}$$

Eq.(11) means that the k-th Chebyshev moment of the Radon transform g is orthogonal to the trigonometric functions of degree n if the absolute value of n is larger than k. In other words, the k-th Chebyshev moment of g does not contain the frequency components higher than or equal to k. Hence, a general sampling theorem for the trigonometric polynomials gives the following finite sum expression to Eq.(11) for any integer $L(\geq (2k+1)/2)$ [11,15]:

$$\sum_{l=0}^{2L-1} g_k(\frac{\pi l}{L}) exp(in\frac{\pi l}{L}) = 0 : k+1 \leq n \leq 2L-k-1. \tag{12}$$

It should be noticed that Eq.(12) is not an approximation of Eq.(11), but the exact expression of Eq.(11) in a discrete form.

If we denote $g_k(\frac{\pi l}{L})$ by g_{kl} for brevity, then Eq.(12) yields

$$\sum_{l=0}^{2L-1} g_{kl} exp(in\frac{\pi l}{L}) = 0 : k+1 \leq n \leq 2L-k-1. \tag{13}$$

Let $\mathbf{G_k}$ be the vector defined as

$$\mathbf{G_k} = (g_{k0}, g_{k1}, \ldots, g_{kL-1}). \tag{14}$$

Eqs.(13) and (7) mean that the vector $\mathbf{G_k}$ is a code word of the DFT code for each k. Hence, we can correct at most $[(2L-2k-1)/2]$ number of errors by using the DFT code. An efficient algorithm for error correction will be proposed in the next section.

4 Error correction algorithm

Error correction algorithms for the DFT code have been discussed in several literatures [2,7,10,17,18]. They are, however, not applied to the current problem because of big size of projection data.

We propose a new practical algorithm for the DFT code. Combining the common techniques such as the FFT, the linear prediction, and the Cholesky decomposition yields an efficient and robust algorithm.

Now we shall describe the algorithm. Let $\hat{g}(X, \alpha)$ be the observed Radon transform which includes errors.

[Algorithm for error correction]

1. Calculate the Chebyshev moments $\hat{g}_{kl}$ by

$$\hat{g}_{kl} = \int_0^{\pi} g(cos\theta, \pi l/L) sin(k+1)\theta d\theta. \tag{15}$$

Substituting Eq.(9) into Eq.(10) yields Eq.(15). The set of Chebyshev moments $\hat{g}_{kl}$ is the code word of the DFT code as mentioned in the previous section. Calculation of Eq.(15) is easily done by using the FFT.

2. Calculate the syndrome s_n by

$$s_n = \sum_{l=0}^{2L-1} \hat{g}_{kl} exp(in\frac{\pi l}{L}) : k+1 \leq n \leq 2L-k-1. \tag{16}$$

Calculation of Eq.(16) is easily done by using the FFT.

3. Solve the AR (Auto-Regressive) equation

$$\sum_{r=0}^{p} a_r s_{n-r} = 0 : a_0 = 1, k+1+p \leq n \leq 2L-k-1, p \leq L-k-1 \tag{17}$$

with p the number of errors to be corrected. We will propose later an efficient method which provides the error number p and hence the solution $\{a_r\}$ of Eq.(17).

4. By using the AR coefficients $\{a_r\}$, construct the error locator equation $h(x)$ as follows:

$$h(x) = \sum_{r=0}^{p} a_r x^{p-r}. \tag{18}$$

5. Each root of the error locator equation $h(x)$ provides an error location. Indeed, if it follows that for an integer l

$$h(exp(-i\frac{2\pi l}{L})) = 0, \tag{19}$$

then $\hat{g}_{kl}$ contains an error, which is denoted by e_l. Otherwise, $\hat{g}_{kl}$ contains no error. Decide the location of errors by getting all roots of the error locator equation (18).

6. Detect all errors e_{l_r} by solving the equation

$$s_n = \sum_{r=0}^{p} e_{l_r} exp(in\frac{\pi l_r}{L}) : k+1 \leq n \leq 2L-k-1. \tag{20}$$

Eq.(20) is easily solved by using the FFT.

7. Correct errors by putting

$$g_{kl_r} = \hat{g}_{kl_r} - e_{l_r}. \tag{21}$$

8. There are many ways to reconstruct the original image $f(x,y)$ from $\{g_{kl}\}$. We will discuss it in Section 6.

The rest of this section will be devoted to the problem mentioned in the item 3. In practical applicaions such as CT we must consider the noise effect. Then, instead of Eq.(17) we discuss the following equation

$$\sum_{r=0}^{p} a_r s_{n-r} = \varepsilon_n : a_0 = 1, k+1+p \leq n \leq 2L-k-1, p \leq L-k-1 \tag{22}$$

with ε_n the noise term. Our problem is to obtain the number, p, of errors and the maximum likelihood estimatin of the AR coefficients $\{a_r\}$ in Eq.(22).

For a fixed p, the maximum likelihood estimatin of the AR coefficients $\{a_r\}$ in Eq.(22) under the assumption of Gaussian noise is obtained as the solution of

$$\begin{pmatrix} & & \\ & r_{ij} & \\ & & \end{pmatrix} \begin{pmatrix} a_1 \\ a_2 \\ a_3 \\ \vdots \\ a_p \end{pmatrix} = \begin{pmatrix} -r_{01} \\ -r_{02} \\ -r_{03} \\ \vdots \\ -r_{0p} \end{pmatrix}, \tag{23}$$

where r_{ij}'s are the auto-correlations of the syndrome $\{s_n\}$ defined as

$$\begin{aligned} r_{ij} &= \sum_{n=k+1+p+j}^{2L-k-1+j} s_{n-i}\overline{s_{n-j}}, \\ r_{ji} &= r_{ij} : i \leq j, \end{aligned} \tag{24}$$

where the bar in (24) denotes the complex conjugate. Eq.(23) is expressed in the following matrix form:

$$Ra = b. \tag{25}$$

Since R is a symmetric matrix, we can solve Eq.(25) by using the Cholesky decomposition of the matrix R:

$$R = SDS^*, \tag{26}$$

where S is a triangular matrix, D a diagonal matrix, and S^* the Hermitian conjugate of S [8].

Since the number p of errors is unknown parameter in our case, we apply the following incremental Cholesky decomposition. Let $R^{(i)}$ be the i-th principal submatrix of R. The Cholesky decomposition of $R^{(i)}$ is

$$R^{(i)} = S^{(i)}D^{(i)}S^{(i)*}. \tag{27}$$

The decomposition (27) is incrementally carried out from $i = 1$ until at least one zero-element appears in diagonal of $D^{(i)}$. If $D^{(i+1)}$ is the first matrix with at least one zero-element in diagonal, then $p = i$. Hence,

$$R^{(p)} = S^{(p)}D^{(p)}S^{(p)*} \tag{28}$$

coincides with Eq.(26). Eqs.(28) and (25) yield

$$S^{(p)}D^{(p)}S^{(p)*}a = b. \tag{29}$$

We can easily solve Eq.(29).

That is a way to obtain the number p of errors and the maximum likelihood estimatin of the AR coefficients $\{a_r\}$ in Eq.(22) at the same time.

5 Pseudo-biorthogonal base (PBOB)

For further discussions, we briefly review the theory of pseudo-biorthogonal bases (PBOB). The concept of the PBOB is origoinally introduced in [12,13] and applied to the image restoration problem in [14] and the general sampling theorems in [15].

Let H be an N-dimensional complex Hilbert space with an inner product $(*, *)$. A set of $2M(M \geq N)$ elements $\{\phi_m, \phi_m^*\}_{m=1}^M$ in H is called a PBOB if it follows that for any f in H

$$f = \sum_{m=1}^{M} (f, \phi_m)\phi_m^*. \tag{30}$$

In this case, it also follows that for any f and g in H

$$(f, g) = \sum_{m=1}^{M} (f, \phi_m)\overline{(g, \phi_m^*)}. \tag{31}$$

If $M = N$ and $\phi_m^* = \phi_m$ for all m, then the PBOB is reduced to an orthonormal base (ONB). If $M = N$ and $\phi_m^* \neq \phi_m$ for some m, then the PBOB is reduced to a biorthonormal base (BONB). if $M > N$ and $\phi_m^* = \phi_m$ for all m, then the PBOB is reduced to a pseudo-orthogonal base (POB)[16].

For any set of M elements $\{\phi_m\}_{m=1}^M$ which spans H, we can always construct the so-called dual base $\{\phi_m^*\}_{m=1}^M$ such that $\{\phi_m, \phi_m^*\}_{m=1}^M$ is a PBOB in H. There exist an infinite number of dual bases if $M > N$. Several methods for constructing the dual bases are given in [12,13].

6 Reconstruction formulae

A method for obtaining the correct Chebyshev moments $\{g_{kl}\}$ from the projection data $\hat{g}(X, \alpha)$ with errors has been proposed in Section 4. We will discuss methods to reconstruct the original image $f(x, y)$ from the corrected Chebyshev moments $\{g_{kl}\}$ in this section.

The first way to reconstruct the original image is to use the traditional methods such as the convolution method and the filtered back-projection methd. Eq.(10) and the orthogonal relation of the Chebyshev polynomials of the second kind yield

$$g(X, \pi l/L) = \frac{2}{\pi}\sqrt{1-X^2}\sum_{k=0}^{\infty} g_{kl}u_k(X). \tag{32}$$

Then, a truncation series of Eq.(32) yields an approximation of $g(X, \pi l/L)$, to which we can apply the traditional reconstruction methods.

The second way is to use the methods introduced in [1,5,9]. For any function $\phi(X)$, Eq.(1) yields

$$\int_{-1}^{1} g(X, \alpha)\phi(X)dX = \int_C f(x, y)\phi(x cos\alpha + y sin\alpha)dxdy \tag{33}$$

with C the unit disk.

Let Π_L be the subspace of functions which are zero outside the unit disk C and coinside with polynomials with degree less than or equal to L on C. Eq.(9) yields the following lemmas.

[Lemma 2] [1] The set of functions $\{\varphi_{kl}(x, y)\}$ defined as

$$\varphi_{kl}(x, y) = u_k(x cos\frac{\pi l}{k+1} + y sin\frac{\pi l}{k+1}) : l = 0, 1, \ldots, k, k = 0, 1, \ldots, L-1 \tag{34}$$

is an orthogonal base in Π_{L-1}. The best approximation, $f_{L-1}(x, y)$, of $f(x, y)$ in Π_{L-1} is given by

$$f_{L-1}(x, y) = \sum_{k=0}^{L-1}\sum_{l=0}^{k}(f, \varphi_{kl})\varphi_{kl}(x, y), \tag{35}$$

$$(f, \varphi_{kl}) = \frac{1}{\pi}\int_C f(x, y)u_k(x cos\frac{\pi l}{k+1} + y sin\frac{\pi l}{k+1})dxdy. \tag{36}$$

[Lemma 3] [1] The set of functions $\{\phi_{kl}(x, y), \phi_{kl}^*(x, y)\}$ defined as

$$\phi_{kl}(x, y) = u_k(x cos\frac{\pi l}{L} + y sin\frac{\pi l}{L}) : l = 0, 1, \ldots, L-1, k = 0, 1, \ldots, L-1, \tag{37}$$

$$\phi^*_{kl}(x,y) = \frac{k+1}{L}\phi_{kl}(x,y) : l = 0,1,\ldots,L-1, k = 0,1,\ldots,L-1 \tag{38}$$

is a pseudo-biorthogonal base in Π_{L-1}. The best approximation, $f_{L-1}(x,y)$, of $f(x,y)$ in Π_{L-1} is given by

$$f_{L-1}(x,y) = \sum_{k=0}^{L-1}\sum_{l=0}^{L-1}(f,\phi_{kl})\phi^*_{kl}(x,y), \tag{39}$$

$$(f,\phi_{kl}) = \frac{1}{\pi}\int_c f(x,y)u_k(x\cos\frac{\pi l}{L} + y\sin\frac{\pi l}{L})dxdy. \tag{40}$$

Eqs.(33), (36), and (40) mean that the expansion coefficients in (35) and (39) are given by the Chebychev moments. Then, the orthogonal expansion (35) yields the following reconstruction formula.

[Lemma 4][1]

$$f_{L-1}(x,y) = \frac{1}{\pi}\sum_{k=0}^{L-1}\sum_{l=0}^{k}\tilde{g}_{kl}\varphi_{kl}(x,y), \tag{41}$$

where

$$\tilde{g}_{kl} = \int_{-1}^{1} g(X,\pi l/(k+1))u_k(X)dX. \tag{42}$$

On the other hand, the pseudo-biorthogonal expansion (39) yields the following reconstruction formula.

[Lemma 5][1,5,9]

$$f_{L-1}(x,y) = \frac{1}{\pi}\sum_{k=0}^{L-1}\sum_{l=0}^{L-1} g_{kl}\phi^*_{kl}(x,y), \tag{43}$$

where

$$g_{kl} = \int_{-1}^{1} g(X,\pi l/L)u_k(X)dX. \tag{44}$$

Eq.(41) uses $k+1$ number of Chebyshev moments for getting the k-th coefficients. On the other hand, Eq.(43) uses L number of Chebyshev moments for getting the k-th coefficients. That means Eq.(43) is a redundant expression of $f_{L-1}(x,y)$. That is why the reconstruction formula (43) is robust against noises [1].

As mentioned in Section 3, the DFT code can correct at most $[(2L-2k-1)/2]$ number of errors. Hence, we can obtain the corrected g_{kl} for k such as $k \le [(2L-2p-1)/2]$. In practical situations, we have no prior knowledge about the number of errors. So we assume that the maximum number of errors is p_{max}. Let $M = [(2L-2p_{max}-1)/2]$. And we reconstruct images by using

$$f_{M-1}(x,y) = \frac{1}{\pi}\sum_{k=0}^{M-1}\frac{k+1}{L}\sum_{l=0}^{L-1} g_{kl}\phi_{kl}(x,y). \tag{45}$$

7 Computer simulations

Two kinds of computer simulations are demonstrated. The first simulations compare the convolution method with the series expansion methods mentioned in Eqs.(43) and (45) (see Figs.1 to 3). The second illustrates how the proposed error correction method performs under different circumstances (see Fig.4). All figures are put on the last pages of this paper.

A common phantom is used for those experiments. It is put together by superimposing a number of elemental objects, i.e., squares and disks, on the unit disk in the (x, y)-plane (cf. Fig.1(a)). The largest square is of size 0.1×0.1 and of density 1. The largest square is multiplied by 0.6 both in size and density, so that the second largest square is created. Such a successive multiplication by 0.6 yields a sequence of elemental squares. A sequence of elemental disks is also created in a similar way.

All reconstructions are shown by 200×200 pixels in Figs.1 to 4.

For those experiments, the Radon transform $g(X, \alpha)$ is expressed by 512×512 pixels. In other words, the Radon transform is sampled at the 512 points in the interval $[-1, 1]$ on the X-axis and at the 512 points in the interval $[0, \pi]$ on the α-axis, respectively. In case of the convolution method, sample points of X are uniformly distributed over $[-1, 1]$. In case of series expansion methods in Eqs.(43) and (45), $X_m = cos\theta_m$ with uniformly distributed θ_m are used.

Fig.1 shows reconstructions from projections without error. (a) is the result using the convolution method with the Shepp-Logan's filter function [5]. (b) is the result using Eq.(43). In Fig.1, the range $[0, 1]$ of brightness of the reconstructions is represented with 8 bits. The brightness over 1 and less than 0 are clipped with 255 and 0, respectively.

Fig.2 shows the linear enhancement of the reconstructions shown in Fig.1. The range $[0, 1/50]$ of brightness of the reconstructions is represented with 8 bits. The brightness over 1/50 and less than 0 are clipped with 255 and 0, respectively.

Fig.3 shows the reconstruction from projections without error using Eq. (45) with $M = 256$. Used is the same scale of brightness as in Fig.1.

Fig.1 shows that there are no big difference between the convolution method and Eq.(43). Both method provide almost the same images as the original phantom. On the other hand, Fig.2 shows that those reconstruction methods have the fairly different detail structure of ripples. Figs.1(b) and 3 show that Eq.(45) provides not so bad approximation to Eq.(43).

Fig.4 shows reconstructions from erroneous projections using the error correction algorithm proposed in Section 4 and Eq.(45) with $M = 256$. Used is the same scale of brightness as in Fig.1. The number of errors is 22, whose locations are randomly chosen. The amount of errors are also randomly chosen from $[0, 1]$.

(a) is the result using Eq.(45) with $\hat{g}_{kl}$ as g_{kl}. That is, Eq.(45) is directly applied to $\hat{g}_{kl}$ without any error correction.

(b) is the result using Eq.(43) with error corrected g_{kl}. In this experiment, instead of Eq.(19) the following is used

$$|h(exp(-i\frac{2\pi l}{L}))| \leq \varepsilon \qquad (46)$$

with $\varepsilon > 0$ a properly chosen small number. A rough choice of ε provides reconstructions with lower quality. Such an example is given in (c). Figs.3 and 4 demonstrate the usefulness of the proposed method.

8 Conclusions

We showed that the redundancy in the Radon transform leads us to the DFT code in a natural way. The DFT code is a typical analog code. Following the theory of DFT code, we proposed an error detection and correction method for erroneous projections. We also proposed to use the series expansion methods developped in [1,5,9] for reconstructing original images after correcting errors, because of their robustness against noises. Those series expansion methods directly provide original images using the Chebyshev moments of the projections. Finally some numerical experiments were demonstrated.

References

[1] I. Kumazawa and T. Iijima : "Redundancy of projection data and its application to improve the quality of reconstructed image", Trans. IEICE Japan, J67-D, 11, pp.1340-1347(1984)(in Japanese).

[2] I. Kumazawa and H. Ogawa : "Evaluation of the stability of analog codes against noise by the theory of pseudo-biorthogonal bases", Trans. IEICE Japan, J72-A, 2, pp.406-413(1989)(in Japanese).

[3] I. Kumazawa, H. Tajima and H. Ogawa : "Image reconstruction from erroneous projections - Radon transform as an analog coding -", Trans. IEICE Japan, J72-A, 2, pp.425-431(1989)(in Japanese).

[4] P. D. Lax and R. S. Phillips : "The Paley-Wiener theorem for the Radon transform", Comm. Pure Appl. Math., 23, pp.409-424(1970).

[5] B. F. Logan and L. A. Shepp : "Optimal reconstruction of a function from its projections", Duke Math. J., 42, 4, pp.645-659(1975).

[6] A. K. Louis : "Picture reconstruction from projections in restricted range", Math. Meth. in the Appl. Sci., 2, pp.209-220(1980).

[7] Y. Maekawa and K. Sakaniwa : "An extention of DFT code and the evaluation of its performance", Trans. IEICE Japan, J69-A, 4, pp.497-508(1986)(in Japanese).

[8] J. K. Markel and H. Gray : "Linear prediction of speech", Springer-Verlag(1976).

[9] R. B. Marr : "On the reconstruction of a function on a circular domain from a sampling of its line integrals", J. Math. Anal. and Appl., 45, pp.357-374(1974).

[10] T. G. Marshall, Jr.: "Real number transform and convolutional codes", Proc. 24th Midwest Symp. on Circuit and Systems, pp.650-653(1982).

[11] H. Ogawa: "On the parity of the number of sampling points via the theory of pseudo-orthogonal bases", Trans. IECE Japan, 60-D, 10, pp.854-860(1977)(in Japanese).

[12] H. Ogawa : "A theory of pseudo-biorthogonal bases", Trans. IECE Japan, J64-D, 7, pp.555-562(1981)(in Japanese).

[13] H. Ogawa : "Pseudo-biorthogonal bases of type O", Trans. IECE Japan, J64-D, 7, pp.563-569(1981)(in Japanese).

[14] H. Ogawa : "Optimal digital iamge restration", in D. D. Majumder, ed., Advances in Information Science and Technology. Indian Statistical Institute, Calcutta, pp.290-297(1984).

[15] H. Ogawa : "A unified approach to generalized sampling theory", Proc. International Conference on Acoustics, Speech and Signal Processing, pp.1657-1660(1986).

[16] H. Ogawa and T. Iijima : "A theory of pseudo-orthogonal bases", Trans. IEICE Japan, 58-D, 5, pp.271-278(1975)(in Japanese).

[17] J. K. Wolf : "Redundancy and the discrete fourier transform and impulse noise cancelation", IEEE Trans. Commun., COM-31, 3, pp.458-461(March 1983).

[18] J. K. Wolf : "Analog Codes", ICC'83, A8.4(1983).

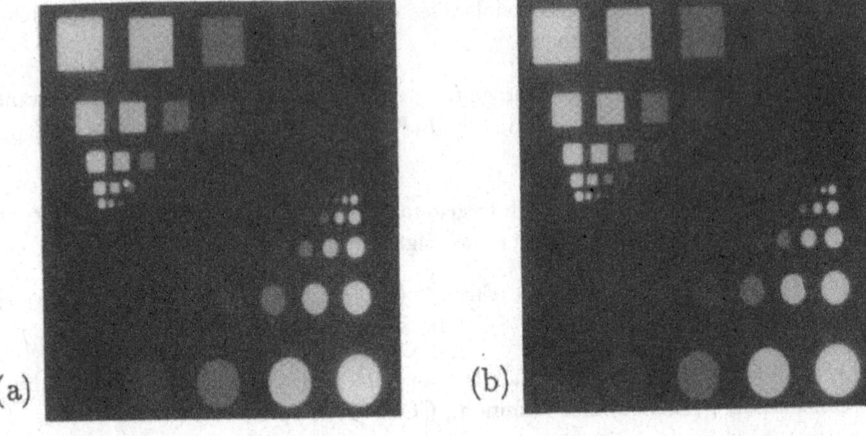

Fig.1. Reconstructions from projections without error. (a) is the result using the convolution method. (b) is the result using Eq.(43).

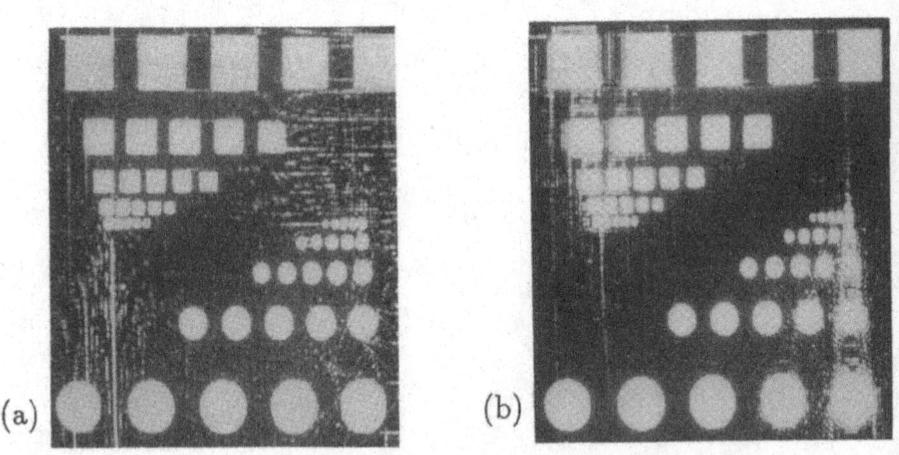

Fig.2. Enhancement of ripples in the reconstructions shown in Fig.1.

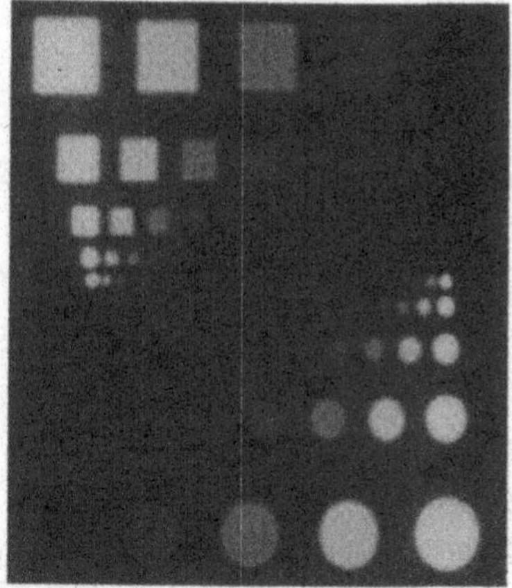

Fig.3. Reconstructions from projections without error using Eq.(45) with $M = 256$.

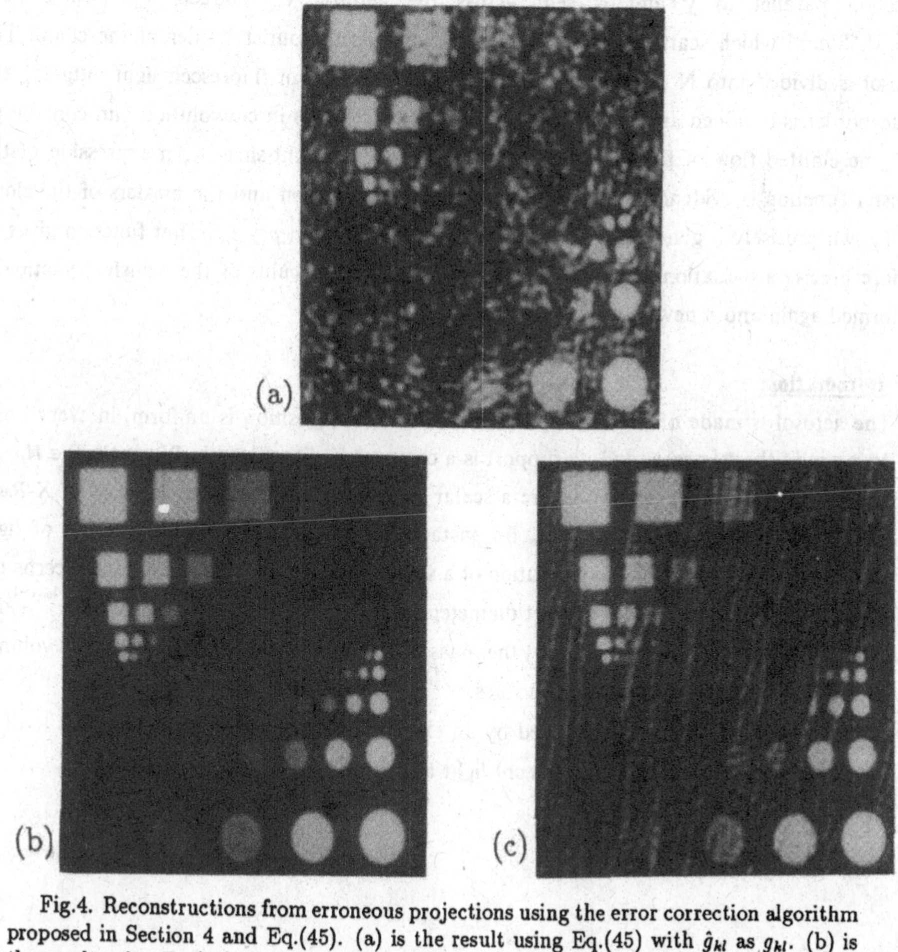

(a)

(b)

(c)

Fig.4. Reconstructions from erroneous projections using the error correction algorithm proposed in Section 4 and Eq.(45). (a) is the result using Eq.(45) with $\hat{g}_{kl}$ as g_{kl}. (b) is the result using Eq.(45) with error corrected g_{kl}. For detecting error locations Eq.(44) is used with a properly chosen ϵ. (c) is the result using a roughly chosen ϵ in Eq.(46).

DETERMINATION OF THE SPECIFIC DENSITY OF AN AEROSOL THROUGH TOMOGRAPHY

Louis R. OUDIN
French-German Research Institute of Saint-Louis
B.P. 34 F68301 Saint-Louis.

Summary:

An aerosol is considered whose droplet diameter distribution, and specific density depend only on two coordinates (y,z). The droplets contain a dilution of fluorescent product sensitive to a light-sheet of green light ($\lambda = 0.504\mu m$). This light-sheet is contained in the plane Oyz , has a direction parallel to y and is sent across the aerosol. It produces an orange light ($\lambda = 0.585\mu m$) which scatters across the aerosol towards the outlet border of the cloud. The aerosol is divided into N parallel equidistant slices. The flow of fluoresced light outgoing the cloud border is obtained as a transfer function iterated N times in convolution and convoluted with the emitted flow of fluoresced light at the level of the light-sheet. An expression of the transfer function is evidenced. Since the droplet size distribution and the borders of the cloud are known precisely it gives the possibility to reach the function $\rho(y,z)$. That function gives us a more precise attenuation function of the light-sheet. The calculus of the transfer function is performed again and a new more precise function ρ is reached.

1. Introduction:

The aerosol is made of liquid droplets; its chemical composition is uniform, in every point M(x,y,z) of the $\mathbf{R}^3$ space ,and its support is a compact K discretized in P^3 voxels, $P \in \mathbf{N}$.
Unlike classical tomographies, where a scalar variable is restituted (in the case of X-Rays and Nuclear Magnetic Resonance, for instance), fluorescence and/or scattering of light across an aerosol involves the restitution of a vector variable in the space $\mathbf{R}^n$. It concerns the distribution function h(D) of droplet diameters D discretized into a vector $\{h(D_i)\}_{i=0}^{i=I_{max}-1}$ for each point $M(x,y,z) \in \mathbf{R}^3$, and $\rho(M)$ the mass of liquid droplets per unit of aerosol volume, with I_{max} the number of discretized values.
We will use the fluorescence induced by an exciting light-sheet inside the compact K of P^3 voxels, and the scattering of fluorescent light to restitute the $I_{max} \times P^3$ unknowns.

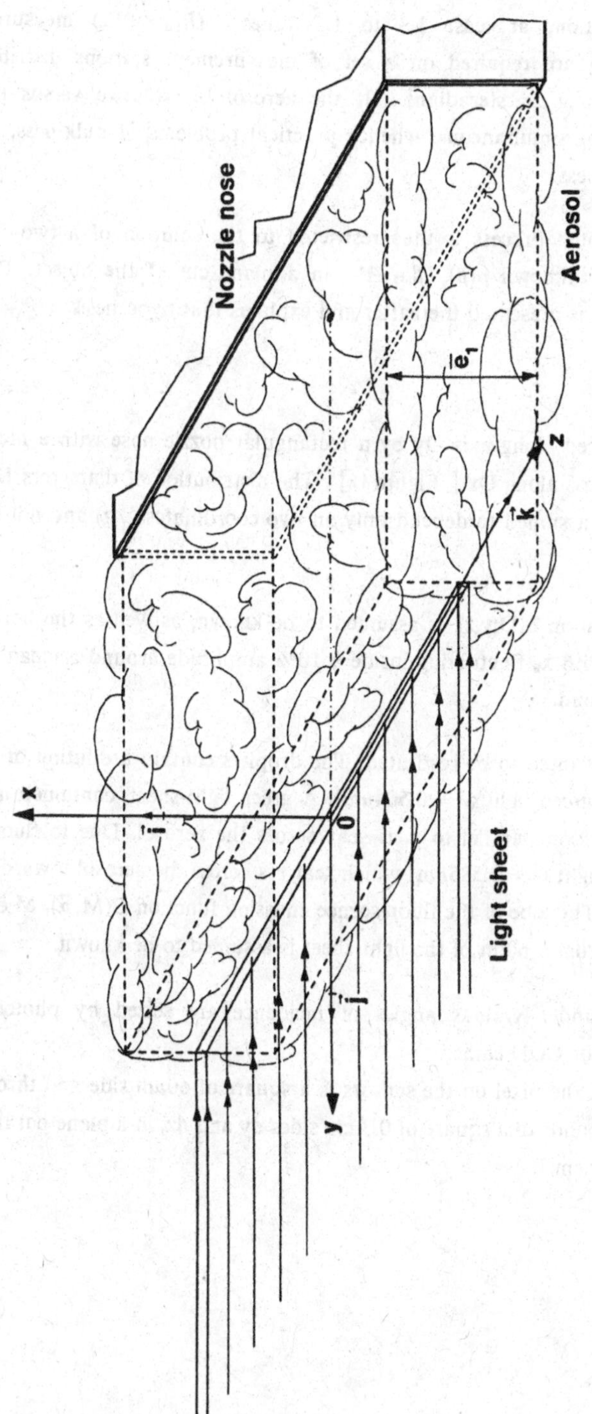

Figure 1

For error compensation, at least 1.3 to 1.5 times $(I_{max} \times P^3)$ measurements of fluorescence/scattering are required on a set of measurement stations distributed in a homogeneous way along 2π steradians. If the aerosol is evolutive versus time, these measurements must be simultaneous, whence practical problems of bulkiness, synchronisation, and expensiveness.

The following descripted process is thus restricted to the solution of a two-dimensional problem with scalar unknown $\rho(\vec{\beta})$, $\vec{\beta} \in \mathbf{R}^2$, in a plane cut of the object. The way of generating the aerosol is presented thereafter and explains that hypothesis.

2. General presentation:

The aerosol is produced along axis Oy by a rectangular nozzle nose with a median plane (yOz), with its thickness along Ox [Figure 1]. The distribution of diameters D for liquid droplets, $\frac{dN}{dD}(y,z)$ is assumed to depend only on two coordinates (y,z) and not on x in the reference Oxyz.

The diameter distribution h(D;y,z) is assumed to be known, as well as the borders of the aerosol $x_B = B(y,z)$, with x_B fluctuating inside a 10% amplitude around a mean value $\mp \frac{\bar{e}}{2}$ on each side of the cloud.

The mass density is wanted to be restituted. The droplets contain a dilution of fluorescent product, sensitive to green light ($\lambda = 0.504\mu m$). A green light-sheet, contained in the plane 0yz, and with a direction parallel to y, is sent across the aerosol. Due to fluorescence, it produces an orange light ($\lambda = 0.585\mu m$) which scatters across the aerosol towards the outlet surface $x_B = B(y,z)$. The lobe of the fluorescence emission function $C(M, \vec{\alpha})$, $M \in \mathbf{R}^3$, $\{\vec{\alpha} \in \mathbf{R}^3 ; |\vec{\alpha}| = 1\}$ from a point of the light-sheet is assumed to be known.

The outlet images under various angles of incidence are seized by photonic sensors (photographic plates or CCD cameras).
To settle the notions, the pixel on the sensors is a square of $60\mu m$ side and through a 1/50 magnification corresponds to a square of 0.3 cm sides dy and dz, in a plane parallel to (yOz) (dy = dz = p = 0.3 cm).

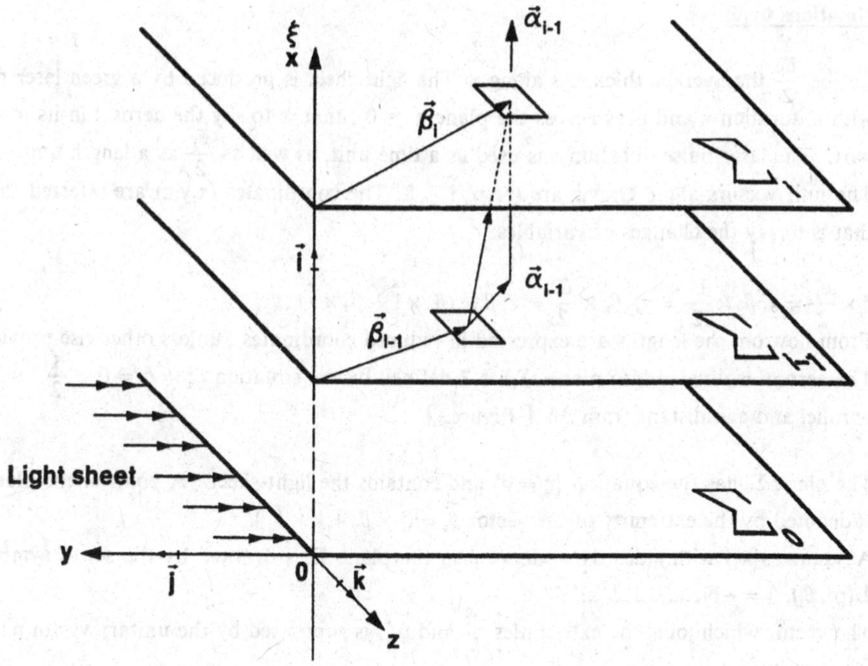
ξ
x
$\vec{\alpha}_{i-1}$
$\vec{\beta}_i$
$\vec{i}$
$\vec{\alpha}_{l-1}$
$\vec{\beta}_{l-1}$
Light sheet
y
$\vec{j}$
0
$\vec{k}$
z

Figure 2

3. Notations used:

Let be $\frac{\overline{e_1}}{2}$ the average thickness along x. The light-sheet is produced by a green laser pulse with a duration τ and goes across the plane $x = 0$, that is to say the aerosol in its median part. The laser pulse duration τ is used as a time unit, as well as $\frac{\overline{e_1}}{2}$ as a length unit.
The unit vectors along Ox,y,z are (resp) $\vec{i}, \vec{j}, \vec{k}$. The coordinates (x,y,z) are referred to $\frac{\overline{e_1}}{2}$, that is to say the changes of variables:

$\xi \times \frac{\overline{e_1}}{2} = x,\ \beta_y \times \frac{\overline{e_1}}{2} = y,\ \beta_z \times \frac{\overline{e_1}}{2} = z;\ \vec{\beta} = (\beta_y \times \vec{j} + \beta_z \times \vec{k})$.
From now on, the lengths are expressed in reduced coordinates, unless otherwise provided.
The aerosol is divided into planes $\Sigma_i, i \in \mathbf{Z}$ defined by the equation $\{\xi = \xi_i = (i - \frac{1}{2}) \times \Delta\xi\}$, parallel and equidistant from $\Delta\xi$ [Figure2]

The plane Σ_0 has the equation $\{\xi = 0\}$ and contains the light-sheet. A point of the plane Σ_i is denoted by the extremity of the vector $\vec{\beta}_i = (\vec{j} \times \beta_y + \vec{k} \times \beta_z)$.
A square pixel with sides $dy = dz = p$ in the plane Σ_i is denoted by the set of symbols : $\Sigma_i(p^2, \vec{\beta}_i)$, $i = -N_e, \ldots, 0, 1, 2, \ldots, N_e$.
The vector which joins the extremities $\vec{\beta}_i$ and $\vec{\beta}_{i+1}$ is supported by the unitary vector $\vec{\alpha}_i$:
$\vec{\alpha}_i = \vec{i} \times \sin\alpha_i + \vec{\alpha}'_i$,
$\vec{\alpha}'_i = \vec{j} \times \alpha_{iy} + \vec{k} \times \alpha_{iz}$, complying with the relations:

$$(1)\quad \begin{cases} \vec{\beta}_1 = \vec{\beta}_0 + \dfrac{\vec{\alpha}'_0 \times \Delta\xi}{2 \times \cos\alpha_0} \\ \vec{\beta}_{i+1} = \vec{\beta}_i + \dfrac{\vec{\alpha}'_i \times \Delta\xi}{\cos\alpha_i} \quad, \forall i \in \mathbf{N}, i \neq 0 \end{cases}$$

4. Description of the model and its construction:

a. Production of fluorescence by a pixel $\Sigma_0(p^2, \vec{\beta}_0)$ in the light-sheet:

The aerosol is met by a plane wave inside the light-sheet, with a reduced thickness ε, carrying during the duration τ an initial exciting energy $(I_0(\beta_{0z}) \times d\beta_{0z})$ for a slice $d\beta_z$, at the value β_{0z} of the coordinate of the light-sheet ($\lambda = 0.504\ \mu m$ green). The quantity of energy which reaches the elementary section of the cloud centered in $\Sigma_0(p^2, \vec{\beta}_0)$ is equal to:
$I(\vec{\beta}_0) = I_0(\beta_z) \times \exp\{-\int_{\beta=\beta_{0y}}^{\beta=\beta_{ymax}} \sigma_f(h_i(\beta_y, \beta_{0z})) \times \rho(\beta_y, \beta_{0z}) \times d\beta_y\}$
with $I(\vec{\beta}_0)$ and $I_0(\beta_{0z})$ in Joule/cm.,
with $\beta_{y\,max}$, the starting coordinate of the light-sheet on the y axis,

$h_1(D, \vec{\beta}_0).dD$ = the number of droplets whose diameters are comprised between D and D+ dD, for 1 gramme of aerosol.

The preceding relation may be written as: $I(\vec{\beta}_0) = I_0 \times (\beta_{0z}) \times \exp(-A(\vec{\beta}_0))$,

with $A = -\int_{\beta_y=\beta_{0y}}^{\beta_y=\beta_{ymax}} \sigma_f(h_1(\bullet, \{\beta_y, \beta_{0z}\})) \times \rho(\beta_y, \beta_{0z}) \times d\beta_y$.

There are the definition relations for $h_1(D, \vec{\beta})$

as well as $h(D, \vec{\beta})$ the droplet distribution :

$$h(D, \vec{\beta}) = \frac{1}{N_{D_{min}}^{D_{max}}(\vec{\beta})} \times \frac{d}{dD}(N_0^D(\vec{\beta}))$$

$N_{D_1}^{D_2}(\vec{\beta})$ = number of droplets/cm³ whose diameters are comprised between D_1 and D_2.

ρ_∞ = mass density of compact liquid, in g/cm³.

$$h_1(D, \vec{\beta}) = \frac{h(D, \vec{\beta})}{\int_{D=D_{min}}^{D=D_{max}} h(D) \times \rho_\infty \times \frac{\pi \times D^3}{6} \times dD}, \text{ in } g^{-1} \times cm^{-1}.$$

Energy emitted by a pixel $\Sigma_0(p^2, \vec{\beta}_0)$ of the light-sheet:

The exciting energy $I(\vec{\beta}_0)$, composed of green photons (λ_0 = 0.504 μm) causes the dye to resonate (Rhodamine B). The latter produces one orange photon (λ_1 = 0.585 μm) for one green photon with an efficiency ϕ_r = 0.92 [1], [2]. The energy produced by the pixel $\Sigma_0(p^2, \vec{\beta}_0)$ is given by:

$$[\rho \times w_0](\vec{\beta}_0, \vec{\alpha}'_0) = \rho(\vec{\beta}_0) \times \sigma_f[h_1(., \vec{\beta}_0)] \times \frac{\lambda_0}{\lambda_1} \times \phi_r \times \exp(-A(\vec{\beta}_0)) \times I_0(\beta_{0z}) \times C(h_1(\bullet, \vec{\beta}_0), \vec{\alpha}'_0) \times p^2$$

$[\rho \times w_0]$ in Joule/steradian, fluoresced at the extremity of $\vec{\beta}_0$ in the direction $\vec{\alpha}_0 = \vec{i} \times \cos\alpha_0 + \vec{\alpha}'_0$.

$C(h_1(\bullet, \vec{\beta}_0), \vec{\alpha}'_0)$ = fluorescence lobe emission at the extremity of $\vec{\beta}_0$, towards $\vec{\alpha}_0$, in steradians⁻¹.

Let A be such that:

$$A = \frac{\lambda_0}{\lambda_1} \times \phi_r \times \exp(-A(\vec{\beta}_0)) \times I_0(\beta_{0z}) \times C(h_1(\bullet, \vec{\beta}_0), \vec{\alpha}'_0) \times p^2.$$

It can be written:

$$[\rho \times w_0](\vec{\beta}_0, \vec{\alpha}'_0) = [\rho \times \sigma_f \times A](\vec{\beta}_0, \vec{\alpha}'_0)$$

σ_f = capture section per gramme.

For a compact slice of liquid with parallel sides there is the relation:

$$\sigma_f = \sigma_s \times N_{av} \times \frac{C_{rh}}{M_{rh}}, \text{ with } C_{rh} = \frac{\text{mass of dye}}{\text{mass of solution}} \simeq 10^{-4},$$

N_{av} = 6.0225 × 10^{23}, Avogadro's number of molecules per mole.

σ_s = 1.02 × 10^{-16} cm² per dye molecule.

M_{rh} = mole mass of dye = 478.5g (for Rhodamine 6G.)

Actually, for an aggregate of liquid balls, σ_f depends on the shape of liquid interfaces constituting the aerosol, and the capture section is about 4.5 times higher. The section σ_f can be found by experiment or by calculation through electromagnetic model of Chew & al.[3], [4].

c. **Exchange of energy between the planes Σ_0 and Σ_1:**

The energy received through the pixel $\Sigma_1(p^2, \vec{\beta}_1)$ is evaluated. It arrives either directly $[\rho \times w_d]$ or by scattering $[\rho \times w_s]$.

The window $\Sigma_1(p^2, \vec{\beta}_1)$ is seen , from the emitting windows $\Sigma_1(p^2, \vec{\beta}_0)$ under the directions $\vec{\alpha}_0$ such that:

$$\vec{\beta}_1 = \vec{\beta}_0 + \frac{\vec{\alpha}'_0}{\cos \alpha_0} \times \frac{\Delta\xi}{2}, \quad \text{and} \quad \vec{\alpha}_0 = \vec{i} \times \sin \alpha_0 + \vec{\alpha}'_0.$$

A part $[\rho \times w_d]$ reaches directly the window $\Sigma_1(p^2, \vec{\beta}_1)$, under the entry direction $\vec{\alpha}_0$ equal to its going out direction $\vec{\alpha}_1$.

$$[\rho \times w_{1d}](\vec{\beta}_1, \vec{\alpha}'_1) = [\rho \times w_0](\vec{\beta}_1 - \frac{\vec{\alpha}'_1 \times \Delta\xi}{2 \times \cos \alpha_1}, \vec{\alpha}'_1) \times K(\vec{\beta}_1 - \frac{\vec{\alpha}'_1 \times \Delta\xi}{2 \times \cos \alpha_1}, \vec{\beta}_1 + \frac{\vec{\alpha}'_1 \times \Delta\xi}{2 \times \cos \alpha_1}, \vec{\alpha}_1),$$

with $\cos \alpha_i = \sqrt{1 - |\vec{\alpha}_i|^2}$, $i \in \mathbf{N}$,
with K = ratio of the surface not occulted by the balls divided by the entire surface of the light beam passage. K is the transmission function between two points $(\vec{\beta}_i + \vec{i} \times \xi_i)$ and $(\vec{\beta}_j + \vec{i} \times \xi_j)$, with $\xi_j = \xi_i + \Delta\xi$, and is given by :

$$K = \mathrm{Max}\left[[1 - \frac{\bar{e}}{2} \times \frac{\Delta\xi}{\cos \alpha_i} \int_{D_{min}}^{D_{max}} \frac{\pi \times D^2}{4} \times \frac{[\rho(\vec{\beta}_i) \times h_1(D, \vec{\beta}_i) + \rho(\vec{\beta}_j) \times h_1(D, \vec{\beta}_j)]}{2} .dD], 0 \right]$$

A part $[\rho \times w_s]$ due to scattering arrives at the window $\Sigma_1(p^2, \vec{\beta}_1)$. It is written as :

$$[\rho w_{1s}](\vec{\beta}_1, \vec{\alpha}'_1) = \iint_{D_{\alpha 0}} [\rho w_0]\left(\vec{\beta}_1 - \frac{\vec{\alpha}'_0 \Delta\xi}{2 \times \cos \alpha_1}, \vec{\alpha}'_0\right) \times Cr\left(\frac{|\vec{\alpha}'_1 - \vec{\alpha}'_0|}{\Delta\alpha}\right) \times$$

$$\times [\rho g'_\xi]\left(\vec{\beta}_1, \frac{|\vec{\alpha}'_1 - \vec{\alpha}'_0|}{\Delta\alpha}\right) \times \frac{\Delta\xi}{2 \times \cos \alpha_1} .d\alpha_{0y}\, d\alpha_{0z} .$$

Let be D_{α_0} the integration domain, a compact of $\mathbf{R}^2$ limited by the crénel function Cr(t), $t \in \mathbf{R}$, such that

$Cr(t) \equiv 1$, for $|t| \leq 1$,

$Cr(t) \equiv 0$, for $|t| > 1$,

$g'_\xi(\vec{\beta}_1, \vec{\alpha}'_1)$ is the scattering function for a diameter distribution $h_1(D, \vec{\beta}_1)$, and the main part of which is :

$$g'_\xi(\vec{\beta}_1, \vec{\alpha}'_1) = \int_{D=D_{min}}^{D=D_{max}} \frac{\bar{e}_1}{2} \times \frac{\pi^2 D^4}{16\lambda_1^2} \times h_1(D, \vec{\beta}_1) \times j_1^2(\vec{\alpha}'_1, D) \times dD \quad [5]$$

with $\rho \times g'_\xi$ dimensionless,

with $j_1^2(\vec{\alpha}'_1, D) = \frac{\cos(2|\vec{\alpha}'_1|) + 3}{4} \times \left(\frac{2J_1(u)}{u}\right)^2$, and $u = \frac{\pi \times D \times |\vec{\alpha}'_1|}{\lambda_1}$.

$J_1(u) = \sum_{k=0}^{\infty}(-1)^k \frac{u^{1+2k}}{2} \times \frac{1}{k!(k+1)!}$ the Bessel function.

(H₀)

The function $Cr\left(\frac{|\vec{\alpha}'|}{\Delta\alpha}\right)$ is used with $\Delta\alpha$ limited to the fourth zero of $J_1(u)$ (the fourth black ring of the Airy light spot), that is to say $\frac{\pi \times D_{min} \times \Delta\alpha}{\lambda_1} \leq 13.34$.

For $D_{min} = 6\mu m$ and $\lambda = 0.585\mu m$ it gives $\Delta\alpha \leq 0.414401$ and Arc sin (0.4144401) = 24°46/100. Inside the four black rings (zero rings) a little more than 96 % of the scattered energy is localized . The sum of the direct and scattered contributions going to the window $\Sigma_1(p^2, \vec{\beta}_1)$ along the direction $\vec{\alpha}_1$ turns to be a convolution * with regard to α_{1y}, α_{1z}.

$$[\rho w_1](\vec{\beta}_1, \vec{\alpha}'_1) = \frac{1}{\cos\alpha_1} \times [\rho \times w_0]\left(\vec{\beta}_1 - \vec{\alpha}'_1 \frac{\Delta\xi}{2\cos\alpha_1}, \vec{\alpha}'_1\right) * \left[Cr\left(\frac{|\vec{\alpha}'_1|}{\Delta\alpha}\right) \times \rho g'_\xi(\vec{\beta}_1, \vec{\alpha}'_1) \times \frac{\Delta\xi}{2}\right]$$

$$+ \frac{1}{\cos\alpha_1}\left[[\rho w_0]\left(\vec{\beta}_1 - \frac{\vec{\alpha}'_1 \times \Delta\xi}{2\cos\alpha_1}, \vec{\alpha}'_1\right) \times K\left(\vec{\beta}_1 - \frac{\vec{\alpha}'_1 \times \Delta\xi}{2\cos\alpha_1}, \vec{\beta}_1 + \frac{\vec{\alpha}'_1 \times \Delta\xi}{2\cos\alpha_1}, \vec{\alpha}'_1\right)\right] * \delta(\vec{\alpha}'_1).$$

The preceding expression, just as it is, does not authorize to get $[\rho \times w_0]$ as a convolution factor . Thus in the preceding expression, let us assume that, in K, the variation of ρ and h_1 is linear with regard to ξ along the segment **(L)** of straight line between the points $(\vec{\beta}_1 - \frac{\vec{\alpha}'_1 \times \Delta\xi}{2 \times \cos\alpha_1} + \vec{i}0)$ and $(\vec{\beta}_1 + \frac{\vec{\alpha}'_1 \times \Delta\xi}{2 \times \cos\alpha_1} + \vec{i} \times \Delta\xi)$,

then it can be written, except for a term $\propto \Delta\xi^3$.:

$$\frac{1}{\cos\alpha_1}\times\left[[\rho\times w_0]\left(\vec{\beta}_1-\frac{\vec{\alpha}'_1\times\Delta\xi}{2\cos\alpha_1},\vec{\alpha}'_1\right)\times K\left(\vec{\beta}_1-\frac{\vec{\alpha}'_1\times\Delta\xi}{2\cos\alpha_1},\vec{\beta}_1+\frac{\vec{\alpha}'_1\times\Delta\xi}{2\cos\alpha_1},\vec{\alpha}'_1\right)*\delta(\vec{\alpha}'_1)\right]=$$

$$\left[\frac{1}{\cos\alpha_1}\left[[\rho\times w_0]\left(\vec{\beta}_1-\frac{\vec{\alpha}'_1\times\Delta\xi}{2\cos\alpha_1},\vec{\alpha}'_1\right)\right]\right]*\left[K(\vec{\beta}_1,\vec{\beta}_1,\vec{0})+\Delta\xi^3\times\frac{|\vec{\alpha}'_1|^2\vec{e}_1\times\pi}{96(1-|\vec{\alpha}'_1|^2)}[D^3]_{D_{min}}^{D_{max}}\times\right.$$

$$\left.\times\left[\frac{dh_1}{d\xi}\times\frac{d\rho}{d\xi}\right]\times\delta(\vec{\alpha}'_1)\right]$$

with $\frac{d}{d\xi}h_1$ and $\frac{d}{d\xi}$ the derivatives along **(L)**.

(H₁)

Let us assume that the light (signal leaving the cloud) is negligible for an exit angle $|\alpha_{Ne}|<24°66/100$; the assimilation of $\frac{1}{\cos\alpha_{Ne}}=\frac{1}{\sqrt{1-|\vec{\alpha}'_{Ne}|^2}}$ to 1 causes an error lower than 10% .

(H₂)

Therefore, the term $\propto\Delta\xi^3$ can be neglected and $[\rho\times w_1]$ can be written in the form :

(2) $$[\rho w_1](\vec{\beta}_1,\vec{\alpha}'_1)=\frac{1}{\sqrt{1-|\vec{\alpha}'_1|^2}}[\rho w_0]\left(\vec{\beta}_1-\vec{\alpha}'_1\times\frac{\Delta\xi}{2\cos\alpha_1},\vec{\alpha}'_1\right)*\psi_1(\vec{\beta}_1,\vec{\alpha}'_1),$$ with

$$\psi_1(\vec{\beta}_1,\vec{\alpha}'_1)=\left[Cr\left(\frac{|\vec{\alpha}'_1|}{\Delta\alpha}\right)\times[\rho g'_\xi](\vec{\beta}_1,\vec{\alpha}'_1)\times\Delta\xi\right]+\left[K(\vec{\beta}_1,\vec{\beta}_1,\vec{0})\times\delta(\vec{\alpha}'_1)\right].$$

d. **Energy exchange between the planes Σ_{i-1} and Σ_i :** [Figure2]

The preceding chain of reasoning can be easily extended to the energy exchange between two consecutive planes Σ_{i-1} and Σ_i, $i = 2,3,\ldots,N_e$

The following direct contribution $[\rho\times w_{id}]$ of the pixels $\Sigma_{i-1}(p^2,\vec{\beta}_{i-1})$ for a window $\Sigma_i(p^2,\vec{\beta}_i)$ is found as:

$$[\rho\times w_{id}](\vec{\beta}_i,\vec{\alpha}'_i)=\frac{1}{\sqrt{1-|\vec{\alpha}'_i|^2}}[\rho\times w_{i-1}\times]\left(\vec{\beta}_i-\frac{\vec{\alpha}'_i\times\Delta\xi}{\sqrt{1-|\alpha'_i|^2}},\vec{\alpha}'_i\right)\times$$

$$\times K\left(\vec{\beta}_i-\frac{\vec{\alpha}'_i\times\Delta\xi}{2\cos\alpha_i},\vec{\beta}_i+\frac{\vec{\alpha}'_i\times\Delta\xi}{2\cos\alpha_i},\vec{\alpha}'_i\right)*\delta(\vec{\alpha}'_i).$$

The scattered energy reaching the window $\Sigma_i(p^2,\vec{\beta}_i)$ from various windows $\Sigma_{i-1}(p^2,\vec{\beta}_{i-1})$ is written as :

$$[\rho w_{is}](\vec{\beta}_i,\vec{\alpha}'_i)=[\rho w_{i-1}]\left(\vec{\beta}_i-\frac{\vec{\alpha}'_i\times\Delta\xi}{\cos\alpha_i},\vec{\alpha}'_i\right)*\left[Cr\left(\left|\frac{\vec{\alpha}'_i}{\Delta\alpha}\right|\right)\times[\rho g'_\xi](\vec{\beta}_i,\vec{\alpha}'_i)\times\Delta\xi\right].$$

Working out the same approximations on K and on $\cos\alpha_i$ as previously, it comes for $[\rho\times(w_s+w_d)]$ the expression:

(3) $[\rho w_i](\vec{\beta}_i, \vec{\alpha}'_i) = [\rho w_{i-1}]\left(\vec{\beta}_i - \frac{\vec{\alpha}'_i}{\cos \alpha_i}, \vec{\alpha}'_i\right) * \psi_i(\vec{\beta}_i, \vec{\alpha}'_i)$, with

(4) $\psi_i(\vec{\beta}_i, \vec{\alpha}'_i) = [\rho g'_\xi](\vec{\beta}_i, \vec{\alpha}'_i) \times \frac{\Delta\xi \times \varepsilon_i}{\cos \alpha_i} + K(\vec{\beta}_i, \vec{\beta}_i, \vec{0}) \times \delta(\vec{\alpha}'_i)$,

with $\varepsilon_i = 1$ for $i \neq 1$ and $\varepsilon_1 = 1/2$.

e. **Presentation of the general formula giving energy exchange from the light-sheet as far as the exit :**

The light-sheet provides the exciting energy $I_0(\beta_{ymax})$ before entry into the cloud. The light-sheet transforms at $\Sigma_0(p^2, \vec{\beta}_0)$ a part of the energy into :

$[\rho w_0](\vec{\beta}_0, \vec{\alpha}'_0) = [\sigma_f\, A\, \rho](\vec{\beta}_0, \alpha'_0)$

with $A = \frac{\lambda_0}{\lambda_1} \times \phi_r \times \exp(-A(\vec{\beta}_0)) \times I_0(\beta_{0z}) \times C(h_1(\bullet, \vec{\beta}_0), \vec{\alpha}'_0) \times p^2$.

It is reminded that,

- each domain $D_{\alpha i}$, $i \in \{1,2,3, \dots N_e\}$ is given by $|\vec{\alpha}'_i| < 1$ in general and $|\vec{\alpha}'_i| <$ Arc sin 25° here ,
- each element of surface $d\alpha_y . d\alpha_z$, $i \in \{1,2,3, \dots N_e\}$ is denoted by $d\vec{\alpha}_i$.

The planes Σ_i ,$i \in \{1,2,3, \dots , N_e\}$ are similar to successive floors. From a floor to the next, there occur the transfers of energy :

$$(5)_1 \quad [\rho w \times_1](\vec{\beta}_1, \vec{\alpha}'_1) = \iint_{\vec{\alpha}'_0 \in D_{\alpha 0}} [\rho \times w_0]\left(\vec{\beta}_0 - \frac{\vec{\alpha}'_0 \times \Delta\xi}{2 \cos \alpha_0}, \vec{\alpha}'_0\right) \times \psi_1(\vec{\beta}_1, (\vec{\alpha}'_1 - \vec{\alpha}'_0), \vec{\alpha}'_1) \times d\vec{\alpha}'_0$$

$$(5)_2 \quad [\rho \times w_2](\vec{\beta}_2, \vec{\alpha}'_2) = \iint_{\vec{\alpha}'_1 \in D_{\alpha 1}} [\rho w_1]\left(\vec{\beta}_1 - \frac{\vec{\alpha}'_1 \times \Delta\xi}{\cos \alpha_1}, \vec{\alpha}'_1\right) \times \psi_2(\vec{\beta}_2, (\vec{\alpha}'_2 - \vec{\alpha}'_1), \vec{\alpha}'_2) \times d\vec{\alpha}'_1$$

$$(5)_3 \quad [\rho \times w_3](\vec{\beta}_3, \vec{\alpha}'_3) = \iint_{\vec{\alpha}'_2 \in D_{\alpha 2}} [\rho w_2]\left(\vec{\beta}_2 - \frac{\vec{\alpha}'_2 \times \Delta\xi}{\cos \alpha_2}, \vec{\alpha}'_2\right) \times \psi_3(\vec{\beta}_3, (\vec{\alpha}'_3 - \vec{\alpha}'_2), \vec{\alpha}'_3) \times d\vec{\alpha}'_2$$

... ...

$$(5)_i \quad [\rho \times w_i](\vec{\beta}_i, \vec{\alpha}'_i) = \iint_{\vec{\alpha}'_{i-1} \in D_{\alpha_{i-1}}} [\rho \times w_{i-1}]\left(\vec{\beta}_{i-1} - \frac{\vec{\alpha}'_{i-1} \times \Delta\xi}{\cos \alpha_{i-1}}, \vec{\alpha}'_{i-1}\right) \times \psi_i(\vec{\beta}_i, (\vec{\alpha}'_i - \vec{\alpha}'_{i-1}), \vec{\alpha}'_i) \times$$

$$\times \, d\,\vec{\alpha}_{i-1}$$

... ...

$$(5)_{N_e} \quad [\rho \times w_{N_e}](\vec{\beta}_{N_e}, \vec{\alpha}'_{N_e}) = \iint_{\vec{\alpha}'_{N_e-1} \in D_{\alpha N_e - 1}} [\rho \times w_{N_e-1}](\vec{\beta}_{N_e-1} - \frac{\vec{\alpha}'_{N_e-1} \times \Delta\xi}{\cos \alpha_{N_e-1}}, \vec{\alpha}'_{N_e-1}) \times$$

$$\times \, \psi_{N_e}(\vec{\beta}_{N_e}, (\vec{\alpha}'_{N_e} - \vec{\alpha}'_{N_e-1}), \vec{\alpha}'_{N_e}) \times d\,\vec{\alpha}'_{N_e-1} \, ,$$

with N_e being dependent on the local thickness.

5. Solution of the system:

a. Conditions on $\Delta\xi$ the step between the planes Σ:

The paths of light beams between two consecutive planes Σ were implicitly assumed until now, sufficiently short to neglect the absorption . If not the case, the function ψ_i would be written as:

$$\psi_i(\vec{\beta}_i, \vec{\alpha}'_i) = [\rho g'_\xi](\vec{\beta}_i, \vec{\alpha}'_i) \times \frac{\Delta\xi \times \varepsilon_i}{\sqrt{1 - |\vec{\alpha}'_i|^2}} \times \exp\left[- \frac{\Delta\xi \times \varepsilon_i}{\sqrt{1 - |\alpha'_i|^2} \times n \times La} \right] +$$

$$+ \, \delta(\vec{\alpha}'_i) \times \text{Max}\left[0 \; , \left\{ 1 - \frac{\varphi \times \Delta\xi}{\sqrt{1 - |\alpha'_i|^2}} \right\} \right]$$

with $n = 10$ and L_a = reduced thickness for an absorption of 10% (given by experience),

with

$$\varphi = \frac{\overline{e1}}{2} \times \int_{D_{min}}^{D_{max}} \frac{\pi D^2}{8} \times \left(\rho(\vec{\beta}_i + \vec{u}) \times h_1(D, \vec{\beta}_i - \vec{u}) + \rho(\vec{\beta}_i - \vec{u}) \times h_1(D, \vec{\beta}_i + \vec{u}) \right) . dD$$

$$\varphi = \varphi(\vec{\beta}_i, \vec{\alpha}'_i) \, , \text{ with } \vec{u} = \frac{\Delta\xi \times \vec{\alpha}'_i}{2\sqrt{1 - |\alpha'_i|^2}} \, .$$

(H_0)

The scattered energy is assumed to be negligible for angles $|\alpha_i| > 24°1/2 = \alpha_{max} = 0.42686$ rad.; $\alpha'_{max} = \sin \alpha_{Max}$.

Thus $\Delta\xi$ is chosen sufficiently small to satisfy the conditions:

1) $$\frac{\Delta\xi}{\sqrt{1 - |\vec{\alpha}'_{max}|^2}} \leq L_a \text{ or } \boxed{\Delta\xi \leq L_a \times \sqrt{1 - |\vec{\alpha}'_{max}|^2}}$$

2) Let φ_s be the lowest over-estimation of $\varphi(\vec{\beta}_i, \vec{\alpha}'_i)$, $\forall \vec{\alpha}'_i \in D_{\alpha i}$.

$$\forall \vec{\beta}_i \in \Gamma_\beta = \{\vec{\beta} \in \mathbf{R}^2 : |\vec{\beta}| < \beta_{max}\},$$

β_{max} being given by the intersection of the cloud and of the plane Σ_i.

An over-estimate of φ_s is given by the condition:

$\varphi_s \leq \bar{e}_1 \times \text{Sup}(\rho \times h_1) \times \frac{\pi}{48} \times (D^3_{max} - D^3_{min})$ as well as

$$\frac{\varphi_s \times \Delta\xi}{\sqrt{1 - |\vec{\alpha}'_{Max}|^2}} \leq 1 \quad \text{that is to say} \quad \boxed{\Delta\xi \leq \frac{\sqrt{1 - |\vec{\alpha}'_{Max}|^2}}{\varphi_s}}$$

The function ψ_i can therefore be written thanks to simplifications:

(6) $$\psi_i(\vec{\beta}_i, \vec{\alpha}'_i) = [\rho g'_\xi](\vec{\beta}_i, \vec{\alpha}'_i) \times \frac{\Delta\xi \times \varepsilon_i}{\sqrt{1 - |\vec{\alpha}'_i|^2}} + \left(1 - \varphi(\vec{\beta}_i, \vec{\alpha}'_i) \times \frac{\Delta\xi}{\sqrt{1 - |\vec{\alpha}'_i|^2}}\right) \times \times \delta(\vec{\alpha}'_i)$$

b. **<u>The transformations T_1 and T_2: [6]</u>**

Let be D ($\mathbf{R}^4$) the space of the functions of compact support, indefinitely derivable, with values in $\mathbf{R}$. Let us consider a function $F \in D$ ($\mathbf{R}^4$) whose support is $\Gamma_\beta \times \Gamma_\alpha$ defined by

$$\Gamma_\beta = \{\vec{\beta} \in \mathbf{R}^2 : |\vec{\beta}| < \beta_{max}\}$$

$$\Gamma_\alpha = \{\vec{\alpha}' \in \mathbf{R}^2 : |\vec{\alpha}'| \leq \alpha'_{Max}\}, \text{ for } F = F(\vec{\beta}, \vec{\alpha}').$$

The Fourier image of a function F is denoted by:

$$\hat{F} = \int_{\mathbf{R}^2} F(\bullet, \vec{\alpha}') \times \exp(-2\pi i(\vec{\alpha}'.\vec{\eta})).d\vec{\alpha}'$$

with $(\vec{\alpha}'.\vec{\eta})$ the scalar product,

with $d\vec{\alpha}'$ the element of integration over $\mathbf{R}^2$.

1) <u>The transformation T_1 is defined by :</u> $\quad T_1(F) = \int_{R^2} F(\vec{\beta}, \vec{\alpha}') \times \exp(-2\pi i(\vec{\alpha}'.\vec{\eta})).d\vec{\alpha}'$

2) <u>The transformation T_2 is defined by :</u>

$$T_2(F) = \int_{R^2} F(\vec{\beta} - \mu \times \vec{\alpha}', \vec{\alpha}') \times \exp(-2\pi i(\vec{\alpha}'.\vec{\eta})).d\vec{\alpha}', \ \mu \in \mathbf{R}$$

Thereafter, it is assumed, thanks to preceding hypothesis, that permutations of sums Σ and integrations $\int$ are valid.

3) <u>Estimation of $[T_2 - T_1](F)$:</u>

Thanks to Taylor's development , the preceding expression of $T_2(F)$ becomes:

$$T_2(F) = \int_{R^2} \sum_{\ell=0}^{\infty} \frac{(-\mu)^\ell}{\ell!} \times (\alpha_y \frac{\partial}{\partial \beta_y} + \alpha_z \frac{\partial}{\partial \beta_z})^\ell \bullet F(\vec{\beta}, \vec{\alpha}') \times \exp(-2\pi i(\vec{\eta}, \vec{\alpha}')).d\vec{\alpha}'$$

The terms $(-2\pi i\alpha_y)$ and $(-2\pi i\alpha_z)$ are evidenced as transforms of derivation operators

$$T_2(F) = \sum_{\ell=0}^{\infty} \frac{(\frac{\mu}{2\pi i})^\ell}{\ell!} \times \int_{R^2} [(-2\pi i\alpha_y)\frac{\partial}{\partial \beta_y)} + (-2\pi i\alpha_z)\frac{\partial}{\partial \beta_z)}]^\ell \bullet F(\vec{\beta}, \vec{\alpha}') \times \\ \times \exp(-2\pi i(\vec{\eta}, \vec{\alpha}')).d\vec{\alpha}'$$

$$T_2(F) = \sum_{\ell=0}^{\infty} \frac{(\frac{\mu}{2\pi i})^\ell}{\ell!} \times (\frac{\partial}{\partial \eta_y}\frac{\partial}{\partial \beta_y} + \frac{\partial}{\partial \eta_z}\frac{\partial}{\partial \beta_z})^\ell \bullet T_1(F)$$

Let be $\mathbf{D}'$ ($\mathbf{R}^4$), the space of the distributions (continuous linear functionals) applied to $\boldsymbol{D}$ ($\mathbf{R}^4$) the space of the testing functions (already defined). The expression of $T_2(F)$ can be written as a convolution with $T_1(F)$ of a distribution of support $\{0\}$ such that :

$\delta^{(\nu_1)}(\vec{\beta}, \vec{\eta}) = \delta^{(1,0,1,0)}(\vec{\beta}, \vec{\eta}) \in \mathbf{D}'(\mathbf{R}^4)$, $\nu_1 \in (\mathbf{R}^4)$

$\delta^{(\nu_2)}(\vec{\beta}, \vec{\eta}) = \delta^{(0,1,0,1)}(\vec{\beta}, \vec{\eta}) \in \mathbf{D}'(\mathbf{R}^4)$, $\nu_2 \in (\mathbf{R}^4)$

$$T_2(F) = \sum_{\ell=0}^{\infty} \frac{(\frac{\mu}{2\pi i})^\ell}{\ell!} \times (\delta^{(\nu_1)}(\vec{\beta}, \vec{\eta}) + \delta^{(\nu_2)}(\vec{\beta}, \vec{\eta}))^{*\ell} \bullet T_1(F)_{(\vec{\beta}, \vec{\eta})},$$

with ' * ' the fourfold convolution and $(\bullet)^{*\ell}$ the ℓ times iterated convolution.

$$T_2(F) = (\delta(\vec{\beta}, \vec{\eta}) + \sum_{\ell=1}^{\infty} (\frac{\mu}{2\pi i})^{\ell} \sum_{p=0}^{\ell} C_p^{\ell} \times \delta^{(p\vec{v}_1 + (\ell-p)\vec{v}_2)}(\vec{\beta}, \vec{\eta})) * (T_1(F)_{(\vec{\beta}, \vec{\eta})})$$

with $C_p^{\ell} = \frac{\ell!}{p! \times (\ell - p)!}$

$$\boxed{[T_2 - T_1](F) = (\frac{\mu}{2\pi i})[\frac{\partial}{\partial \beta_y}\frac{\partial}{\partial \eta_y} + \frac{\partial}{\partial \beta_z}\frac{\partial}{\partial \eta_z}] \bullet T_1(F) + O(\frac{-\mu^2}{4\pi^2})}$$

4) Influence on the discretization of $\vec{\beta}$ if μ is assimilated to zero:

The pixels are sized to squares $p \times p$. A priori, the location of the extremity of $\vec{\beta}$ is approximated in a square $p \times p$

Let be $F, G \in \boldsymbol{D}(\mathbf{R}^4)$. Let be $\bullet$ the operation

$$F \bullet G = \int_{|\vec{\tau}'| < \alpha'_{Max}} F(\vec{\beta} - \mu\vec{\tau}', \vec{\tau}') \times G(\vec{\beta}, \vec{\alpha}' - \vec{\tau}').d\vec{\tau}'.$$

For each $\vec{\alpha}'$, there exists a vector $\vec{\theta} \in (\mathbf{R}^2)$. , $|\vec{\theta}| < 1$ such that

$$F \bullet G = \int_{|\vec{\tau}'| < \alpha'_{Max}} F(\vec{\beta} - \vec{\theta}\mu\alpha'_{Max}, \vec{\tau}') \times G(\vec{\beta}, \vec{\alpha}' - \vec{\tau}').d\vec{\tau}'$$

Assuming that $F = \rho(\vec{\beta}) \times w(\vec{\beta}, \vec{\alpha}')$, and knowing that $\rho(\vec{\beta})$ is the sought quantity, the actual discretization of the extremity of $\vec{\beta}$ will be a disk of radius

$$[\mu \times \alpha'_{Max}] = \left(\frac{\Delta\xi}{\sqrt{1 - |\vec{\alpha}'|^2}} \times \alpha'_{Max} \right).$$

c. **The approximation upon the general relation of energy exchange:**

Let the general relation be

$$[\rho \times w_i](\vec{\beta}_i, \vec{\alpha}'_i) = \int_{D_{\alpha_{i-1}}} [\rho \times w_{i-1}] (\vec{\beta}_{i-1}, \vec{\alpha}'_{i-1}) \times \psi_i(\vec{\beta}_i, \vec{\alpha}'_i - \vec{\alpha}'_{i-1}, \vec{\alpha}'_i).\, d\vec{\alpha}'_{i-1}\,.$$

Let be $\mathbf{E}'(\mathbf{R}^2)$ the space of distributions with compact support, with variable $\vec{\alpha}'$, and with parameter $\vec{\beta}_i$. It appears that $\psi_i \in \mathbf{E}'(\mathbf{R}^2)$. The T_1 transform of ψ_i is a Fourier transform, with unbounded support, indefinitely derivable with respect to the $\vec{\eta}$ variable. It is allowed to exchange the convolution of ψ_i with $[\rho \times w_{i-1}]$ of bounded support, with the product when applying the T_1 transformation:

$$\psi_i(\vec{\beta}_i, \vec{\alpha}'_i - \vec{\alpha}'_{i-1}, \vec{\alpha}'_i) = [\rho g'_{\xi}](\vec{\beta}_i, \vec{\alpha}'_i - \vec{\alpha}'_{i-1}) \times \frac{\Delta\xi\varepsilon_i}{\cos\alpha_i} + K\left(\vec{\beta}_i - \frac{\vec{\alpha}'_i \times \Delta\xi}{2\cos\alpha_i}, \vec{\beta}_i + \frac{\vec{\alpha}'_i \times \Delta\xi}{2\cos\alpha_i}, \vec{\alpha}_i\right) \bullet$$

$$\bullet\, \delta(\vec{\alpha}'_i - \vec{\alpha}'_{i-1})\,.$$

Let the hypothesis be recalled briefly:

(H_0) limits the scattering angle Arcsin ($|\vec{\alpha}'_i - \vec{\alpha}'_{i-1}|$) to 24°46/100 = 0.427 rad.

(H_1) limits α_i to 24° 6/10 , that is to say $|\vec{\alpha}'_i| < 0.4166 = \alpha'_{Max}$.

(H_2) $\frac{1}{\cos\alpha_i}$ is assimilated to 1 with an relative error lower than 10% .

(H_3) The function $K(\vec{\beta}_i - \frac{\vec{\alpha}'_i\Delta\xi}{2\cos\alpha_i}, \vec{\beta}_i + \frac{\vec{\alpha}'_i\Delta\xi}{2\cos\alpha_i}, \vec{\alpha}'_i)$ is assimilated to $K(\vec{\beta}_i, \vec{\beta}_i, \vec{0})$

The third argument of K depends only on $\frac{1}{\sqrt{1-\vec{\alpha}'^2_i}}$. Now K will be written as $K = K(\vec{\beta}_i)$.

The relation $(5)_i$ can be written as a convolution with respect to $\vec{\alpha}'_i$. The Fourier transform of both members can be expressed by applyings of T_1 and T_2:

$$[\rho \times w_i](\vec{\beta}_i, \vec{\alpha}'_i) = [\rho \times w_{i-1}]\left(\vec{\beta}_i - \frac{\vec{\alpha}'_i \times \varepsilon_i}{\cos\alpha_i} \times \Delta\xi, \vec{\alpha}'_i\right) \underset{\vec{\alpha}'_i}{*} \psi_i(\vec{\beta}_i, \vec{\alpha}'_i)\,.$$

$$,\ \varepsilon_1 = 1/2, \varepsilon_2 = \varepsilon_3 = \cdots = \varepsilon_{N_e} = 1$$

That is to say, by Fourier transformation and exchange between convolution and product:

(6) $T_1[\rho \times w_i] = T_2[\rho \times w_{i-1}] \times T_1[\psi_i]$.

It is known that $T_2[\rho \times w_{i-1}]$ converges uniformly towards $T_1[\rho \times w_{i-1}]$ when $\frac{\vec{\alpha}'_i\Delta\xi}{\cos\alpha_i}$ converges towards $\vec{0}$, and that $\rho \times w_{i-1} \in \boldsymbol{D}$ ($\mathbf{R}^4$) has a Fourier Transform which is analytical and rapidly decreasing.

Therefore $$|T_2[\rho \times w_{i-1}] - T_1[\rho \times w_{i-1}]| \leq \frac{|\vec{\alpha}'_i|\Delta\xi \times M}{\sqrt{1-|\vec{\alpha}'_i|^2}}$$ with

$$M \leq \frac{1}{\pi} \times \mathrm{Sup}\left|\left[\frac{\partial}{\partial\beta_y}\frac{\partial}{\partial\eta_y} + \frac{\partial}{\partial\beta_z}\frac{\partial}{\partial\eta_z}\right] \bullet T_1[F]\right|$$

$$(\vec{\beta}, \vec{\eta}) \in \Gamma_\beta \times R^2(\vec{\eta})$$

There occurs the fourth hypothesis:

H_4

Assimilation of $T_2[\rho \times w_{i-1}]$ to $T_1[\rho \times w_{i-1}]$ is allowed.

That assimilation amounts to search $\rho(\vec{\beta})$ as a mean value on the disk centred upon the extremity of $\vec{\beta}$ and with reduced radius $[\alpha'_{Max} \times \Delta\xi]$. Because of the recurrence on the N_e aerosol slices, the resultant approximation is a mean value of $\rho(\vec{\beta})$ on the disk centred upon the extremity of $\vec{\beta}$ and with reduced radius $\alpha'_{Max} \times \Delta\xi \times N_e = \alpha'_{Max} = 0.4166$.

d. **Extraction of the function ρ:**

Thanks to these approximations, the relation (6) is written :

$$T_1[\rho \times w_i] = T_1[\rho w_{i-1}] \times T_1[\psi_i] + 0(\Delta\xi)$$

That remainder is neglected because of H_4 cited in 5.c . Considering the relation (5), there comes :

$$(7) \quad T_1[\rho \times w_{N_e}] = T_1[\rho w_0] \times T_1[\psi_1] \times \prod_{k=2}^{k=N_e} T_1[\psi_k] .$$

Each of the terms $T_1[\psi_k]$ $k = 2, 3, \dots, N_e$ corresponds to the same transfer function for aerosol slices having the same thickness. The term $T_1[\psi_1]$ corresponds to the transfer function of an aerosol slice having a thickness $\frac{\Delta\xi}{2}$. Finally, the general relation (7) gives, taking as arguments $\vec{\beta}$ and $\vec{\eta}$:

$$(8) \quad T_1[\rho \times w_{N_e}] = T_1[\rho \times w_0] \times (T_1[\psi])^{N_e - 1/2} .$$

There is $T_1[\rho \times w_0] = \rho \times T_1[w_0]$,

$$(9) \quad T_1[\psi] = a \times \rho \times \Delta\xi + 1 - b \times \rho \times \Delta\xi$$

with $\boxed{a = T_1[g'_\xi]}$ and $\boxed{b = \left[\frac{\bar{e}_1}{2} \times \int_{D_{min}}^{D_{max}} \frac{\pi \times D^2}{4} \times h_1(D, \vec{\beta}).dD \right]}$.

From (8) and (9) an equation which gives $\rho(\vec{\beta})$, is drawn

$$(10) \quad [\rho(\vec{\beta}) \times \Delta\xi \times (a - b) + 1] \times \rho(\vec{\beta})^{\frac{1}{N_e - 1/2}} = \frac{T_1[\rho w_{Ne}]}{T_1[w_0]} .$$

The right member $\frac{T_1[\rho \times w_{N_e}]}{T_1[w_0]}$ is known. Indeed:

- $[\rho \times w_{N_e}]$ is given by optical sensors

- w_0 is known through the image of light sensors set inside the plane yOz, and watching the cloud with an optical axis parallel with Oz.

The function $T_1[w_0]$ is known, except for a noise function $B = B(\vec{\eta})$. The roots of $T_1[w_0]$ create poles in the right members. To avoid this, several artful algorithms are available, [7],[8]$_1$ ... [8]$_4$ Either the noise in the photonic receptor can be considered as dependent on the signal or not. If the noise $B(\vec{\eta})$ is independent of it, one of these algorithms is:

$$(11) \quad [\rho \times \Delta\xi \times (a - b) + 1]\rho^{\frac{1}{N_e - 1/2}} = \frac{T_1[\rho w_{N_e}] \times \overline{T_1[w_0]}}{|T_1[w_0]|^2 + B^2}.$$

Let be c the known quantity:

$$c = \frac{T_1[\rho w_{N_e}] \times \overline{T_1[w_0]}}{|T_1[w_0]|^2 + B^2}$$

The function B is given in an empirical way. The relation (11) can be written as the product of two inverse numbers:

$(\delta\xi \times \rho \times (a - b) + 1) \times (\frac{\rho^{\frac{1}{N_e - 1/2}}}{c}) = 1$

It is reminded that, as the Fourier Transform of an even function, 'a' is a real function. In the same manner, as the integral of a real function, 'b' is a real function. The function ρ is not negative . The phase of the function c must be weak, that is to say the correlation function

$\int_{\vec{\alpha}'' \in \Gamma_\alpha} [\rho \times w_{N_e}](\vec{\beta}, \vec{\alpha}'') \times [w_0](\vec{\beta}, \vec{\alpha}' + \vec{\alpha}'').d\vec{\alpha}''$

must be (nearly) even with respect to the variable $\vec{\alpha}'$. Let be Ξ the sign of c which must satisfy the relation for a pertinent solution ρ_0:

$\Xi = \text{Sign}(c) = \text{Sign}(\rho_0 \times \delta\xi \times (a - b)) = \mp 1$. For that reason c is written as : $c = \Xi \times |c|$

Two kinds of a relevant initialization function $\rho_0(\vec{\beta})$ (corresponding respectively to two cases) will be shown thereafter as available. Let be assumed that such an initialization function $\rho_0(\vec{\beta})$ is available for solving the preceding equation. Then, a refined solution $\rho_1 = \rho_0 + \delta\rho$ is also available with $\delta\rho$ given by:

$$\delta\rho = \left(\frac{[\Xi \times |c| \times \rho_0^{\frac{1}{N_e - 1/2}} - \rho_0\Delta\xi \times (a - b) - 1]}{\Delta\xi \times (a - b) + \Xi \times |c| \times \rho_0^{\frac{N_e + 1/2}{N_e - 1/2}}/(N_e - 1/2)} \right)$$

Two cases arise:

1) In the product of the two inverse numbers, the left one is the lowest:

$$|[\rho \times \Delta\xi \times (a-b)+1]| < \frac{\rho^{\frac{1}{N_e-1/2}}}{\Xi \times |c|}$$

In that case, initialization is taken with

$$\boxed{\rho_0 = \Xi \times |c|^{N_e-1/2}}$$

2) In the product of the two inverse numbers, the right one is the lowest:

$$|[\rho \times \Delta\xi \times (a-b)+1]| > \frac{\rho^{\frac{1}{N_e-\frac{1}{2}}}}{\Xi \times |c|}$$

In that case, initialization is taken with

$$\boxed{\rho_0 = \mathrm{Max}\left\{\frac{\Xi \times |c|-1}{\Delta\xi \times (a-b)}, 0\right\}}$$

The value of $\rho(\vec{\beta})$ is introduced again in the calculation of $I(\vec{\beta}_0)$ given by 4.a that is to say:

$$I(\vec{\beta}_0) = I_0(\beta_z) \times \exp\left\{-\int_{\beta=\beta_{0y}}^{\beta=\beta_{ymax}} \sigma_f(h_1(\beta_y, \beta_{0z})) \times \rho(\beta_y, \beta_{0z}) \times d\beta_y\right\}$$

The calculus of the transfer function is performed again and a new more precise function ρ is reached.

6. Conclusions:

An attempt has been made to approximate conditions analogous to those met in classical Radon's Tomography for extraction of mass density distribution. That extraction was performed in the two-dimensional case. For that purpose, a part of the face of the cloud, near the entry of the light-sheet, as well as the average plane of it are parallel to this light-sheet. Upon the centre of that part of the face of the cloud a cone is built whose axis is normal to the face, whose vertex is on the face, and whose aperture angle is 50 °. Inside the cone are distributed in an angular homogeneous way, some photographic sets, all aiming at the centre of that part of the cloud face. The data provide the function $[\rho \times w_{N_e}]$. Other set-up can be substituted , which use neither a light-sheet nor the fluorescence: indeed, for a cloud with two sides roughly plane and parallel, a large plane wave sprung from a light source , parallel to the cloud rear face crosses and scatters across the cloud. The sensors, at the same time detect the signals in the cone already described , before the front face.

REFERENCES

1. A. HIRTH , Contribution au développement du laser à colorants dans le proche infra-rouge. Application à l'étude des propriétés du laser d'une série de Cyanines Thèse de Doctorat, Université Pasteur, 67 Strasbourg (F), 1974.
2. F. P. SCHAEFER, Dye Lasers, Springer Verlag, 1974
3. H. CHEW, P.J. NULTY, and M. KERKER, Model for Raman and fluorescent scattering by molecules embedded in small particles, Physical Review, A, volume 13, Number 1, Jan. 1976, pp. 396 - 404.
4. W.H. MARLOW, Aerosol Microphysics I, Particle interaction. Volume 16, Springer Verlag, 1980.
5. R.H. GIESE, Tabellen von Mie-Streufunktionen I, Gemische dielektrischer Teilchen, (Ruhr Universtät Bochum) Max-Planck Institut für Physik und Astrophysik, München, MPI-PAE Extraterr. 40, Dezember 1970.
6. Vo-Khac-KHOAN, Distributions, Analyse de Fourier, Opérateurs aux dérivées partielles, Tomes I and II, Vuibert éditeur, 1972.
7. A. GIRARD, L'inversion du produit de convolution en physique. Mise au point bibliographique, Note Technique 121, Office National d'études et de recherches Aérospatiales (29, Av. Div. Lecleclerc 92 Châtillon (F)) 1967.

8.1 O. FAUGERAS, Déconvolution aveugle par des techniques homomorphiques Journées d'étude du 24 Mars 1977, " Déconvolution, Filtrage inverse, Imagerie ", (SEE 48 r. de la Procession 75724 Paris) Reference 7725128 (1977).

8.2 J.RONSIN, Déconvolution en temps réel par filtrage inverse de Wiener. Application au traitement d'image, Reference 7725129, idem SEE (1977).

8.3 J.F. ABRAMATIC, Modèles récurrents de filtres biindiciels, Reference 7725132, idem SEE (1977).

8.4 E. ROSENCHER, Un algorithme de synthèse de filtres biindiciels par une méthode hilbertienne, Reference 7725133, idem SEE (1977).

COMPUTED TOMOGRAPHY AND ROCKETS

Eric Todd Quinto

Department of Mathematics
Tufts University
Medford, MA 02155 USA

1. Introduction.

X-ray tomography is an effective technique for the non-destructive evaluation of rocket parts [Schneider, *et al.*, Shepp and Srivastava]. Because defects are shown precisely in CT reconstructions, engineers can assess the magnitude and nature of failures. However, there are cases in which a complete data set (X-ray data over uniformly distributed lines passing through all parts of the object) is not efficient or even possible to acquire. In these cases, standard tomographic reconstruction algorithms will not be appropriate.

In this article we describe our *exterior reconstruction algorithm* that reconstructs the outer shell of an object using only X-ray tomographic data that passes through the shell and not the center of the object. Such data are called *exterior tomographic data*. We will present results on rocket motor simulations using fan beam data.

Rocket exit cones and rocket motors have similar areas of interest for non-destructive evaluation. A rocket exit cone is can be made of as many as fourty laminated layers and each crossection is an annulus with a hollow center. The most common defects in exit cones are very thin separations, or delaminations, between the layers. A rocket motor is made up of a metal or composite shell that surrounds a thin insulating layer that surrounds rocket fuel. Tiny air pockets on either side of the insulator or separations in composite cases are common defects. In both exit cones and motors, the defects run along circumferences and have sharp boundaries in the radial direction. In both cases, the centers of these objects are not of structural interest.

Standard computed tomographic algorithms require X-ray data over lines passing through all parts of the object, including the center. However, even the most penetrating of X-rays are attenuated so highly when travelling through the center

The author was partially supported by NSF grant MCS 8901203. The author is indebted to Paul Burstein of Skiametrics for much support and practical information including pointing out the application to large rocket motors, suggesting appropriate phantoms to test and appropriate amount of data to take, as well as useful comments to the manuscript. The author thanks Charles Dunkl for the suggestion to use Cesaro summability to help get rid of Gibbs phenomenon in polynomial sums. The author is indebted to the Institut für Numerische und instrumentelle Mathematik der Universitat Münster for the display programs for figures 1 and 2, to Tufts University undergraduate Scott Turner for his help testing the algorithm, as well as to Peter Maass for clever suggestions about the algorithm and display programs.

of very large diameter rocket motors that they provide little useful data for fine spatial resolution [Burstein, 1989].

Reconstruction algorithms using exterior data have advantages. The exterior data acquisition method can be used on large diameter rockets where the standard data acquisition method fails. Data acquisition time will be lower than with normal C.T. scans because less data are required; on large diameter rocket motors, the acquisition time for standard CT data can be 100 minutes or longer for a single slice [Burstein, 1989]. Smaller scanners can be designed to work on site because of the smaller amount of data to be acquired. Recent tragedies demonstrate the utility of such on site scanners for detecting defects in rocket motors. There are even mathematical reasons why exterior data are ideally suited to detect common defects [Quinto 1988] (see §3). Exterior data are also useful for astronomical studies of the solar corona [Altschuler] and in medical tomography [Shepp and Kruskal].

In [1963] Cormack showed reconstruction from exterior data is possible for compactly supported functions (see also Helgason [1965] for rapidly decreasing functions on $\mathbb{R}^n$). Lewitt and Bates [1978, 1988], Louis [1988], and Natterer [1980] have developed good reconstruction algorithms that use exterior data.

The author's exterior reconstruction algorithm [Quinto 1983, 1988, 1990] employs a singular value decomposition [Perry; Quinto 1983 for $\mathbb{R}^n$] and *a priori* information about the shape of the object to be reconstructed. Specifically it uses the fact that the part of the object of interest is an annulus of known shape and that the object density is known in a thin band just inside the annulus of interest (for rocket bodies: the band is in the fuel just inside the rocket shell, for exit cones: the hollow center).

As with other limited data problems [Davison, Finch, Louis 1986, 1989], reconstruction from exterior data is much more highly ill-posed (that is, much more difficult and more sensitive to noise) than standard tomography. In fact, reconstruction from exterior data is continuous in no range of Sobolev norms. By comparision, reconstruction with complete data is continuous of order $+1/2$ in Sobolev norms. Thus, reconstruction from exterior data takes away an "infinite number of derivatives" from the data, but reconstruction from complete data takes away only one-half derivative from the data.

Section 2 of this article provides the definitions and the inversion procedure. Reconstructions and discussion are in §3.

2. The algorithm.

First let $\cdot$ denote the standard inner product on $\mathbb{R}^2$; let $|\ |$ be the induced norm, and let dx be Lebesgue measure on $\mathbb{R}^2$. Let $\theta \in [0, 2\pi]$, and let $p \in \mathbb{R}$. Now let $d\theta$ and dp denote the standard measures on $[0, 2\pi]$ and $\mathbb{R}$, respectively. In order to define the Radon transform let $L(\theta, p) = \{x \in \mathbb{R}^2 | x \cdot \overline{\theta} = p\}$, the line with normal vector $\overline{\theta} = (\cos\theta, \sin\theta)$ and directed distance p from the origin. The points (θ, p) and $(\theta + \pi, -p)$ parametrize the same line $L(\theta, p)$, so we will always assume $p \geq 0$ in this article. Let dx_L be arc length, the measure on $L(\theta, p)$ induced from Lebesgue measure on $\mathbb{R}^2$. The *classical Radon transform* is defined for an integrable function f on $\mathbb{R}^2$ by

$$Rf(\theta, p) = \int_{L(\theta,p)} f(x) dx_L. \tag{2.1}$$

$Rf(\theta,p)$ is just the integral of f over the line $L(\theta,p)$.

Let E be the exterior of the unit disc in $\mathbb{R}^2, E = \{x \in \mathbb{R}^2 \mid 1 \leq |x|\}$, and let $E' = [0,2\pi] \times [1,\infty)$. E' corresponds to the set of lines $L(\theta,p)$ that lie in E.

The *exterior Radon transform* is the transform R as a map from integrable functions on E, the area outside the center of the object to be reconstructed, to integrable functions on E', the set of lines that do not meet the center of the object. Let $L^2(E)$ be the Hilbert space of functions on E defined by weight $(1/\pi)|x|(1-|x|^{-2})^{1/2}dx$ and let $L^2(E')$ be the Hilbert space of functions on E' defined by weight $(\pi p)^{-1}d\theta dp$. One part of the author's algorithm is the following singular value decomposition (SVD) (see [Quinto, 1988, Propositions 3.1-2] for a precise statement).

Proposition 2.1. *There are orthonormal bases $\{h_m | m \in \mathbb{Z}\}$ of $L^2(E)$ and $\{g_m | m \in \mathbb{N}\}$ of $L^2(E')$ such that the exterior Radon transform $R: L^2(E) \to L^2(E')$ satisfies*

$$Rh_m(\theta,p) = 0 \text{ for } m \leq 0 \tag{2.2}$$

and,

$$Rh_m(\theta,p) = C_m g_m(\theta,p) \text{ for } m > 0 \tag{2.3}$$

where the constants C_m satisfy

$$C_m = \mathcal{O}(1/\sqrt{m}) \text{ for } m > 0. \tag{2.4}$$

Each basis function $h_m(r\overline{\theta})$ is an orthogonal polynomial in $1/r$ multiplied by $e^{i\ell\theta}$ for some $\ell \in \mathbb{Z}$; thus each h_m has only one non-zero term in its polar Fourier expansion (the Fourier expansion in the polar coordinate θ).

Proposition 2.1 is R. M. Perry's singular value decomposition for the exterior Radon transform on $\mathbb{R}^2$ and is proved using identities in [Perry] involving orthogonal polynomials. See [Maass 1990] for a unified treatment of singular value decompositions. This decomposition is *not* an inversion method because of the presence of the non-trivial null space (2.2). Thus, any successful reconstruction algorithm must use more than just the SVD.

An immediate corollary of the SVD is the null space characterization:

Proposition 2.2. *A function $f_N \in L^2(E)$ is in the null space of $R: L^2(E) \to L^2(E')$ iff for each $\ell \in \mathbb{Z}$ the ℓth polar Fourier coefficient, $(f_N)_\ell(r)$, is a polynomial in $1/r$ of the same parity as ℓ, of degree less than $|\ell|$, and with lowest order term in $1/r$ of degree at least 2.*

The SVD is one key to the author's algorithm. Let $f(x) \in L^2(E)$ be the density to be reconstructed, then the singular value decomposition gives f_R, the projection of f onto the orthogonal complement of the null space of the exterior Radon transform. Because of the slow decrease of singular values in (2.4), recovering f_R is only as mildly ill-posed as inversion of the Radon transform with complete data (compare with the singular values in [Cormack 1964]). Let f_N be the projection of f onto the null space of the exterior transform. Of course, $f = f_R + f_N$ and f_N is not recovered by the SVD.

The other key to the algorithm is the fact that rocket bodies and exit cones have *a priori* known (homogeneous) inner structure and known outer radius, $K > 1$. For rocket motors, we scale distances so the thin band $1.0 \le |x| \le 1.03$ lies in the fuel just inside the insulator. In the case of a rocket exit cone, we scale so $|x| = r \in [1, 1.03]$ is just inside the hollow center of the cone. Thus, one knows $f(x) = 0$ for $|x| > K$ and one knows $f(x) = const$ for $|x| \in [1, 1.03]$. For exit cones $const = 0$ and for motors, $const$ is the density of fuel. Even if the density of the area containing rocket fuel is not constant, it is still known accurately enough to be used by the algorithm.

This *a priori* information is used to recover f_N. Because the basis functions are expressed in terms of trigonometric monomials, the algorithm is performed on each Fourier coefficient. Let $(f_N)_\ell$ be the ℓth polar Fourier coefficient of f_N. We take $\ell \in \mathbb{Z} \setminus \{0\}$ as, according to Proposition 2.2, $(f_N)_0 \equiv 0$. As f is constant near $r = 1$, the polar Fourier coefficients f_ℓ for $\ell \neq 0$ will be zero for $r \in [1, 1.03]$, and as $f = f_N + f_R$, we have the *a priori* condition

$$(f_N)_\ell(r) = -(f_R)_\ell(r) \text{ for } r \in [1, 1.03] \cup [K, \infty). \tag{2.5}$$

This restriction uniquely determines $(f_N)_\ell(r)$ for $r \ge 1$ by [Quinto, 1988].

The basic algorithm to recover f_ℓ is to use the SVD to recover $(f_R)_\ell(r)$ for $r \ge 1$ and then use equation (2.5) and the null space restriction, Proposition 2.2, to find $(f_N)_\ell(r)$. A polynomial of degree less than $|\ell|$ is least-square fit to the data, $-(f_R)_\ell(r)$, for $r \in [1, 1.03] \cup [K, \infty)$. This polynomial, the reconstruction for $(f_N)_\ell$, is interpolated to $[1.03, K]$ using the explicit knowledge of its coefficients. This gives the reconstruction of the Fourier coefficient f_ℓ, and the reconstruction of f is a smoothed sum of the Fourier coefficients (see [Quinto 1988] for details).

The unstable part of the algorithm is the recovery of $(f_N)_\ell$. The interpolation procedure using (2.5) has been tested on data for which the values of f are not known near $r = 1$, and the reconstructions are acceptable without accurate *a priori* information [Quinto 1988].

This algorithm is easily adapted to any rotationally invariant data acquisition scheme such as fan beam geometry. The only part of the algorithm that depends explicitly on the data set is the calculation of $(f_R)_\ell$. The algorithm first must calculate the polar Fourier coefficient, $(Rf)_\ell$ and then perform numerical integrals in p to get the coefficients of $(f_R)_\ell$ in the basis functions. Since the data set is rotationally invariant, the scanner rotates through an evenly spaced number of angles $\theta_1, \theta_2, ..., \theta_n$ and for each θ_j; the lines in the data seta are at are the same fixed distances from the origin, $p_0, p_1, ..., p_m$, that do not depend on j. Because of rotation invariance, for each p_i, there is a number $\Delta\theta_i$ *that depends only on* i *and the data acquisition geometry* such that all lines of distance p_i from the origin are parameterized by: $L(\theta_k + \Delta\theta_i, p_i)$ for $k = 1, 2, ..., n$. This observation simplifies the calculation of Fourier coefficients. Then an interpolation is done in p to perform the integrals in p.

3. Reconstructions and discussion.

Figure 1 shows a part of the phantom, and figures 2a&b give the reconstruction in polar coordinates $x = (r, \theta)$ with $\theta \in [\pi/8, 3\pi/8]$ on the horizontal axis and $r \in [1, 1.10]$ on the vertical axis ($r = 1.10$ at the bottom). The first quadrant is displayed, $\theta \in [\pi/8, 3\pi/8]$, because the defect is in that quadrant. In order to provide sufficiently fine radial resolution the scale in r is magnified by a factor of 7.85.

Figure 1 shows a phantom of a rocket motor with fuel of density 1.7 inside the circle of radius $r = 1.052$, an insulator of density 1.1 from $1.052 < r < 1.056$, and a shell of density 1.5 and outer radius $r = 1.093$. The defect rests against the inside boundary of the insulator and extends for 0.06 radians and is 0.0014 units thick (it is seen tangentially by only three detectors). It is centered at $\pi/4$ radians and has density zero.

Figure 2a-b shows the reconstruction with 1% multiplicative L^∞ noise. Fourty-five polar Fourier coefficients are recovered ($0 \leq |\ell| < 45$). For each coefficient, 220 polynomials in $1/r$ are reconstructed. Data are collected in a fan beam with 200 rays from $p = 1.0$ to $p = 1.10$ that emanate from the source in evenly spaced angles. The source and fan beam rotate around the object in 512 equally spaced angles. Figure 2a is without postprocessing, and figure 2b sets density values near (−3% to +6%) the density of the shell, 1.5, to become 1.5 and density values near (−3% to +5%) the density of the fuel, 1.7, to become 1.7. The rationale for this postprocessing is that defects are almost always densities near zero, not near 1.5 or 1.7. Two hundred and fifty-six levels of grey from are displayed between densities 0.57 and 1.71. Reconstructions of other parts of the phantom are at least as good.

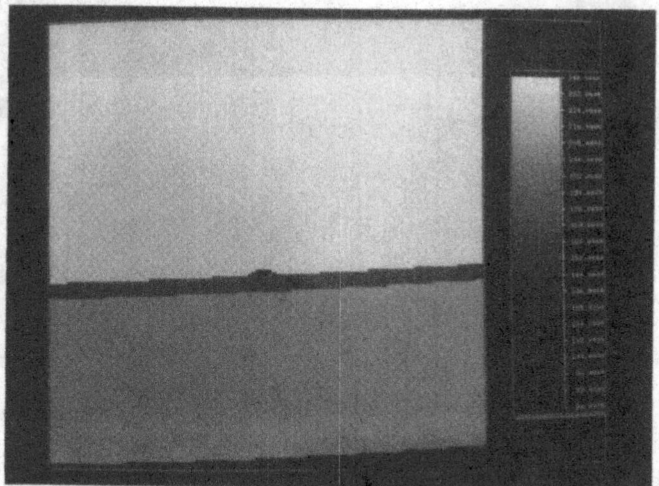

Figure 1. *Polar coordinate display of rocket motor phantom.* The horizontal axis corresponds to $\theta \in [\pi/8, 3\pi/8]$, the vertical corresponds to $r \in [1, 1.10]$ (magnified by a factor of 7.85). The "wedge" near $r = 1.10$ (at the bottom of the display) occurs because of the offset.

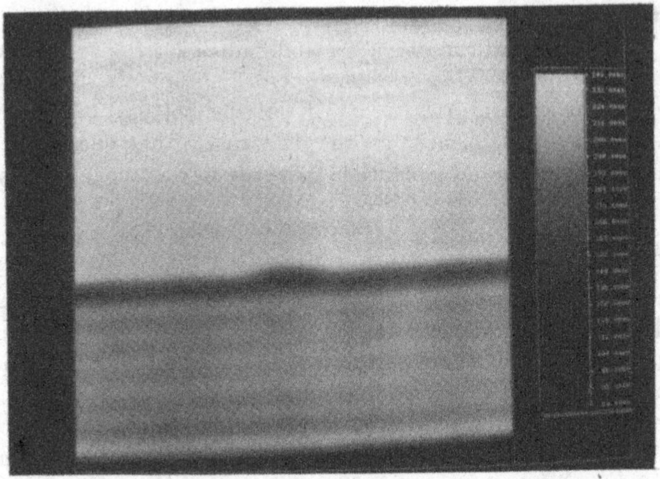

Figure 2a. *Polar coordinate display of rocket motor reconstruction without processing and using the same scale as in figure 1.* The magnification in r exaggerates the smoothing of the defect.

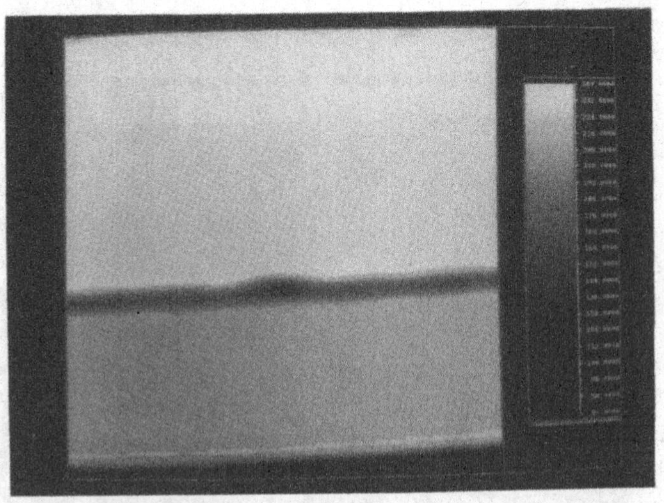

Figure 2b. *Polar coordinate display of rocket motor reconstruction with postprocessing and using the same scale as in figure 1.*

To decrease Gibbs phenomenon in the polynomial and Fourier coefficient sums and to decrease the effects of noise, the algorithm multiplies the coefficients of the basis functions by weight factors, much like in Cesaro sums. The reconstruction of the defect is thereby smoothed, and this smoothing is exaggerated by the increased radial resolution of the displays. Reconstructions of the other quadrants are at least as good as that shown, and reconstructions of rocket exit cones from fan beam data are as good as the reconstructions from parallel beam data in [Quinto 1990].

The phantom was chosen to be similar to real defects and to be difficult for the author's algorithm. The rocket body is offset by 1/140 units in the positive x−direction from the center of the coordinate system in order to give it high polar Fourier coefficients, ones that are less well reconstructed by the algorithm. If the rocket were centered, its Fourier coefficients for $\ell \neq 0$ would all be zero, and they wouldn't mask the Fourier coefficients of the defect. The offset is chosen to be at the outer limit of tolerence for scans of large rocket motors.

Common defects are seen well from exterior data. Shepp and Srivastava [p. 78] argue that CT is ideally suited to detecting delaminations in rocket exit cones because of the *tangent casting effect* associated with sharp material density differences that occur tangent to X-rays in the data set. Simply put, an X-ray that travels tangent to a defect will detect it easily (especially if it is tangent along a major axis). Exterior data are tangent to delaminations (along major axes) as well as separations in rocket motors and, therefore, detect these common defects clearly. This is true because of an anlytic property of the Radon transform; the Radon transform easily detects boundaries of f that are tangent to lines in the data set, but not boundaries in other directions. Delaminations and separations are easy for exterior data to detect because their boundaries are generally along the curve of the annulus–they are tangent to the lines in the exterior data set and, therefore, they are easy to detect. The rigorous mathematical reason for this analytic property is that R is an elliptic Fourier integral operator of a special form (this discussion can be made precise using wave front sets, see [Quinto, 1980, 1988]).

References

M. D. Altschuler 1979, Reconstruction of the global-scale three-dimensional solar corona, *in* "Image Reconstruction from Projections, Implementation and Applications"(G. T. Herman, Ed.), pp. 105-145, Topics in Applied Physics, Vol. 32, Springer-Verlag, New York/Berlin.

P. Burstein 1989, private communication.

A. M. Cormack 1963, Representation of a function by its line integrals with some radiological applications, *J. Appl. Phys.* **34**, 2722-2727.

A. M. Cormack 1964, Representation of a function by its line integrals with some radiological applications, **II** *J. Appl. Phys.* **35**, 2908-2913

M. Davison 1983, The ill-conditioned nature of the limited angle tomography problem, *SIAM J. Appl. Math.*, **43**, 428-448.

D. V. Finch 1985, Cone beam reconstruction with sources on a curve, SIAM J. Appl. Math. 45, 665-673.

R. M. Lewitt 1988, Overview of inversion methods used in computed tomography, in Advances in Remote Sensing Retrieval Methods, Deepak Publishing, Hampton, VA.

R. M. Lewitt and R. H. T. Bates 1978, Image reconstruction from projections. II, Projection completion methods (theory), *Optik* **50**, 189-204, **III**: Projection completion methods (computational examples), Optik **50**, 269-278.

A. Louis 1986, Incomplete data problems in X-ray computerized tomography 1. Singular value decomposition of the limited angle transform, *Numer. Math.* **48**, 251-262.

A. Louis 1988, private communication.

A. Louis 1989, Incomplete data problems in X-ray computerized tomography 2. truncated projections and region-of-interest tomography, *Numer. Math.* **56**, 371-383.

P. Maass 1990, The interior Radon transform, submitted.

F. Natterer 1980, Efficient implementation of "optimal" algorithms in computerized tomography, *Math. Meth. Appl. Sci.* **2**, 545-555.

R. M. Perry 1977, On reconstruction a function on the exterior of a disc from its Radon transform, *J. Math. Anal. Appl.* **59**, 324-341.

E. T. Quinto 1980, The dependence of the generalized Radon transform on defining measures, *Trans. Amer. Math. Soc.* **257**, 331-346.

E. T. Quinto 1983, The invertibility of rotation invariant Radon transforms, *J. Math. Anal. Appl.* **91**, 510-522.

E. T. Quinto 1988, Tomographic reconstructions from incomplete data–numerical inversion of the exterior Radon transform., *Inverse Problems* **4**, 867-876.

E. T. Quinto 1990, Limited data tomography in non-destructive evaluation, *Signal Processing Part II: Control Theory and Applications*, IMA Volumes in Mathematics and its Applications, Vol. 23, 347-354, Springer-Verlag 1990.

R. J. Schneider, P. Burstein, F. H. Seguin, and A. S. Kreiger 1986, High-spacial-resolution computed tomography for thin annular geometries, Review of progress in qualitative non-destructive evaluation, Vol 5a, Donald O. Thompson and Dale E. Chimenti editors, Plenum Press.

L. A. Shepp and J. B. Kruskal 1978, Computerized tomography: The new medical X-ray technology, *Amer. Math. Monthly* **85**, 420-439.

L. A. Shepp and S. Srivastava 1986, Computed tomography of PKM and AKM exit cones, *A. T & T. Technical Journal*, **65**, 78-88.

Vol. 1411: B. Jiang (Ed.), Topological Fixed Point Theory and Applications. Proceedings. 1988. VI, 203 pages. 1989.

Vol. 1412: V.V. Kalashnikov, V.M. Zolotarev (Eds.), Stability Problems for Stochastic Models. Proceedings, 1987. X, 380 pages. 1989.

Vol. 1413: S. Wright, Uniqueness of the Injective III₁ Factor. III, 108 pages. 1989.

Vol. 1414: E. Ramirez de Arellano (Ed.), Algebraic Geometry and Complex Analysis. Proceedings, 1987. VI, 180 pages. 1989.

Vol. 1415: M. Langevin, M. Waldschmidt (Eds.), Cinquante Ans de Polynômes. Fifty Years of Polynomials. Proceedings, 1988. IX, 235 pages.1990.

Vol. 1416: C. Albert (Ed.), Géométrie Symplectique et Mécanique. Proceedings, 1988. V, 289 pages. 1990.

Vol. 1417: A.J. Sommese, A. Biancofiore, E.L. Livorni (Eds.), Algebraic Geometry. Proceedings, 1988. V, 320 pages. 1990.

Vol. 1418: M. Mimura (Ed.), Homotopy Theory and Related Topics. Proceedings, 1988. V, 241 pages. 1990.

Vol. 1419: P.S. Bullen, P.Y. Lee, J.L. Mawhin, P. Muldowney, W.F. Pfeffer (Eds.), New Integrals. Proceedings, 1988. V, 202 pages. 1990.

Vol. 1420: M. Galbiati, A. Tognoli (Eds.), Real Analytic Geometry. Proceedings, 1988. IV, 366 pages. 1990.

Vol. 1421: H.A. Biagioni, A Nonlinear Theory of Generalized Functions, XII, 214 pages. 1990.

Vol. 1422: V. Villani (Ed.), Complex Geometry and Analysis. Proceedings, 1988. V, 109 pages. 1990.

Vol. 1423: S.O. Kochman, Stable Homotopy Groups of Spheres: A Computer-Assisted Approach. VIII, 330 pages. 1990.

Vol. 1424: F.E. Burstall, J.H. Rawnsley, Twistor Theory for Riemannian Symmetric Spaces. III, 112 pages. 1990.

Vol. 1425: R.A. Piccinini (Ed.), Groups of Self-Equivalences and Related Topics. Proceedings, 1988. V, 214 pages. 1990.

Vol. 1426: J. Azéma, P.A. Meyer, M. Yor (Eds.), Séminaire de Probabilités XXIV, 1988/89. V, 490 pages. 1990.

Vol. 1427: A. Ancona, D. Geman, N. Ikeda, École d'Eté de Probabilités de Saint Flour XVIII, 1988. Ed.: P.L. Hennequin. VII, 330 pages. 1990.

Vol. 1428: K. Erdmann, Blocks of Tame Representation Type and Related Algebras. XV. 312 pages. 1990.

Vol. 1429: S. Homer, A. Nerode, R.A. Platek, G.E. Sacks, A. Scedrov, Logic and Computer Science. Seminar, 1988. Editor: P. Odifreddi. V, 162 pages. 1990.

Vol. 1430: W. Bruns, A. Simis (Eds.), Commutative Algebra. Proceedings. 1988. V, 160 pages. 1990.

Vol. 1431: J.G. Heywood, K. Masuda, R. Rautmann, V.A. Solonnikov (Eds.), The Navier-Stokes Equations – Theory and Numerical Methods. Proceedings, 1988. VII, 238 pages. 1990.

Vol. 1432: K. Ambos-Spies, G.H. Müller, G.E. Sacks (Eds.), Recursion Theory Week. Proceedings, 1989. VI, 393 pages. 1990.

Vol. 1433: S. Lang, W. Cherry, Topics in Nevanlinna Theory. II, 174 pages.1990.

Vol. 1434: K. Nagasaka, E. Fouvry (Eds.), Analytic Number Theory. Proceedings, 1988. VI, 218 pages. 1990.

Vol. 1435: St. Ruscheweyh, E.B. Saff, L.C. Salinas, R.S. Varga (Eds.), Computational Methods and Function Theory. Proceedings, 1989. VI, 211 pages. 1990.

Vol. 1436: S. Xambó-Descamps (Ed.), Enumerative Geometry. Proceedings, 1987. V, 303 pages. 1990.

Vol. 1437: H. Inassaridze (Ed.), K-theory and Homological Algebra. Seminar, 1987–88. V, 313 pages. 1990.

Vol. 1438: P.G. Lemarié (Ed.) Les Ondelettes en 1989. Seminar. IV, 212 pages. 1990.

Vol. 1439: E. Bujalance, J.J. Etayo, J.M. Gamboa, G. Gromadzki. Automorphism Groups of Compact Bordered Klein Surfaces: A Combinatorial Approach. XIII, 201 pages. 1990.

Vol. 1440: P. Latiolais (Ed.), Topology and Combinatorial Groups Theory. Seminar, 1985–1988. VI, 207 pages. 1990.

Vol. 1441: M. Coornaert, T. Delzant, A. Papadopoulos. Géométrie et théorie des groupes. X, 165 pages. 1990.

Vol. 1442: L. Accardi, M. von Waldenfels (Eds.), Quantum Probability and Applications V. Proceedings, 1988. VI, 413 pages. 1990.

Vol. 1443: K.H. Dovermann, R. Schultz, Equivariant Surgery Theories and Their Periodicity Properties. VI, 227 pages. 1990.

Vol. 1444: H. Korezlioglu, A.S. Ustunel (Eds.), Stochastic Analysis and Related Topics VI. Proceedings, 1988. V, 268 pages. 1990.

Vol. 1445: F. Schulz, Regularity Theory for Quasilinear Elliptic Systems and – Monge Ampère Equations in Two Dimensions. XV, 123 pages. 1990.

Vol. 1446: Methods of Nonconvex Analysis. Seminar, 1989. Editor: A. Cellina. V, 206 pages. 1990.

Vol. 1447: J.-G. Labesse, J. Schwermer (Eds), Cohomology of Arithmetic Groups and Automorphic Forms. Proceedings, 1989. V, 358 pages. 1990.

Vol. 1448: S.K. Jain, S.R. López-Permouth (Eds.), Non-Commutative Ring Theory. Proceedings, 1989. V, 166 pages. 1990.

Vol. 1449: W. Odyniec, G. Lewicki, Minimal Projections in Banach Spaces. VIII, 168 pages. 1990.

Vol. 1450: H. Fujita, T. Ikebe, S.T. Kuroda (Eds.), Functional-Analytic Methods for Partial Differential Equations. Proceedings, 1989. VII, 252 pages. 1990.

Vol. 1451: L. Alvarez-Gaumé, E. Arbarello, C. De Concini, N.J. Hitchin, Global Geometry and Mathematical Physics. Montecatini Terme 1988. Seminar. Editors: M. Francaviglia, F. Gherardelli. IX, 197 pages. 1990.

Vol. 1452: E. Hlawka, R.F. Tichy (Eds.), Number-Theoretic Analysis. Seminar, 1988–89. V, 220 pages. 1990.

Vol. 1453: Yu.G. Borisovich, Yu.E. Gliklikh (Eds.), Global Analysis – Studies and Applications IV. V, 320 pages. 1990.

Vol. 1454: F. Baldassari, S. Bosch, B. Dwork (Eds.), p-adic Analysis. Proceedings, 1989. V, 382 pages. 1990.

Vol. 1455: J.-P. Françoise, R. Roussarie (Eds.), Bifurcations of Planar Vector Fields. Proceedings, 1989. VI, 396 pages. 1990.

Vol. 1456: L.G. Kovács (Ed.), Groups – Canberra 1989. Proceedings. XII, 198 pages. 1990.

Vol. 1457: O. Axelsson, L.Yu. Kolotilina (Eds.), Preconditioned Conjugate Gradient Methods. Proceedings, 1989. V, 196 pages. 1990.

Vol. 1458: R. Schaaf, Global Solution Branches of Two Point Boundary Value Problems. XIX, 141 pages. 1990.

Vol. 1459: D. Tiba, Optimal Control of Nonsmooth Distributed Parameter Systems. VII, 159 pages. 1990.

Vol. 1460: G. Toscani, V. Boffi, S. Rionero (Eds.), Mathematical Aspects of Fluid Plasma Dynamics. Proceedings, 1988. V, 221 pages. 1991.

Vol. 1461: R. Gorenflo, S. Vessella, Abel Integral Equations. VII, 215 pages. 1991.

Vol. 1462: D. Mond, J. Montaldi (Eds.), Singularity Theory and its Applications. Warwick 1989, Part I. VIII, 405 pages. 1991.

Vol. 1463: R. Roberts, I. Stewart (Eds.), Singularity Theory and its Applications. Warwick 1989, Part II. VIII, 322 pages. 1991.

Vol. 1464: D. L. Burkholder, E. Pardoux, A. Sznitman, Ecole d'Eté de Probabilités de Saint- Flour XIX-1989. Editor: P. L. Hennequin. VI, 256 pages. 1991.

Vol. 1465: G. David, Wavelets and Singular Integrals on Curves and Surfaces. X, 107 pages. 1991.

Vol. 1466: W. Banaszczyk, Additive Subgroups of Topological Vector Spaces. VII, 178 pages. 1991.

Vol. 1467: W. M. Schmidt, Diophantine Approximations and Diophantine Equations. VIII, 217 pages. 1991.

Vol. 1468: J. Noguchi, T. Ohsawa (Eds.), Prospects in Complex Geometry. Proceedings, 1989. VII, 421 pages. 1991.

Vol. 1469: J. Lindenstrauss, V. D. Milman (Eds.), Geometric Aspects of Functional Analysis. Seminar 1989-90. XI, 191 pages. 1991.

Vol. 1470: E. Odell, H. Rosenthal (Eds.), Functional Analysis. Proceedings, 1987-89. VII, 199 pages. 1991.

Vol. 1471: A. A. Panchishkin, Non-Archimedean L-Functions of Siegel and Hilbert Modular Forms. VII, 157 pages. 1991.

Vol. 1472: T. T. Nielsen, Bose Algebras: The Complex and Real Wave Representations. V, 132 pages. 1991.

Vol. 1473: Y. Hino, S. Murakami, T. Naito, Functional Differential Equations with Infinite Delay. X, 317 pages. 1991.

Vol. 1474: S. Jackowski, B. Oliver, K. Pawałowski (Eds.), Algebraic Topology, Poznań 1989. Proceedings. VIII, 397 pages. 1991.

Vol. 1475: S. Busenberg, M. Martelli (Eds.), Delay Differential Equations and Dynamical Systems. Proceedings, 1990. VIII, 249 pages. 1991.

Vol. 1476: M. Bekkali, Topics in Set Theory. VII, 120 pages. 1991.

Vol. 1477: R. Jajte, Strong Limit Theorems in Noncommutative L_2-Spaces. X, 113 pages. 1991.

Vol. 1478: M.-P. Malliavin (Ed.), Topics in Invariant Theory. Seminar 1989-1990. VI, 272 pages. 1991.

Vol. 1479: S. Bloch, I. Dolgachev, W. Fulton (Eds.), Algebraic Geometry. Proceedings, 1989. VII, 300 pages. 1991.

Vol. 1480: F. Dumortier, R. Roussarie, J. Sotomayor, H. Żoładek, Bifurcations of Planar Vector Fields: Nilpotent Singularities and Abelian Integrals. VIII, 226 pages. 1991.

Vol. 1481: D. Ferus, U. Pinkall, U. Simon, B. Wegner (Eds.), Global Differential Geometry and Global Analysis. Proceedings, 1991. VIII, 283 pages. 1991.

Vol. 1482: J. Chabrowski, The Dirichlet Problem with L^2 Boundary Data for Elliptic Linear Equations. VI, 173 pages. 1991.

Vol. 1483: E. Reithmeier, Periodic Solutions of Nonlinear Dynamical Systems. VI, 171 pages. 1991.

Vol. 1484: H. Delfs, Homology of Locally Semialgebraic Spaces. IX, 136 pages. 1991.

Vol. 1485: J. Azéma, P. A. Meyer, M. Yor (Eds.), Séminaire de Probabilités XXV. VIII, 440 pages. 1991.

Vol. 1486: L. Arnold, H. Crauel, J.-P. Eckmann (Eds.), Lyapunov Exponents. Proceedings, 1990. VIII, 365 pages. 1991.

Vol. 1487: E. Freitag, Singular Modular Forms and Theta Relations. VI, 172 pages. 1991.

Vol. 1488: A. Carboni, M. C. Pedicchio, G. Rosolini (Eds.), Category Theory. Proceedings, 1990. VII, 494 pages. 1991.

Vol. 1489: A. Mielke, Hamiltonian and Lagrangian Flows on Center Manifolds. X, 140 pages. 1991.

Vol. 1490: K. Metsch, Linear Spaces with Few Lines. XIII, 196 pages. 1991.

Vol. 1491: H. Gillet, E. Lluis- Puebla, J.-L. Loday, V. Snaith, C. Soulé, Higher Algebraic K-theory: an overview. VI, 164 pages. 1991.

Vol. 1492: K. R. Wicks, Fractals and Hyperspaces. VIII, 168 pages. 1991.

Vol. 1493: E. Benoît (Ed.), Dynamic Bifurcations. Proceedings, Luminy 1990. VII, 219 pages. 1991.

Vol. 1494: M.-T. Cheng, X.-W. Zhou, D.-G. Deng (Eds.), Harmonic Analysis. Proceedings, 1988. IX, 226 pages. 1991.

Vol. 1495: J. M. Bony, G. Grubb, L. Hörmander, H. Komatsu, J. Sjöstrand, Microlocal Analysis and Applications. Montecatini Terme, 1989. Editors: L. Cattabriga, L. Rodino. VII, 349 pages. 1991.

Vol. 1496: C. Foias, B. Francis, J. W. Helton, H. Kwakernaak, J. B. Pearson, H_∞-Control Theory. Como, 1990. Editors: E. Mosca, L. Pandolfi. VII, 336 pages. 1991.

Vol. 1497: G. T. Herman, A. K. Louis, F. Natterer (Eds.), Mathematical Methods in Tomography. Proceedings 1990. X, 268 pages. 1991.